ETHNOPSYCHIATRY

MCGILL-QUEEN'S/ASSOCIATED MEDICAL SERVICES STUDIES
IN THE HISTORY OF MEDICINE, HEALTH, AND SOCIETY

SERIES EDITORS: J.T.H. CONNOR AND ERIKA DYCK

This series presents books in the history of medicine, health studies, and social policy, exploring interactions between the institutions, ideas, and practices of medicine and those of society as a whole. To begin to understand these complex relationships and their history is a vital step to ensuring the protection of a fundamental human right: the right to health. Volumes in this series have received financial support to assist publication from Associated Medical Services, Inc. (AMS), a Canadian charitable organization with an impressive history as a catalyst for change in Canadian healthcare. For eighty years, AMS has had a profound impact through its support of the history of medicine and the education of healthcare professionals, and by making strategic investments to address critical issues in our healthcare system. AMS has funded eight chairs in the history of medicine across Canada, is a primary sponsor of many of the country's history of medicine and nursing organizations, and offers fellowships and grants through the AMS History of Medicine and Healthcare Program (www.amshealthcare.ca).

ETHNOPSYCHIATRY

HENRI F. ELLENBERGER

Edited by Emmanuel Delille
Translated by Jonathan Kaplansky

McGill-Queen's University Press
Montreal & Kingston • London • Chicago

ISBN 978-0-2280-0384-7 (cloth)
ISBN 978-0-2280-0385-4 (paper)
ISBN 978-0-2280-0445-5 (ePDF)
ISBN 978-0-2280-0446-2 (ePUB)

Legal deposit fourth quarter 2020
Bibliothèque nationale du Québec

Printed in Canada on acid-free paper that is 100% ancient forest free
(100% post-consumer recycled), processed chlorine free

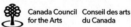

Funded by the Government of Canada   Financé par le gouvernement du Canada   Canada Council for the Arts   Conseil des arts du Canada

We acknowledge the support of the Canada Council for the Arts.
Nous remercions le Conseil des arts du Canada de son soutien.

Library and Archives Canada Cataloguing in Publication

Title: Ethnopsychiatry / Henri F. Ellenberger ; edited by Emmanuel Delille ;
   translated by Jonathan Kaplansky.
Other titles: Ethno-psychiatrie. English
Names: Ellenberger, Henri F. (Henri Frédéric), 1905–1993, author. |
   Delille, Emmanuel, editor. | Kaplansky, Jonathan, 1960– translator.
Series: McGill-Queen's/Associated Medical Services studies in the history
   of medicine, health, and society ; 56.
Description: Series statement: McGill-Queen's/Associated Medical Services
   studies in the history of medicine, health, and society ; 56 | Translation of:
   Ethno-psychiatrie. | Includes bibliographical references and index.
Identifiers: Canadiana (print) 20200302914 | Canadiana (ebook) 20200302965
   | ISBN 9780228003854 (softcover) | ISBN 9780228003847 (hardcover)
   | ISBN 9780228004455 (PDF) | ISBN 9780228004462 (ePUB)
Subjects: LCSH: Cultural psychiatry. | LCSH: Psychiatry, Transcultural. |
   LCSH: Cultural psychiatry—History. | LCSH: Psychiatry, Transcultural
   History. | LCSH: Ellenberger, Henri F. (Henri Frédéric), 1905–1993.
Classification: LCC RC455.4.E8 E4513 2020 | DDC 616.890089—dc23

This book was typeset in 10.5/13 Sabon.

Contents

PART THREE | APPENDICES

Decentralizing the Main Narrative of Transcultural Psychiatry

This critical edition of Henri Ellenberger's *Ethnopsychiatry* arose from the observation that the main narrative imposed until now on cultural psychiatry has been distorted, excessively centred around individual figures such as Georges Devereux and other "pioneers" so as to neglect the social, cultural, and political contexts that contributed to the emergence of an international postwar research network. In reality, this network only became established through collective work: academic journals, collective publications, teachings, and conferences. Throughout the 1950s and 1960s, in the context of the independence years, several medical and scientific communities emerged in the field of cultural psychiatry. They were connected to one another through academic activities and no longer simply through colonial administrations. My objective therefore is to bring to light an author relatively unknown in cultural psychiatry – despite his having written the first French-language synthesis of the discipline – and dialogically reconstruct his involvement in the field.

The isolated genius is a persistent myth in the history of medicine. Overall, it could be said that the history of cultural psychiatry (cross-cultural psychiatry, transcultural psychiatry, or *ethnopsychiatrie* in French) does not take into account the diversity of documentation that can be found on the subject, and even less so the available archives. Historiographical thinking is lacking, despite abundant sources – public archives exist, are open to researchers, and make it possible to question the past and reconstruct a variety of discourses and practices.

The idea of beginning with Ellenberger's own archives does not come from the need to defend a forgotten figure in cultural psychiatry. Rather, my goal is to introduce the reader to a multitude of figures (prosopography) and narratives that reveal the hidden ties between yesterday's colonial medical practice and the challenges postcolonial studies face today. To complete this editorial work, I have explored at length the archives left by Eric Wittkower, Brian Murphy, and their colleagues at McGill University and conducted a historical analysis of the scientific works of another North American team leader, the ambitious Alexander Leighton. A book will soon be published that will examine the young Ellenberger's work in folk medicine[1] in France. I will not address this here as it bears no relation to madness and would require an entirely separate analysis.

The historical essay that precedes Ellenberger's *Ethnopsychiatry* focuses on the postwar period, at the junction between psychiatry and anthropology, a combination inherited by the following generations despite the development of other scientific fields (psychiatric epidemiology, medical anthropology, and so on). As I will further explore in the first part of this this book, I chose to adopt the perspective of the American historian Alice Bullard, who treats cultural psychiatry as a knowledge of transition and/or in transition. The synthesis published by Ellenberger in 1965–67 illustrates this process well, as it continues to draw from knowledge gathered under colonial rule, while relativizing Western knowledge and avoiding the racist representations of his predecessors. On no account do I present here the history of a single discipline, but rather that of a body of knowledge that has been successively reworked.

To give but one example, in the 1960s there was no single therapeutic practice in cultural psychiatry. Wittkower himself, under whose direction Ellenberger worked, practised standard psychoanalysis in an "orthodox" fashion until the end of his life. By contrast, Ellenberger's practice throughout his life was eclectic, closer to Janet than to Freud, though it did not exclude any branch of clinical psychology. Thanks to his biographer Andrée Yanacopoulo, we also know that Ellenberger interpreted his dreams according to the principles of C.J. Jung, and I should add that his concept of criminology included Adler's ideas. Murphy renounced medical practice to focus entirely on science and became one of Canada's foremost specialists in psychiatric epidemiology. Ellenberger maintained a lasting friendship with him when he left McGill to join the Université de Montréal.

Evidently, we are far removed from the representations of the early 2000s, when cultural psychiatry was often presented as therapeutic practice for migrants, centring on the question of trauma. Truth be told, nothing is further from this recent transformation than the paths of the postwar figures of this book: the migrants were in fact therapists who fled Nazi Germany or later the Cold War, and who found in North America the means to satisfy their intellectual ambitions after their academic careers had been cut short in their native countries or in emerging states finally freed from colonial rule. This makes for a strange reversal of representations, since these exiled psychiatrists more often than not had North American patients, including Native Americans: the foreigners were the healers, not the healed. Above all, it must be taken into consideration that Ellenberger and his colleagues were themselves the bearers of a transcultural history, and that transcultural means transnational as much as it does transdisciplinary.

Another question emerges: Is Ellenberger's ethnopsychiatry a true product of Canadian academia? Not quite, since it relies on his first academic works put together in France, Switzerland, and the United States. That said, his synthesis does espouse certain specificities of the Canadian or *Montréalais* way of life: setting aside that it was written for a French public and published in Paris, it was still produced at an English-speaking university. It encompasses the teaching that Ellenberger dispensed in English to his students. Most of all, it is the synthesis of the work of a bilingual team – that is to say, Ellenberger speaks on behalf of a collective of researchers. The individual disappears somewhat behind the research he presents.

Yet Ellenberger's voice does surface on several occasions. As I am the first to point out, his ethnopsychiatry relies on his own clinical experience and showcases patients he saw as a doctor in the United States. This is not insignificant, as Ellenberger has often been presented as a simple historian of psychoanalysis or psychology, and thus has been arbitrarily cut off from his professional context, which was first that of a psychiatrist providing consultations until he retired. His psychiatric and psychotherapeutic practice is even more interesting in that it creates a bridge to Indigenous studies, religious history, and the history of psychedelic drugs: on this last topic, I refer the reader to the work of historian Erika Dyck.[2]

Finally, this research has also greatly impacted knowledge of Ellenberger and widened the perception of his scientific range. In North America, historian Mark Micale did outstanding historiographical work, demonstrating Ellenberger's contribution to the cultural history of psychiatry to a large audience. In France, first taken up by psychoanalysts, Ellenberger was presented as a historian of Freudian ideas. Then, as psychoanalysis lost its aura in contemporary culture, historians of psychology took over and presented him as an epigone of Janet. Removed from the nostalgia for Freud and Janet, this critical edition aims to corroborate that Ellenberger was above all a comparatist. His impressive work titled *The Discovery of the Unconscious* (1970) is not a long history according to the school of the *Annales* (Marc Bloch and Lucien Febvre), nor is it a Foucauldian genealogy; rather, it is a historical essay comparing the evolution of four contemporary psychodynamic systems – those of Adler, Janet, Jung, and Freud – without favouring one or the other, and considering them from the viewpoint of history and comparative literature. Ellenberger was a great reader of the comparatists, particularly Fernand Baldensperger and Paul Van Tieghem, both close to the Geneva school of Romance philology. A student of ethnographer Arnold Van Gennep, Ellenberger read folklorists, anthropologists, Africanists, Americanists, *Literaturwissenschaftler*, and so on. Therefore it seems only natural that he should be interested in a field that psychiatrist Emil Kraeplin named comparative psychiatry. The strong ties between his *Ethnopsychiatry* and *The Discovery of the Unconscious* show that Ellenberger can now be read differently: as a comparatist, his interest in the methods of hermeneutics is part of a multi-generational practice in a family of Protestant pastors.

One further remark concerning terminology: after editorial discussions, it was decided to keep Ellenberger's terminology so as not to alter his text. Nonetheless, it was tempting to rename the book *Transcultural Psychiatry*, as this terminology became internationally established thanks to Wittkower's team at McGill. The decision is difficult: Ellenberger himself wrote that he considered the expressions *ethnopsychiatrie* (in French) and transcultural psychiatry (in English) to be equivalent in the bilingual context of Montreal. For him, the two terms did not refer to two different concepts, but rather to two ways of referring to the same field of research in the two languages he spoke on a daily basis. As the term "ethnopsychiatry" is frequently used in his text, it was not possible to transform the title of the book without also modifying its other occurrences. Out of respect for the original text, I have thus decided to retain the term ethnopsychiatry, which gives a somewhat dated feel to the writing. I will therefore end with this final remark: while, as a general rule, editors of the classics present authors as timeless, is it not the historian's task to examine a fifty-year-old corpus as a source from another time,[3] now foreign to us, and whose context has become inaccessible and requires exegetic logic to understand? I urge the reader to take part in this critical challenge.

Emmanuel Delille
Montreal, 2019

NOTES

1 Emmanuel Delille, *À la découverte d'Henri Ellenberger. De l'ethnographie folklorique à l'histoire culturelle de la psychiatrie* (forthcoming).

2 E. Dyck, "Introduction," in F. Kahan, *A Culture's Catalyst: Historical Encounters with Peyote and the Native American Church in Canada*, ed. E. Dyck (Winnipeg: University of Manitoba Press, 2016), ix–xxxv.

3 This also holds true for the terminology: medical terms such as *cretin*, *mongoloid idiot*, and *retarded children* are no longer used today. Modern equivalent terms are indicated intermittently in the endnotes. The same applies to anthropological terminology: terms such as *tribe*, *Indian*, *Negro*, *Eskimo*, and *primitive* were still commonplace in social sciences in the 1960s. Today they are clearly considered racist and are no longer acceptable. Terminology also varies depending on the country: for example, *First Nations* designates certain Indigenous peoples of Canada, but not of other English-speaking countries.

Acknowledgments

The Éric de Dampierre Library (Université Paris Ouest Nanterre), Library of the Max-Planck-Institute for History of Science (MPIWG, Berlin), the Henri Ey Medical Library, François Bordes and the Institut mémoires de l'édition contemporain (IMEC), the Centre d'archives de philosophie, d'histoire et d'édition des sciences (CAPHES, ENS-Paris / PSL), the Centre de documentation Henri Ellenberger, the Centre Marc Bloch (CMB, Humboldt Universität zu Berlin), Alessandra Cerea, René Collignon, Ivan Crozier, Maurice Dongier, Irène Ellenberger, Michel Ellenberger, and Michael Ghil (ENS-Paris), Mary K.K. Hague-Yearl, the Japan Society for the Promotion of Science (JSPS), Jonathan Kaplansky, Médéric Kerhoas, Laurence Kirmayer, Arthur Kleinman, Catherine Lavielle, Éric Le Grossec, Samuel Lézé, Anne Lovell, Christopher Lyons and the Osler Library, McGill University, Marie Satya McDonough, McGill University Archives, Médiathèque of Musée du Quai Branly, Jane Murphy, Tanya Murphy, André Normandeau, Pivnicki Award Committee, Richard Rechtman, Nadine Rodary, Pascale Skrzyszowski-Butel, Nicolas Tajan, Kosuke Tsuiki, and the Jinbunken (Institute for Research in Humanities, Kyoto University), Andrée Yanacopoulo, Allan Young and the Department of Social Studies of Medicine (SSOM, McGill University), and András Zempléni. The translation of this book was made possible by a grant from the Collegium-Lyon Institute for Advanced Studies.

PART ONE

From Exotic Psychiatry to the University Networks of Cultural Psychiatry: Toward a History of Ethnopsychiatry as a Corpus of Knowledge in a Transitional Period (1945–1965)

Emmanuel Delille

This new edition reproduces the texts that Henri Ellenberger (1905–1993) wrote for the *Traité de psychiatrie* in the *Encyclopédie medico-chirurgicale* (EMC)[1] collection in 1965 and 1967, to which I have added selected archival materials so as to critically present their relevance for the shared history of psychiatry and ethnology from a social, political, and cultural point of view.

SITUATING THE PROBLEM

After a series of definitions and a brief biographical note, this new edition of Henri Ellenberger's texts aims to offer the reader elements for reflection on transcultural psychiatry so as to better understand the history of the knowledge surrounding this corpus and assess its construction of medical, human, and social sciences today. Why? This corpus, published fifty years ago in the EMC, constitutes the first French-language synthesis on transcultural psychiatry. In particular, here we wish to shed light on the connections that unite or distinguish a series of contemporaries who wrote these texts, such as Roger Bastide, Henri Collomb, Georges Devereux, Henri Ellenberger, and Frantz Fanon among the francophones, but also Erwin

H. Ackerknecht, Alexander H. Leighton, Brian Murphy (he used his middle name Brian as first name in daily life, but signed H.B.M. Murphy), and Eric Wittkower among the anglophones, most often cited individually with a view toward a professional history. For example, Erwin Ackerknecht (1906–1988), in the third edition of his history of psychiatry (1985), scorned the craze for transcultural psychiatry and qualified it as "trendy."[2] At the same time, too often one may forget that he himself was trained in French ethnology before beginning an American career and that his historical narrative opens with a chapter on ethnological considerations, which is unusual for a history of medicine. That means there is a historiographical issue to define, which is not at all simple or obvious at first glance. For time passes, and the outlines of certain figures that used to be familiar blurs; new generations ask questions and no longer accept pat answers or simplifications.[3] That is why this general presentation does not linearly follow the chapters of Henri Ellenberger's "Ethnopsychiatry" (1965) and instead provides cross-disciplinary analyses, emphasizing the role of the scientific participants and networks in the phenomena of the circulation of knowledge.

After the 1980s and the death of "pioneering" figures, the history of French-language transcultural psychiatry and English-language cultural psychiatry was the subject of a variety of historical narratives and biographical essays. As examples, we note various genres since the 1990s and the first decade of the twenty-first century: portraits of pioneers (by Gilles Bibeau and Ellen Corin,[4] Brian Murphy,[5] and Raymond Prince[6]); autobiographies (Georges Devereux[7] and Raymond Prince[8]); monographs devoted to influential figures (for example, Robert Arnaud[9] on Henri Collomb, and Georges Bloch[10] and Alessandra Cerea[11] on Georges Devereux); institutional appraisals (Anne E. Becker and Arthur Kleinman,[12] René Collignon,[13] Laurence Kirmayer,[14] Brian Murphy,[15] and András Zempléni[16]); the place of cultural psychiatry in the internal history of English-language psychiatry;[17] the putting into perspective based on colonial history (the influential essay by Richard Keller,[18] Frantz Fanon's biography,[19] Waltraud Ernst's essay on India,[20] Catherine Coleborne's essay on Australia,[21] the recontextualizing work by François Vatin on Octave Mannoni);[22] and the role of transcultural psychiatry networks in the globalization of mental health policies (Matthew Heaton).[23] We must also cite studies that broach this history via mental disorders that prevail locally (Ivan

Crozier[24] and Howard Chiang[25] on the history of *koro*), as well as social science researchers (anthropology, sociology, political science, etc.) who stress the postcolonial issues of transcultural psychiatry (Didier Fassin and Richard Rechtman).[26] But it would be naive to believe that doctors[27] waited for historians to wonder what to think about the history of this hybrid knowledge: there is no shortage of questioning about the colonial origins of exotic psychiatry and the professionalization of the field in universities.

This list is not exhaustive; above all it highlights the sheer variety of narratives, spaces, and frames of reference. Concerned about redefining these developments in a long-term perspective, I will adopt the analytical framework of Alice Bullard,[28] who approaches the professionalization of the field of transcultural psychiatry as an academic discipline in terms of "transition," driven by intellectuals who favoured decolonization and by policies for integrating refugees and migrants during the period of economic boom and rapid modernization of postwar society (this period has several designations: the pop years in English, *Trente Glorieuses* in French, *Wirtschaftswunder* in German). One cannot understand Henri Ellenberger's "Ethno-psychiatrie" (1965–67), the first French-language synthesis of this field of research and medical and psychological practices, without placing it in a context of the transition between the exotic psychiatry that thrived in colonial empires and the birth of transnational academic networks. This corpus avoids the canon of colonial medicine but does not yet belong to a well-established academic field: it illustrates this time of transition in its own way.

We will see later on that many participants in transcultural psychiatry such as Henri Ellenberger went through transcultural experiences themselves, most often due to the war. Some are known by the public, others not. In reality, in-depth knowledge of the eth-nopsychiatric corpus through archival materials and intersecting readings in English, French, and German (some English-language authors after 1945 were former German-speaking scientists[29] of the 1930s, and the reader can verify the considerable number of German-language sources in Henri Ellenberger's bibliography) offers a solid alternative to the classic portrait of the isolated genius, father or mother of a discipline produced with difficulty. The way in which Georges Devereux is remembered (1908–1995) is a good example of historiographical impasse. Critical research urgently needs to examine not only colonial[30] and postcolonial history but also the history of knowledge mobilized during the Cold War, as well as an intellectual history able to formulate the problem beyond the inherent limitations of the history of health care. For medicine and psychoanalysis are not always at the heart of professional narratives; that is also the case with intellectual networks, especially in terms of journals founded in the immediate postwar period in a context of "scientific migrations."[31] Moreover, a field such as social anthropology has its own arc of history,[32] which does not always cross paths with medicine or psychoanalysis, but often more with religious history.

The terminology is important and varies according to scientific culture: the term *ethnopsychiatrie* (often translated as transcultural psychiatry) became established in French to describe most often ethnopsychoanalysis, a hybrid knowledge that combines ethnology, medicine, and psychoanalysis, due to the cultural importance it had in France in the twentieth century. In English-speaking countries, psychoanalysis was not at the heart of discussions, though its use in the colonial context was not ignored.[33] In the face of this inhibiting legacy, the term ethnopsychiatry was abandoned at the same time as the British Empire, which was not the case in France. Other terms are used in English; the semantic field is varied, made up of competing expressions, used sometimes as synonyms or literal translations, the nuances of which are sometimes difficult to understand in French and or in English: comparative psychiatry (in German: *vergleichende Psychiatrie*), cross-cultural psychiatry, cultural psychiatry, *ethnopsychiatrie* (in German: *Ethnopsychiatrie*), folk psychiatry, *psychiatrie exotique*, *psychologie coloniale*, *psychologie des peuples*, transcultural psychiatry, and so on. One encounters many false friends when going from one language to another: remember, for example, that the terms *ethnologie* and social anthropology are used as correct translations when going from French science to American science. Some authors radically oppose a whole series of terms (the position of Georges Devereux), so it is necessary to specify as much as possible the use the participants involved make of this terminology. We will provide a series of definitions a little later on.

The period that interests us is the one extending from the 1940s to the 1970s. Why? The professional and intellectual biographies of the main participants involved in this field of science in the twentieth century together demonstrate that most of them carried out the first fieldwork or published books during this period. Before the

Second World War, American anthropologists and psychoanalysts of the "culture and personality" school had a decisive influence on the emergence of a postwar cultural psychiatry. American anthropologists often took advantage of their military service to become officers in charge of observing minorities, refugees, prisoners, or enemies of the United States during the 1940s, publishing monographs with the support of the US army and administration. The transition identified by Alice Bullard is closely linked to the policies applied during the Second World War and the Cold War.

In Europe, doctors and social science researchers continued to work in the context of colonialism until the late 1950s and the independence of Algeria: the France of the Fourth Republic violently began the period that saw the end of colonial psychiatry as well as the institutional foundations of a psychiatry of immigrants and refugees in mainland France. But it is not possible to address the history of this field beyond the 1970s and 1980s in the same way, as the participants and the socio-political context were no longer the same. Here I concur with the chronology of Richard Rechtman and Didier Fassin, who note that a new "culturalist reductionism" took hold in psychiatry from 1980 to 2010. Certainly this was based on the knowledge of the 1950s, 1960s, and 1970s, but it henceforth confronted head-on the French values of republican universalism. Moreover, between the 1980s and the first decade of the twenty-first century, new, unorthodox psychiatric care, focusing on cultural differences, was incorporated, putting into perspective the standards of biomedical medicine[34] – which was not yet the case in the France of the Trente Glorieuses (the glorious thirty years from 1945 to 1975).

Alongside the EMC, we find other French encyclopedias that by the 1950s and 1960s already included chapters on the knowledge. To cite but one example, the "Encyclopédie de la Pléiade," edited by Raymond Queneau and published by Gallimard, includes in its *Histoire de la science* (1953) volume a chapter titled "Psychiatrie sociale et ethnologie,"[35] a project augmented fifteen years later by Roger Bastide with his chapter on "Psychiatrie sociale"[36] in the volume *Ethnologie* (168). These encyclopedia articles already emphasize the central role of psychoanalysis in France, which made it possible to link social sciences and mental medicine in the mid-century through learned societies and scholarly journals.

Today, an updated narrative of the developments in ethnopsychiatry is needed, because no historian would now limit his or her history to the framework of psychoanalysis, which is increasingly marginalized in the academic world, and also because it is now possible to work with historic methods using archival holdings, which have been declassified and are open to researchers. Even so, today these documents remain underused. Consulting them and comparing them to one another puts an end to the idea that transcultural psychiatry was merely a matter for misunderstood pioneers. Nor is Paris the only place to explore for this history: the terminology indicates that today, almost by implicit imitation, we can follow the knowledge of comparative psychiatry among German universities (*vergleichende Psychiatrie*) and North American, Asian, and British universities (comparative psychiatry) without going through French-language ethnopsychology and ethnopsychoanalysis. Moreover, it is entirely possible to take Dutch, Spanish, Italian, and even Japanese medicine as an observation point for thoroughly updating the history of transcultural psychiatry. Other avenues are also conceivable, even desirable: we can take an interest in the history of the teaching of social sciences, in representations of the normal and the pathological that they convey, and in the transformation of these norms as these colonial empires disappeared and European countries became "provincialized."[37] Algiers, Java, Montreal, Munich, New York, São Paulo, and even Topeka (Kansas) are among the places featured in this history, no more and no less than Paris, but these stages are less linked to a process of professional specialization than to huge migration flows[38] resulting from a tragic century of successive wars.

BRIEF BIOGRAPHY OF HENRI ELLENBERGER

Andrée Yanacopouló[39] recently published a clear, well-documented biography of Henri Ellenberger based on archival documents held in Paris and Montreal, and also on unpublished family documents. Readers wishing additional biographical data will want to consult it. Henri Frédéric Ellenberger was born in Nalolo on 6 November 1905, in the Zambezi region, at the time the British possession of Northern Rhodesia, currently Zambia. A descendant of Swiss Protestant missionaries (Ellenberger on his father's side, Christol on his mother's), he belonged to a family of prolific intellectuals. His father, Victor Ellenberger (1879–1974), a member of the Société des missionnaires évangéliques de Paris (the Paris Evangelical Missionary Society), authored or translated works of anthropology and natural history.[40] Note that the Ellenberger family had been French-speaking for several generations. As a child, Henri Ellenberger first went to Paris (1914) to study, then to Mulhouse (1921), and then Strasbourg (1924), where he obtained his baccalaureate. He began studying medicine in Strasbourg and continued these studies in Paris, where he was admitted as a resident at the psychiatric hospitals of the Seine as a foreigner (1932). At that time, Henri Baruk (1897–99) had a significant influence on his thesis topic, which he defended in 1933:[41] the psychology of catatonia, a particularly serious deficiency syndrome of schizophrenia. In 1930 he married Esther von Bachst, known as Émilie,[42] of Russian origin, with whom he had four children. The religious ceremony in the Orthodox church of Saint-Serge de Paris caused some turmoil in the Ellenberger family, who were steeped in Protestantism.

In 1934, Henri Ellenberger set up practice as a doctor of nervous disorders in Poitiers, where he became interested in local folklore in the family tradition; in this, he followed the methods of the scholar Arnold Van Gennep (1873–1957),[43] with whom he became friends. He then published a series of articles on folk medicine based on material he gathered in Poitou.[44] In these first scholarly texts, he does not really explain his method or the conclusions he draws from his observations. Predominantly interested in narratives, he kept a record of the known variants of beliefs, magic rituals, and pilgrimages, struck by the people's defiance of official medicine and by their recourse to traditional healers. His data collection was interrupted by the war; he would start it up again afterwards.[45] In the late 1930s, he also worked with Spanish refugees who had flooded into France during the civil war and learned their language.

Henri Ellenberger, his wife, and their children were granted French citizenship in 1939, but in 1941 they made the urgent decision to leave France for Switzerland, faced as they were with the imminent danger of losing their French citizenship under Vichy (as well as the authorization to practise medicine). After a period in Bern (his family's native canton), Ellenberger was appointed assistant physician to the director at Breitenau, in the German-speaking canton of Schaffhausen, near the Rhine Falls. The family settled there from 1943 to 1953. In Switzerland, Henri Ellenberger met some great names in dynamic psychiatry and pioneers of psychoanalysis: Manfred Bleuler (son of Eugen Bleuler), Ludwig Binswanger, Carl G. Jung, Alphonse Maeder, Leopold Szondi, and also Pastor Oskar

Pfister (a friend and frequent correspondent of Sigmund Freud),[46] with whom he underwent training analysis in Zurich in the immediate postwar period. He was also interested in local characteristics of mental disorders, gathering information on the methods of ethnology and publishing an article about "cleaning mania" (*Putzwut*),[47] which he described as a distinctive Swiss characteristic. It was this reflection on the socio-cultural aspects of mental health that he later reinterpreted, in North America, as one of the points of departure for his passion for ethnopsychiatry.

The years 1945 to 1952 were critical for Henri Ellenberger: he learned to use his networks to launch his academic career. After the Liberation, he reconnected with the psychiatrists in Paris whom he had known during his years as an *interne* (medical resident) in psychiatric hospitals of the Seine, particularly with the second generation of the Évolution psychiatrique group, in whose journal he published his first articles on the psychotherapy of Pierre Janet (1859–1947)[48] and a series of articles on the history of Swiss psychiatry, which he collected in a volume published at his own expense.[49] Henri Ey (1900–1977) was then the Secretary General of the Évolution psychiatrique group, at the centre of one of the largest French-language psychiatry networks.[50] Henri Ellenberger was named a corresponding member of the Évolution psychiatrique group in 1951, after agreeing to take part in the *Traité de psychiatrie* (psychiatric treatise), which had been started by Henri Ey and which led to three large volumes of the EMC, a collection published by Éditions techniques (today Elsevier). On the basis of that network and his psychoanalytic training, in 1952 Henri Ellenberger left for the United States to observe American psychotherapies for schizophrenia.[51] At the end of the trip, he was offered a teaching and research position at the Menninger Foundation in Topeka, Kansas, which he took up in September 1953. At that time, the Menninger Foundation was one of the largest psychiatry training centres in North America, where renowned psychotherapists practised. As for cultural psychiatry, we note in particular the presence of Georges Devereux, who published an account of psychoanalytic psychotherapy of Native American patients[52] – and that of Louis Mars (1906–2000),[53] who spent time there in 1954. We will discuss this in more detail later, for Henri Ellenberger cites his two colleagues in his contribution to the EMC and also leaves testimony of his psychotherapeutic experience with Native American patients,[54] which was radically different from that of Georges Devereux, in that he favoured the approach of Pierre Janet rather than that of Sigmund Freud.

Henri Ellenberger remained in the United States for five years. In the context of the Cold War, he could not bring over his wife, who was of Russian origin, and remained separated from his family. In 1958–59 he was offered a position at the University of Honolulu, but seized an opportunity in Montreal: the transcultural psychiatry division[55] that had recently been founded at the anglophone McGill University was recruiting to develop research and teaching of the discipline in the university's Department of Psychiatry (Allan Memorial Institute). Henri Ellenberger settled in Canada in July 1959 as an assistant professor. He was joined by his wife and his youngest daughter, and remained at McGill until 1962, when he entered the francophone Université de Montréal as a professor in the Department of Social Sciences. In 1965 he obtained a chair in criminology[56] in the same department, while practising part-time as a psychiatrist in various hospitals and penitentiaries.

The 1970s brought him international recognition as a historian of medicine, when he published in English a book he had undertaken based on his teaching at the Menninger Foundation on the history of dynamic psychiatry: *The Discovery of the Unconscious: The History and Evolution of Dynamic Psychiatry* (1970).[57] Better known in American historiography than in France, this book contrasted strongly with the then existing literature thanks to its abundant documentation and his critical reading of sources. Neither a conceptual history nor a history of the mechanisms of psychiatric power, Henri Ellenberger's monograph focused on the transmission, reception, and reformulation of knowledge that allowed for the construction of psychological doctrines and knowledge of the psychological unconscious at the end of the nineteenth century. In it he emphasized the role of four major figures without favouring any one: Alfred Adler, Sigmund Freud, Pierre Janet, and Carl G. Jung. His vast scholarship – bordering at times on pointillism – may have been criticized, but his sense of accuracy and his work on the primary sources contrasted strongly with the histories of psychiatry and psychoanalysis of his time, in which Freud was presented as exceptional. Henri Ellenberger chose instead to position his impact in relation to that of three of his contemporaries.

Henri Ellenberger continued his academic career in North America while maintaining strong ties with French psychiatry. He contributed to the EMC's *Traité de psychiatrie* edited by Henri Ey until 1977 (the year of Ey's death). That same year, he retired and gave up several plans for books already well under way, due to the Parkinson's disease that increasingly affected him and the general deterioration of his health. Nevertheless, his rigorous and demystifying historical articles on famous patients of Sigmund Freud and Carl G. Jung, such as Anna O. (1972),[58] Emmy von N. (1977),[59] and Helene Preiswerk (1991),[60] confirm that he blazed a trail for the history of dynamic psychiatry that was not simply a celebration of the genius of Sigmund Freud. He edited a *Précis de psychiatrie* (1981) with Robert Duguay – for which he wrote the chapter "Psychiatrie transculturelle"[61] and contributed to the *Traité d'anthropologie médicale* (Treatise of Medical Anthropology) by Jacques Dufresne.[62] He also published stories for children under the pseudonym Fred Elmont.[63] However, he stopped work a reference book on ethnopsychiatry, begun several times, an outline of which exists[64] in the archives: a few chapters were published during his lifetime in the form of articles.

His last years were a time of rediscovery and belated recognition, marked by critical editions on the initiative of Mark Micale[65] in the United States and by Élisabeth Roudinesco[66] in France. In 1992, a few months before his death, the Centre de recherche et de documentation Henri Ellenberger was founded next to the Henri Ey medical library at the Sainte-Anne Hospital in Paris. It gathered together Ellenberger's documentation, his professional correspondence, his library, and other minor collections from donations (from other French psychiatrists and psychoanalysts), non-inventoried or in the midst of being inventoried. The place, designed mainly by Paris psychoanalysts, is unfortunately seldom consulted by social scientists. Yet we must stress the richness of the collection, which can also be used to cross-check information from other contemporary archives or to stimulate new research or examine Henri Ellenberger's work from a new perspective. To give but one example, Andrée Yanacopulo's recent biography convincingly demonstrates the significance of the religious dimension in Henri Ellenberger's work and intellectual journey: note that he quotes the Bible in his "Ethno-psychiatrie" (1965). But we could expand the analysis to the journeys of his relatives who became missionaries and/or academics. The practice of history,[67] of fiction,[68] and of writing about the self (or auto-fiction)[69] in the Ellenberger family could also be the subject of a comparative study; in addition, the role of women in the family is largely unknown, whereas Andrée Yanacopoulo's biography reveals the existence of major autobiographical sources: there is no shortage of avenues to explore.

THE MONTREAL–PARIS COMMUNICATION ZONE AND THE *ENCYCLOPÉDIE MEDICO-CHIRURGICALE*

To understand Henri Ellenberger's original contribution to ethnopsychiatry, we must first point out that it was part of the series of booklets he published in the 1950s, 1960s, and 1970s in the EMC's *Traité de psychiatrie*. Compiled by Henri Ey, this was one of the many medical treatises published by Éditions techniques. What is the value of a medical encyclopedia specializing the history of science?[70] At a time when it appeared impossible to encompass through thought all the publications devoted to a scientific field, the encyclopedia served as a medium that helped set down knowledge in memory; moreover, it made it possible to centralize the ramifications of knowledge and to experience their historicity in the face of the dispersion of scientific data. It is easier to record the gaps between encyclopedia articles and other documents because encyclopedias provide an overview of the knowledge of their time.

The form the EMC took was inspired by specialized legal publications, which are regularly updated based on the topicality of jurisprudence and the codification of laws. The EMC was founded as a collection in 1929 by Francis Durieux, a jurist, and Professor Armédée Laffont, Dean of the Faculty of Medicine in Algiers. The *Juri-classurs* (1907) are the archetype of this. This model also inspired the publishers of *Techniques de l'ingénieur*, founded after the war by Casimir Monteil, Maurice Postel, and Francis Durieux. Pierre Courtin was the editor of the EMC, as well as a relative of Maurice Postel, whom Francis Durieux knew during the First World War. This editorial venture thus was created by a small circle of close friends and relatives, almost a family undertaking.

The EMC, as a book-object, is comprised of file folders and detachable booklets that are sold by subscription. The collection published regularly to this day: in the first decade of the twenty-first century, the medical treatises of the EMC for a time included CD-ROMs and then DVDs as supporting material, before moving to online publication, which has the advantage of offering subscribers supplementary illustrations and multimedia content not limited to two-dimensional paper or by printing costs. The new texts are joined to the rest of the information contained on the internet through hypertext links but mainly via electronic databases[71] that the current publisher, Elsevier, has created to network its scientific publications and sell them to a globalized public. That public consists of doctors of the Latin culture, in that the EMC is published in French, Spanish, and Italian – but almost not at all in English.

The "Psychothérapie de la schizophrénie"[72] booklet that Henri Ellenberger published in 1955 in the EMC played a pivotal role in his career in North America, for it was his project of gathering the documentation needed for this topic that brought him to the Menninger Foundation.[73] Also very important are his "Analyse existentielle"[74] booklet, which heralded one of his earliest books,[75] and his articles "Castration des pervers sexuels"[76] and "Criminologie,"[77] which should be included in the long bibliography of his work dedicated to the history and practices of criminology. These last two articles already have a place in the "Socio-psychiatrie" chapter of the EMC's *Traité de psychiatrie*, to which the "Ethno-psychiatrie" series was added in 1965.

Yet it is not certain that the two long "Ethnopsychiatrie" booklets played a role in Henri Ellenberger's career. In 1965, he was already a full professor, so we should be wary of retrospective illusions. I am thinking specifically that Raymond Prince's[78] interpretation should be qualified; he sees ethnopsychiatry as the driving force in Henri Ellenberger's intellectual evolution. The truth is that he came to Montreal above all to start an academic career that he was unable to begin in Europe or truly carry out in the United States, be it in ethnopsychiatry, general psychiatry, history of medicine, or criminology. As with other psychiatrists trained in France, a French-speaking country was the preferred choice for Henri Ellenberger: we are thinking of Hassan Azima in Montreal, Paul Sivadon in Brussels, Maurice Dongier in Liège and later in Montreal, Julian de Ajuriaguerra in Geneva, and Henri Collomb in Dakar. Some members of Henri Ellenberger's generation gave up teaching (Henri Ey), and others failed (Jacques Lacan). In the end, while Henri Ellenberger's interest in ethnopsychiatry went back a long way – as Raymond Prince has aptly pointed out – it is nevertheless useful to divide his scholarly output into periods: the summaries of Poitiers folklore from the 1930s and 1940s bear no relation to the methodology he used in his later historical articles from the 1970s to the 1990s.

At the time Henri Ellenberger published his articles on Poitiers folklore, his father and grandfather, ministers in Africa, already had pastoral and ethnological work to their credit.[79] We can certainly establish their ties with Henri Ellenberger's writing before establishing those between him and known specialists in ethnopsychiatry. Archival material indicates that Henri Ellenberger's first attempts were in the ethnological tradition: in particular, he corresponded with (1950–52) with French ethnologist Maurice Leenhardt (1878–1954), a professor at the École pratique des hautes études as well as a Protestant minister. The two families were friendly; Henri Ellenberger knew Maurice Leenhardt through his father. Leenhardt later edited a journal, *Le monde non chrétien*, for which Henri Ellenberger would write a review of a translation.[80] Their correspondence is worth quoting, inasmuch as Henri Ellenberger speaks in it of his documentation research, in which he connects folklore, North American culturalist anthropology, and ethnopsychoanalysis in the Swiss context. Here is an excerpt of the first letter written by Henri Ellenberger to Maurice Leenhardt:

Following my visit to you last December, I subscribed to your most interesting journal "Le Monde non-Chrétien," a few issues of which I had read at my father's. You once kindly suggested that I send you an article on a topic regarding the limits of ethnology and psychiatry. I thought of a very topical subject: "ethnopsychoanalysis." Meanwhile, I tried to obtain the already vast bibliography on the subject. I regret to note that it is virtually impossible to do so in Switzerland. Even the works of Margaret Mead and Ruth Benedict are impossible to find here, and unfortunately, I do not have the financial means to obtain the works at my own expense. But perhaps "Le Monde non-Chrétien" could obtain them as press copies and review them? The only work I have found is "People of Alor," which you have already analyzed!

Allow me to also mention a book that recently was published in South Africa:

A.T. Bryant: "The Zulu People," Pietermaritzburg, 1949.

It was loaned to me by a South African staying in Basel: I read it with keen interest. It is a model monograph, although unillustrated, unfortunately. It provides a detailed description, but with a philosophical interpretation such as your "Do Kamo" (which, sincerely speaking, I find far superior to everything I know about ethnopsychoanalysis: your point of view is far more general and comprehensive).

I also have a request to make. The next Swiss conference of psychiatry has as its general theme "Psychiatry and Folklore." I have agreed to give a paper on exotic mental disorders[,] a topic that I have studied for a long time (I mean, I am trying to find documentation about it, not having been out in the field). I have already collected some, but my documentation is still very incomplete, e.g.[,] on Madagascar. I would be most grateful to you if you could help me in my research, for example by indicating to me the libraries where I could find information.[81]

In the end, Henri Ellenberger never contributed to Maurice Leenhardt's journal, for he soon departed for the United States. In any case, the transcultural psychiatry developed in Canada was not a medical science of folklore as could still be imagined in Switzerland in 1950: Henri Ellenberger's intellectual journey was therefore not a linear one. What's more, when he sought a publisher in the 1960s, he was insistent with those he liaised with, taking the opposite view of his letter to Maurice Leenhardt: academic ethnopsychiatry could not be an exotic psychiatry.

Another correspondence, this one with Eric Wittkower, midway through his process of intellectual development on the American continent, indicates that Henri Ellenberger in fact did not have very clear ideas on the methodology used by researchers in transcultural psychiatry at McGill: Wittkower had him rewrite his research project several time before it was finally adopted in 1959.[82] He then obtained the rank of associate professor at the Allan Memorial Institute (McGill's Department of Psychiatry), where he taught alongside Eric Wittkower and Brian Murphy (1915–1987). His first major transcultural study was titled "The Impact of a Severe, Prolonged Physical Illness of a Child upon the Family" (research conducted from 1 April 1961 to 31 March 1962). That was his first academic research project in the strict sense of the term: a study of the impact of serious and chronic organic diseases on families of various socio-cultural origins. His paper to the World Congress of Psychiatry in Montreal (1961) may be viewed as representative of his work at McGill[83] and attests to a shift in methodological approach (surveys based on interviews, questionnaires, and tests, qualitative and quantitative analyses, etc.) in relation to the Swiss years.

But Henri Ellenberger did not keep his position at McGill for very long. Raymond Prince and Lionel Beauchamp[84] point out that his situation at that time was precarious: first, as a foreigner, he encountered significant difficulties in obtaining administrative approval to practise medicine in tandem with his research activities; and second, the balance of power between anglophones and francophones was unequal at McGill.[85] The Allan Memorial Institute, founded in 1943, next to the Montreal Neurological Institute directed by Wilder Penfield, became, through its first director, Professor Ewen Cameron (1901–1967), one of the largest psychiatric research centres in North America. Ewen Cameron had been trained at Johns Hopkins Hospital in Baltimore under the direction of Adolf Meyer and later became chair of psychiatry at McGill and then President of the American Psychiatric Association (1952), of the Canadian Psychiatric Association (1959), and of the World Psychiatric Association (1961). He played a seminal role in the entire field of mental medicine, from psychoanalysis to biological psychiatry. Ewen Cameron had a number of psychiatrists from Europe and the United States come to Montreal – Miguel Prados[86] in 1944, Eric Wittkower in 1950, Alastair MacLeod in 1951, and Clifford Scott in 1954 – and developed psychoanalysis in order to forestall a brain drain to the United States. Henri Ellenberger and Brian Murphy were recruited in 1959, at a time when McGill's Department of Psychiatry was becoming one of the largest in North America in terms of medical residents.

It is also important to mention that the same psychiatry department was at the heart of a scandal shortly afterwards, during Ewen Cameron's time – a scandal that called into question medical ethics and therapeutic experimentation without the consent of patients. During the Cold War, some of the activities of the Allan Memorial Institute were funded by the United States, which carried out brainwashing experiments there.[87] This matter, which received wide media coverage and has long been public knowledge, led to studies of and testimonies from the victims, and also to literary and television fiction, and so on. It had a direct impact on the emergence and dissemination of transcultural psychiatry. For as unlikely as it may appear, the journal *Transcultural Newsletter* launched by Eric Wittkower was funded through a smokescreen: the Society for the Study of Human Ecology (1957–65). There are no sources that indicate whether Henri Ellenberger spoke about this matter or whether it played a role in his departure from McGill.[88] The university archives there have no records for the Society for the Study of Human Ecology in the archival holdings of the Department of Transcultural Psychiatry.

At the Université de Montréal, Henri Ellenberger continued to teach psychiatry and criminology[89] while also practising at the Hôtel Dieu and the Institut Philippe Pinel. The two booklets he published on ethnopsychiatry in France for the EMC in 1965 were, paradoxically, a kind of summary of the knowledge he had accumulated and the experience he had acquired at McGill, with an English-speaking team, but written in French, at a time when ethnopsychiatry had only a limited place in his medical practice, his teaching, and his publications on the history of psychiatry.

DEFINITIONS AND FOUNDATION MYTH

The current edition of *Le Petit Robert*, a dictionary of the French language, defines ethnopsychiatry (1951) as the "study of the influence of ethnic factors on the genesis and manifestations of mental disorders"; ethnopsychology (1970) is "the study of the psychological characteristics of communities and ethnic groups."[90] However, *Le Petit Robert* does not include the term *ethnopsychoanalysis* (used by Henri Ellenberger in his letter to Maurice Leenhardt), even though that term is used more often that *ethnopsychology* in France. These nouns are viewed as specialized terms connected to teaching (didactics); they point to the need to establish distinctions among subdisciplines and types of knowledge at universities, and in the professional training of psychiatrists and psychologists. They are relatively recent neologisms: *ethno-* refers directly to ethnology, "the study of facts and documents collected by the ethnographer"; and *-logy* to the project of making science. In the same word "family" are disciplines such as *ethnomusicology* (1955).

Having made these semantic clarifications, what is Henri Ellenberger's definition of ethnopsychiatry? It is not very different from the one in the dictionary, though it places more emphasis on mental illnesses, and thus on medicine, than on the complementary sciences that study them, by defining ethnopsychiatry more narrowly in relation to other subdisciplines of the social sciences:

> *Ethno-psychiatry* is the study of mental illness according to the ethnic or cultural groups to which patients belong. This definition delimits ethnopsychiatry in relation:

1 to the *psychology of peoples*, which, as Miroglio (1958) demonstrates, is one of the branches of descriptive sociology;
2 to "*cultural anthropology*," which may be considered as a branch of ethnology in the broadest sense of the term;
3 to *social psychiatry*, which is the study of mental illness according to the social (but not ethnic) groups to which the patients belong.

These distinctions may be rapidly explained according to the participants present in the field when Henri Ellenberger wrote: (1) the psychology of peoples is a genre[91] that enjoyed much success from the late nineteenth century to the mid-twentieth, but in very different, even oppositional forms: Wilhelm Wundt (1832–1920), professor of psychology at the University of Leipzig,[92] sought to develop general laws, while in postwar France, Abel Miroglio (1895–1978)[93] was interested in the distinct psychological traits of Westerners, based on racial theories that led to his marginalization (and that of colonial psychiatry); (2) cultural anthropology is a well-established social science in international academia, which doctors cannot "take over," and which is not founded on medical practice; (3) social psychiatry is not at all easy to differentiate from ethnopsychiatry; quite the contrary, for this was the terminology used by Roger Bastide, professor at the Sorbonne[94] at the time when Henri Ellenberger wrote, both an academic authority and an important link in the construction of this field for francophones. The same year, Roger Bastide published a sociology book (*Sociologie des maladies mentales,* 1965) in which he too established a distinction among three disciplines: social psychiatry, sociology of mental illnesses, and ethnopsychiatry. Although the division proposed by the sociologist has points in common with that of the doctor, it is not entirely the same thing (ethnopsychiatry and social psychiatry should not be confused); we will return to the sociological contribution later on. Finally, the three distinctions established by Henri Ellenberger aim to defend ethnopsychiatry within the medical sciences, by taking a naturalistic and universalist approach, albeit one that is open to the social sciences.

Other terminological distinctions relate to language, in that there exists a vocabulary in English as well as in French – though there is no vocabulary specific to German, perhaps for reasons of chronology (Germany's colonial era came to an end with the First World War). The two common expressions in the postwar years were cross-cultural psychiatry and transcultural psychiatry; new cross-cultural psychiatry and cultural psychiatry are more recent, but I have chosen to use this last one (cultural psychiatry) when I speak of trends in English-speaking countries, because it is more neutral and was already in use in some publications of the 1950s (by Eric Wittkower, for example).

Cross-cultural psychiatry is probably the oldest term in English, but it has not been clearly defined. Transcultural psychiatry was the terminology used by Eric Wittkower at McGill and in his international journal, which is why it was generally adopted in the English-speaking world, but it appears that it was borrowed from Georges Devereux – who claimed to have coined it.[95] "New cross-cultural psychiatry" is the term that the anthropologist and doctor Arthur Kleinman[96] has promoted in recent decades as an alternative to the Canadian model; however, his work extends beyond our chronology, for its began to have an impact after 1977,[97] thus there will be little discussion of it here.

Alice Bullard has noted the importance of technical vocabulary and the differences between French and English that contributed to the creation of distinct semantic fields, from the root *ethno-* in French and *culture* in English. This twofold dual structure is not always easy to use. Alice Bullard's solution is to limit the use of the term *ethnopsychiatry* to local work: "I use the term transcultural mental health care or transcultural psychiatry to refer to practices in which practitioner and patient are from different cultures, which was the case with the Ortigues' work in Senegal. Ethnopsychiatry refers to local psychiatric systems of knowledge, such as detailed in Zempléni (1968) or Devereux (1961)."[98]

She specifies in another essay: "Transcultural psychiatry here is distinguished from 'ethnopsychiatry,' understood as the project launched by Georges Devereux of appropriating entire healing systems from non-Western cultures."[99] Alice Bullard elucidates this type of transition as a reversal of knowledge transfer between imperial and colonized powers. From the point of view of the history of science, if we stand back, this distinction between ethnopsychiatry and transcultural psychiatry is close to the analytic dichotomy that science historian Simon Schaffer[100] introduced for the phenomena of the circulation of knowledge: location versus spatialization of knowledge. Indeed, Schaffer develops a history of knowledge that takes into account a twofold problem: (1) the local roots of scientific experiments (location of facts, first connected to the laboratory for experimental sciences), and (2) their replication in other areas of scholarly sociability and, therefore, the circulation of knowledge in a multi-use place of reception (spatialization of facts, which circulate beyond the laboratory). Certainly, medical and social sciences are not founded on laboratory experiments, as is the case with the sciences Simon Schaffer examines. But the distinctions he makes are invaluable for taking things into account. Besides, in the case of transcultural psychiatry, while knowledge circulated from the former colonies to the former metropoles in the postcolonial period, the ethnocentrism of the former did not disappear, and as Alice Bullard reports, the power relationships remained stable despite the inclusion of this knowledge: "Colonial psychiatry generally produced knowledge while intentionally ignoring or dismissing local beliefs and practices; post-colonial transcultural psychiatry has reversed this, so that local beliefs and practices including culturally specific healing practices inform and sometimes guide transcultural therapeutic interventions. This transformation is rooted in ways of knowing, in evolving scientific practices and codes of ethic."[101]

However, without fundamentally disagreeing with Alice Bullard, I think that the semantic differentiation she proposes cannot be strictly adhered to for the text corpus of Henri Ellenberger and his collaborators at the EMC. Indeed, for practical reasons, Henri Ellenberger uses the terms "ethnopsychiatry" and "transcultural psychiatry" for equivalent concepts, both in his writing and in his correspondence. The explanation is very simple, and rooted in quotidian life: in the bilingual context of Montreal, the two terms do not refer to two distinct scientific concepts, nor do they refer to opposed approaches; rather, they simply refer to how the same academic discipline is named, alternatively, in the working languages of two scientific communities that exist side by side in the same field of communication. That is why Matthew M. Heaton and Alice Bullard's choice to reserve the term ethnopsychiatry when speaking of colonial psychiatry or local knowledge up until the 1950s, and the term transcultural psychiatry to speak of academic and transnational networks after decolonization, is, in my opinion, incorrect: the second distinction may be true for English, but that is not the case in French, and it is an error to believe that the English language consistently held sway during the second half of the twentieth century. Montreal is not simply a bilingual city; it is also a space of acute political tensions between

the two linguistic communities – and this was especially true in the
1960s, which were a time of emancipation in French Canada known
as the Quiet Revolution. Matthew M. Heaton's analysis is apt for his
Nigerian case study, but the vocabulary is different elsewhere: the
terminology used in Romance-language countries is an alternative to
and a shield against the hegemony of the English language.

But it is also important to emphasize what brings us together:
the questioning of postcolonial psychiatry. In an enlightening essay
on the work edited by Neil Lazarus, *The Cambridge Companion
to Postcolonial Literary Studies*,[102] Emmanuelle Sibeud defines
postcolonial as a questioning that completes and confirms other
critical questioning: "Postcolonial refers to objects: traces left by
multiple experiences arisen from colonial domination but also
to theoretical and political positions regarding the study of these
objects."[103] Postcolonial psychiatry is not an origin point to which
to return in order to construct the genealogy of a science; rather, it is
a set of representations and practices as well as a corpus to question
using the tools of historical analysis.

To understand the distinctions made by Henri Ellenberger in his
definition of ethnopsychiatry, we must return to the context of the
humanities and social sciences in the 1950s and 1960s. The issue is
of course one of universalism and cultural relativism, a point that
Didier Fassin and Richard Rechtman have noted in critical publications in recent years alerting people to the reversal of perspective,
as relativism came to prevail over universalism in French ethnopsychiatry. In the EMC in 1965, Henri Ellenberger advocates a balanced
point of view, one that is closer to universalism than to relativism.
The way he addresses this point is extremely interesting: he does not
resolve it head-on with a cut-and-dried judgment, but rather analyzes
it and divides it into six distinct problematics: (1) cultural relativism,
(2) cultural specificity, (3) cultural nuances of mental illnesses, (4)
differentiations within the same cultural group, (5) pathogenic cultural factors, and (6) biocultural interactions.

This approach to the problem should be compared to those of
other participants in the field of ethnopsychiatry – for example, that
of the ethnologist Georges Devereux, whose universalist point of
view is connected to the psychoanalysis of Sigmund Freud and the
sociology of Émile Durkheim and Marcel Mauss, and not to medical science. His position is to present himself as a Durkheimian by
invoking a principle of "social polysegmentation," and therefore

a multiplicity of social "niches" in which diagnosis and remission of an illness only make sense in relation to a given social environment: one's own tribe. For Georges Devereux, in terms of the social analysis of mental disorders, distinctions should be made among the following: (1) sacred disorders, (2) ethnic disorders, (3) typical disorders, and (4) idiosyncratic disorders.[104] At the same time, he is opposed to any form of cultural relativism, indeed more firmly than Henri Ellenberger. He thus aligns himself with the classic position of orthodox psychoanalysts, in accordance with the biological and universalist principles of Sigmund Freud, whereas Henri Ellenberger is more eclectic and takes the position of an encyclopedist.

Today, thirty-five years after his death, Georges Devereux has a central place in the way the history of ethnopsychiatry in France is written. Yet if we focus on the definitions, it is difficult to find in his work stable points of reference. Not because he made an about-face regarding his works, but because he made a point of revising his concepts and annotating his theory with each new edition of his books, a use of the footnote reminiscent of Sigmund Freud's style. Thus, in his *Basic Problems of Ethnopsychiatry*, Georges Devereux speaks freely of psychoanalytic ethnopsychiatry and cross-cultural psychiatry, but also develops other terms to distinguish himself from his contemporaries. In an article titled "L'ethnopsychiatrie comme cadre de reference" (1952), for example, he included terminological notes subsequent to the first edition of the text, in particular regarding the term *metacultural psychiatry*, which he opposes to *transcultural psychiatry*. In this way, he calls for "the creation of an authentic *metacultural* and meta-ethnographic psychiatry, based on a real understanding of the nature and the generalized function of Culture in of *itself*."[105] A note then explains his choice of term: "I remember that I first qualified this type of psychiatry as 'transcultural,' but I must give up this term that I had made up to designate solely this type of psychotherapy, for it has since been appropriated by others who use it to designate all of ethnopsychiatry. I am therefore replacing it with the term 'metacultural.'"[106]

Did Georges Devereux and Henri Ellenberger have an opportunity to discuss in depth the methodological issues of ethnopsychiatry? Their correspondence between 1954 and 1974 (reproduced in the appendix to this book) mainly indicates that Henri Ellenberger regretted Georges Devereux's departure from the Menninger Foundation, that they both suffered from a lack of professional recognition, and that both wondered about the origin of the word *ethnopsychiatry* – not without irony. Georges Devereux thought he could ascribe it to Louis Mars, who was using the term by the early 1950s.[107] In fact, we know today that the word already existed in colonial medicine[108] during the interwar years.

FROM MUNICH TO MONTREAL: COLONIAL MEDICINE, ORIENTALISM, AND COMPARATIVE PSYCHIATRY

What are the beginnings of ethnopsychiatry as a scholarly discipline, or rather, what chronology can be assigned to it? If we must give a symbolic date of creation, the journey of German psychiatrist Emil Kraepelin (1856–1926) seems ideal for establishing a broad consensus among specialists. Emil Kraepelin hoped and prayed for the creation of a "comparative psychiatry"[109] (in much the same way that people at the time were by then speaking of comparative history and comparative literature), on the basis of his stay in Java in 1903 (during a four-month journey to Asia, a written account of which was published in 1904). This already dealt with academic knowledge: Emil Kraeplin was a professor in Munich, and his remarks were limited to known nosological categories: on the basis of *in situ* observations and local statistics at the Buitenzorg mental hospital, which treated both Dutch and Javanese patients, he noted a greater number of Javanese patients suffering from dementia praecox and epilepsy than in Europe, fewer depressives and alcoholics, and little general paralysis (although the syphilis that caused it was then widespread among the inhabitants of Java).

Emil Kraepelin was interested in the local names for mental disorders – that is, in indigenous categories. The best-known examples were *latah* and *amok*, jointly described in the nineteenth century.[110] *Latah* in Malaysia refers to a neurotic behaviour, generally in a woman, characterized by unrestrained imitation of the behaviour of her close circle and excessive obedience to orders. *Amok*[111] describes a fit of indiscriminate and unrestrained violence in a man, which ends only when he is shot. According to Emil Kraepelin, *latah* may boil down to a local socio-cultural form of hysteria, whereas *amok* cannot be considered an illness; it is a morbid composite behaviour that partly resembles psychosis and partly resembles epilepsy.

Ethnopsychoanalysis, which by then had been developed by Hungarian anthropologist Géza Róheim (1891–1953),[112] a student of the psychoanalyst Sándor Ferenczi (1873-1933), is contemporaneous with the comparative psychiatry of Emil Kraepelin. It also rapidly attained university status, starting with the Chair of Anthropology of the University of Budapest (1919).

It is interesting that Henri Ellenberger notes less-known names among the pioneers of the genre: for instance, a German doctor, Heinrich Obersteiner, who in 1889 published a kind of general review of mental disorders among ten or so "exotic" peoples throughout the world, basing his work on medical observations of his time. Beyond that, Henri Ellenberger established in his bibliographical references a genealogy that often goes back to colonial medicine and the explorers' accounts, and not to strictly psychiatric publications. Thus, Emil Kraepelin's journey can only be considered a symbolic, arbitrary date. Before him there already existed a multitude of descriptions written by colonial doctors, but also accounts of travellers, adventurers, sailors, and missionaries, far older, who guided them. Emil Kraepelin's articles on Java, conquered by the Dutch East India Company by the early eighteenth century, followed a whole body of literature in Dutch,[113] little-known because it was untranslated. Henri Ellenberger, who could read the language, cites Dutch sources. In the final analysis, to be unaware of the incidence of this literature of comparative psychiatry before Emil Kraeplin is to deny an entire component of colonialism.

For we must admit: the emergence of academic cultural psychiatry is not so much connected to the figure of Emil Kraepelin, who followed in the tradition of colonial medicine, as to the postwar period, that incredible time of transition, well identified by Alice Bullard, that saw the end of the colonial empires and the beginnings of the postcolonial era – as well as the Cold War. The development of postcolonial studies is generally traced back to the seminal monograph by Edward Said (1935–2003), *Orientalism*. The colonial discourse he analyzed spanned the beginning of European philological studies at the end of the eighteenth century up to American area studies, developed early in the Cold War. Edward Said demonstrated that knowledge of the Orient was closely connected to European colonial expansion in Africa, the Near East, and India; in all these places, science was placed in the service of administrations set up by France, England, Germany, and Russia. From this perspective, Orientalists may be viewed as a professional body of scholars in the service of a discourse of domination. From the new human sciences, they took first philology, then geography, history, and ethnology, and then founded institutes of Oriental languages and culture in order to study, observe, watch over, and, in the final analysis, rectify the image that Orientals had of themselves by imposing Western standards upon them. Of course, medical knowledge was a party to this process; we must take into account this dimension of ethnopsychiatry.

One great contribution of Edward Said was to convincingly demonstrate that orientalism was a type of narration that forged extremely strong ties of intertextuality between knowledge about the Orient and the romantic literature that preceded it, inasmuch as scholars drew more upon travel narratives of the nineteenth century than upon local, indigenous sources. Edward Said relies on the narratives of romantic writers such as Chateaubriand, Lamartine, Nerval, and Flaubert. Remember that the first medico-psychological assertions about "Orientals" were contemporary; we need only mention the name of French psychiatrist Joseph Moreau de Tours.[114] In other respects, this process is not specific to orientalism; historian Mark Micale[115] demonstrated in a landmark article on the history of psychiatry that literary descriptions of hysteria, such as those of Flaubert, preceded and modified medical descriptions. To sum up, we should be wary of this influence in ethnopsychiatry and must also examine the works of fiction and various other accounts that are cited by Henri Ellenberger.

Orientalism was analyzed by Edward Said as a doctrine whose goal is to establish a power relationship over peripheral and heterogeneous peoples by treating them only as a fictitious scholarly object, the Orient, both absolute otherness with no comparison to Western countries, and as fiction completely fabricated by these countries, using stereotypical representations and tired metaphors of inferiority (the Orient as a woman, child, irrationality, flesh rather than spirit, and so on, taken in hand by the male West, mature, rational, spiritual, and so on). Edward Said's observation is that orientalism is always based on surface representations and never on profound or well-documented facts. The position of Western scholars has long been to consider their science as superior, and this made it possible for them to speak on behalf of colonized peoples. Edward Said turned this around, asserting it was always necessary to question the relationship to the colonial past of any exotic representation purporting to be scholarly.[116]

Edward Said's discourse analysis applies to surface representations circulating in the scholarly literature of ethnopsychiatry. There is an important question to raise in relation to Henri Ellenberger's booklets in the EMC: as they are text summaries, stereotypes that were already rather old, like the exotic forms of mental illness described and told about for several centuries, do they not fall under Edward Said's criticism? *Amok* and *latah* are good examples, but there are others. I will return to this in regard to culture-bound syndromes[117] – a term that became commonly used in medicine as of the 1960s and 1970s, attributed to Pow-Meng Yap (1921–1971), professor of psychiatry in Hong Kong and Toronto. This list of exotic mental disorders, the descriptions of which most often (but not always) date back to colonial medicine, has been the focus of special attention from anthropologists and doctors trained in medical anthropology, both to rethink these phenomena from the point of view of the social sciences, and also, on the whole, to call into question the Western psychiatric nomenclature that was imposed on the rest of the world. The dissemination and codification of culture-based syndromes in the form of an international nomenclature is not the result of the mere circulation of ideas, it is knowledge constructed by participants in academic institutions who are linked together by structured networks. In particular, the teaching of ethnopsychiatry must be the focus of all our attention, inasmuch as it is likely to be interpreted as falling under oriental studies.

The first university Department of Cultural Psychiatry (the Division of Social and Transcultural Psychiatry) was founded at McGill, by the doctor and psychoanalyst Eric Wittkower (1899–1983) and anthropologist Jacob Fried, in 1955.[118] So that is another fundamental date, one that justifies declaring that the narrative framework of the history of ethnopsychiatry includes Montreal, after Munich, and not only Paris. Moreover, the naming of Montreal in this regard allows us to emphasize the importance of scientific migrations in this history.

Eric David Wittkower (Erich was his German first name) was born in Berlin on 4 April 1899 into a Jewish family of merchants of British and German origin. He served in the German army at the end of the First World War, then studied medicine at Friedrich-Wilhelm University in Berlin. He specialized in internal medicine at the Berlin university hospital, Charité, which did not at first indicate his future inclination toward psychiatry and the social sciences. But by the late 1920s, his publications revealed an interest in psychotherapy and the role played by emotions in internal medicine. His university career brutally ended in Germany after Hitler came to power: he was fired on 28 March 1933,[119] even before the promulgation of the antisemitic laws of 7 April 1933 (Gesetze zur Wiederherstellung des Berufsbeamtentums), which were aimed at public servants of Jewish origin. This purge, which came especially early and emphatically at the Charité, happened in time for him to make the necessary arrangements to leave for Switzerland with his wife in late March 1933. He soon reached London, where he completed a new specialization in psychiatry (Maudsley Hospital);[120] he then joined the team at the Tavistock Clinic, under the direction of John R. Rees (1890–1969), who had significant responsibilities during the war (Directorate of Army Psychiatry). Eric Wittkower helped develop the program for the psychological selection of British officers. At this institute he earned his international reputation as a specialist in psychosomatic medicine and as a psychoanalyst. He was recruited by McGill University in 1951.

Besides the collaboration between Jacob Fried and Eric Wittkower, there already existed well-known examples of cooperation among anthropologists and physicians – for example, Abram Kardiner (1891–1981) and Ralph Linton (1893–1953)[121] in the Anglo-American world. François Laplantine[122] also mentions Arthur Ramos (1903–1949) and Melville J. Herskovitz (1885–1963), two anthropologists who focused on mental medicine. We can go back even further than this and generalize about the ties between anthropologists and doctors in the nineteenth century surrounding the controversies raised by evolutionism, especially given that some anthropologists were doctors by training. This was a largely transnational phenomenon: for instance, Franz Boas (1858–1942) followed the teaching of the pathologist Rudolph Virchow (1858–1942)[123] in Germany before developing anthropology in the United States. But in terms of mental medicine and social anthropology, in their time this type of collaboration was not yet symmetrical or even a project of pooling information: for a long time, these exchanges involved ethnologists bringing material to psychiatrists, who then interpreted it from a psychopathological point of view. This imbalance led Alfred Louis Kroeber (1876–1960) and Erwin Ackerknecht to point out that possibilities for rapprochement between psychiatrists and anthropologists had their limits. Abundant literature on this type of collaboration exists.[124]

Henri Ellenberger's work is interesting in part because it presents analyses developed in the department of a university, McGill, where there was a real team of doctors and social science researchers who had acquired professional experience in various countries in the world. They mastered several working languages (mainly French, German, and English) and were themselves were mostly refugees or migrants. Their teaching, research seminars, conference presentations, and co-authored articles compel us to rethink Henri Ellenberger's synthesis published in 1965 as also being the result of a "thought collective."

This type of collaboration also reflects the long-term history of the humanities and social sciences. It is necessary to draw a parallel between "comparative psychiatry" and "comparative history," for comparative studies is not a new idea, far from it. French historians Henri Berr (1863–1954), Marc Bloch (1886–1944), and Lucien Lebvre (1878–1956), first at the *Revue de synthèse* and then in the *Annales d'histoire économique et sociale*, paved the way for new works in cultural history, the imagination, and emotions thanks to this type of fruitful exchange. Henri Berr himself wrote in 1911: "History, in fact, is psychology itself: it is the creation and the development of the psyche."[125] Marc Bloch championed the cause of comparative history in the early twentieth century (Oslo, 1928), and, with Henri Berr and Lucien Febvre, embodied the very type of historian open to the psychological sciences, a participant in the great transdisciplinary publishing initiatives, and so on. Sociologist Maurice Halbwachs (1877–1945), author of *The Psychology of Social Class* (1958) and penetrating analyses on collective memory, and historian Georges Lefebvre (1874–1959), author of a history of fear (*The Great Fear of 1789*, 1973), are authors from the Annales School.

The creation of new concepts involves the transfer of knowledge across disciplines: one famous example, according to Hans-Dieter Mann, was Lucien Febvre, who was inspired by linguist Antoine Meillet when he introduced the concept of *outillage mental* or mental toolbox in analogy with Saussure's concept of "language," defined as a "keyboard of possibilities"[126] (as opposed to speech, which is individual). The "history of mentalities," developed by historians who were readers of the psychological medicine of their era, defended the virtues of comparative history. Lucien Febvre's work abounds with analytic tools for interpreting the symbolic world, and individual and collective mental representations, that is, mental structures and categories in the social context of an era.

Subsequently, philosopher and anthropologist of the imagination Michel Durand (1921–2012) took from Carl G. Jung (1875–1961) the very controversial notion of "archetype"; as we will see, Henri Ellenberger, was quite ambivalent in relation to these types of loan words: he criticized excessive usage of them in 1965 but nevertheless used the Jungian concept in 1967 regarding "collective psychoses."

Other avenues exist that do not borrow from psychoanalysis, but more from a historical anthropology. Georges Duby (1919–1996), a specialist in medieval history, wrote excellent studies in which he placed "mental habits" and "mindsets" at the heart of the feudal phenomenon, without freeing them from the socio-economic phenomena specific to that period. Generally speaking, an entire school of medievalists became famous in France in the history of mentalities, integrating it into a total history, the best-known representative of which was Jacques Le Goff (1924–2014). After the Second World War, some researchers in the social sciences – in particular the specialists in ancient Greece Jean-Pierre Vernant (1914–2007) and Pierre Vidal-Naquet (1930–2006), preferred to speak of their field in terms of historical anthropology. Jean-Pierre Vernant was close to Ignace Meyerson (1888–1983), a doctor and psychologist trained notably by Pierre Janet at Salpêtrière, the first French translator of Sigmund Freud's *The Interpretation of Dreams*, a promoter of historical psychology. Other orientations led historians toward the history of private lives and close friends.

Ethnopsychiatry's development needs to be examined alongside these well-known hybrid disciplinary ventures, for it often draws on the same sources. We are thinking in particular of the reinterpretations of pathological psychology described by Marcel Mauss in two of his most famous essays, "The Gift" (Essai sur le don) (1923–24) and "The Physical Effect on the Individual of the Idea of Death Suggested by the Collectivity, (Australia, New Zealand)" (1926),[127] which themselves were inspired by developments in mental medicine and at the same time contested knowledge in the field and disputed the sociological causality of certain phenomena understood in terms of psychological suggestion. It was typically this analytical framework that Henri Ellenberger used in 1965, alongside structuralism and culturalism, which also crossed the boundaries of ethnology and enriched the field of psychiatry in the long term.

AREA STUDIES, STRUCTURALISM, AND THE COLD WAR

When the Department of Transcultural Psychiatry was founded at McGill in 1955, the landscape of the social sciences was undergoing new developments greatly affected by the Cold War. Another type of transversality then became recognized between the social sciences and medicine in North America: area studies – that is, research on cultural areas developed in North American universities. Having been implemented in the United States and then in Canada, this new paradigm had a notable influence on how Henri Ellenberger conceived the possibilities for ethnopsychiatry. Indeed, he clearly emphasized the metaphor of a cultural area, that of psychiatric geography. "There is still considerable work to be done before we are in possession of a psychiatric geography extending over the entire surface of the Earth and encompassing all peoples," he concluded midway through his 1965 presentation, prophesying the revision of "many current concepts regarding the respective frequency and value of symptoms of mental illnesses."

Up until the Second World War – when epidemiology was not yet well developed as an authoritative science[128] – the term medical geography was in common use though vague in its methods. It indeed designates a transnational field of scholarly research, but it was most often limited to literary accounts. Historian Mirko Grmek,[129] who wrote an article on the history of this chapter of medical science, points out that cartographic methods were not used before the middle or the end of the nineteenth century. Yet up until that time,

> people firmly believed that epidemic outbreaks of certain
> illnesses were the result of telluric and cosmic influences on
> a given region and that the nature of the epidemic depended
> basically on a *genius loci*. Despite its etymology and its animist
> resonance, the "spirit of the place" was not considered to be a
> spiritual factor. It was simply the technical term for the set of
> geographic and astral conditions.[130]

After the end of the nineteenth century, there were medical geographical societies in France, Germany, the British Isles, the United States, and elsewhere, that debated the regional specificities of neuropsychiatric disorders, mental retardation, and dementia:

ethnopsychiatry was only a distant heir of these, in large part ignorant of its own origins. There is work that remains to be done that
would involve going through journals[131] of medical geography, proceedings of international conferences (1931, 1934, 1937, 1952, and
1954), and the teachings in that field.[132] Henri Ellenberger, who liked
to maintain correspondence with the great historians of his time, did
not correspond with Henry E. Sigerist (1891–1957), who nevertheless produced influential writing[133] on the history of illnesses, which
partly inherited the project of medical geography in the sense that
migrations and imperial expansion were vectors of contagious diseases. But to better focus here on the specific context of Montreal, it
should be stressed that the field was entirely recast after the Second
World War based on the American paradigm of area studies. The US
administration and army promoted this field as the European colonial administrations had done previously, having been exposed to
new diseases on unknown territory, particularly in Asia. During the
Cold War, Soviet authorities of course did the same thing.

Around that time, area studies were thought of as transdisciplinary
synergies, with the classic academic disciplines cross-fertilizing one
another. Large American foundations such as Ford and Rockefeller
did much to promote this field of research after the war. The political driver behind this field was the US government's perceived need
to understand what was happening in the Soviet Union, China, and
the other states in the Communist Bloc, but also in Africa and Asia,
which were then undergoing decolonization and were deliberating on
which "camp" to join in a now bipolar world. And even if this view of
the humanities was largely American, we can nevertheless state that
this reconfiguration of the humanities had powerful effects in France
on the local administration of knowledge. For example, Fernand
Braudel and Clemens Heller relied on research programs of this type
to develop the sixth section of the École pratique des hautes études.[134]

Before structuralism took hold in the social sciences, area studies
relied heavily on the culturalist movement represented by American
anthropologists like Ruth Benedict, Ralph Linton, and Margaret
Mead, and so on, as well as on doctors such as Abram Kardiner,
a psychiatrist and psychoanalyst. The goal of culturalism was to
demonstrate the impact of culture – and of education in particular – on the "basic personality," through the study of traditional
societies. We cannot state that Henri Ellenberger was a culturalist,
and he denied being one in his correspondence with the editorial

representatives of the EMC, but his articles may be considered as in contact with this prevailing paradigm in North America and as a form of compromise with other types of borrowings, in particular with the French-language social sciences.

When we look at the context in which Henri Ellenberger wrote his articles, with the war and the immediate postwar years as a backdrop, it is important to bear in mind at least one iconic work in area studies that was both prototypical and renowned: the famous and controversial study by American anthropologist Ruth Benedict (1887–1948) on the cultural identity of Japan, *The Chrysanthemum and the Sword* (1946), commissioned by the US War Department during the war as a guide to understanding the enemy's culture. This monograph was widely criticized by the scientific community[135] because in it Ruth Benedict defended her hypotheses without any investigative fieldwork. But it also, unexpectedly yet logically, rapidly became an object of fascination: Benedict's essay would be used by the Japanese under the American occupation as a distorting mirror of American interests in their country. Henri Ellenberger had read Ruth Benedict and would quote from her from time to time.

After the Cold War, area studies became obsolete, or rather their funding came to an end. The decline of the culturalist school, the sudden emergence of postcolonial studies (and subaltern studies, and so on),[136] the enthusiasm with which the great figures of French structuralism were received in the United States, the economic crisis, the end of the bipolar world, the creation of new states, and the enlargement of the European Union also help explain the wrapping up of this approach. Edward Said's authoritative criticism dealt the final blow: "A vast web of interests now links all parts of the former colonial world to the United States, just as a proliferation of academic subspecialties divides (and yet connects) all the former philological and European-based disciplines like Orientalism. The area specialist, as he is now called, lays claims to regional expertise, which is put at the service of government or business or both."[137]

And it fell to Edward Said to demonstrate, with quotations to back him up, how representations by American specialists in cultural areas were laden with racist prejudices of the past, which most often only rehashed the representations of previous European philologists and writers without allowing a voice for individuals among the peoples observed. The archetype of this type of obscurantism was Hamilton A.R. Gibb (1895–1971). But Edward Said also quotes counter-examples, such as the American anthropologist Clifford Geertz and Jacques Berque in France, who broke with the stereotypes of the past. In the final analysis, the decline of area studies does not mean that they did not survive in disciplines carrying other names, but it is important to provide a balance and follow the participants on a case-by-case basis. For example, Henri Ellenberger made personal observations about the environment of Native American reserves in the United States, and not in a colonial context. Native Americans were not affected by decolonization; their status was that of a "minority" – part of the American melting pot and its assimilationist project.

The American careers of Henri Ellenberger and Georges Devereux were closely linked to one institution: the Menninger Foundation. As we have already mentioned, that foundation administered one of the largest private psychiatric complexes of the postwar years and was a training facility dominated by psychoanalysis.[138] Many professionals who fled or left Europe during the 1930s, 1940s, and 1950s found a place there. The therapists and teachers who worked there strongly influenced the dissemination of psychoanalytic ideas in the United States. The Menninger was run by several generations of the Menninger family, and in the 1950s the central figure in that family was Karl Menninger.

The period that Henri Ellenberger spent at the Menninger Foundation allowed him to make his way to academia. While Georges Devereux is renowned for his psychoanalytic and psychotherapeutic work with Native American patients, it is not widely known that Henri Ellenberger also worked with Native Americans in the same institution. Their activities did not entirely overlap: Georges Devereux published his book *Reality and Dream: Psychotherapy of a Plains Indian* in 1951,[139] then left the institution shortly after, whereas Henri Ellenberger arrived in Topeka in 1952 and only settled there in 1953. They actually were only colleagues during 1952.

To complete this picture, remember that Erwin Ackerknecht had been trained at the same school of ethnology as Georges Devereux in Paris and wrote on the health practices of the Plains Indians (the Cheyenne) in the 1940s. While working on the history of malaria along the Mississippi, he wrote articles in the 1940s that dealt with both medicine and ethnology[140] in which he strongly criticized the methods and results of Georges Devereux, well before *Reality and Dream* was published. But at that time, area studies were not part of their contention, nor were they taken into consideration in the arguments that Erwin Ackerknecht and Georges Devereux put forward; it was the intrusion of psychoanalysis that was the subject of debate between the two ethnologists. Yet we are justified in wondering what Edward Said would have thought of the use of psychoanalysis for the study of the Plains Indians; in particular, in the article "Psychopathology, Primitive Medicine, and Primitive Culture,"[141] published in 1943, Erwin Ackerknecht accuses Georges Devereux of not managing to go beyond the old argument of Freudian psychopathology, which structures religion as a neurosis; he also qualifies his model of schizophrenia as a "speculative sociological theory"[142] but acknowledges the value of "primitive psychopathology."[143] Ackerknecht condemns the metaphoric use of the technical vocabulary of psychopathology as "paranoid" and "schizoid" and unhesitatingly declares that this "part of the history of psychopathological labels is tragicomic."[144]

Georges Devereux responded to the criticisms levelled at his 1939 article[145] in a new preface to his book *Mohave Ethnopsychiatry and Suicide*,[146] seeing in them only a culturalist oversimplification, the simplified hypotheses of which he had always condemned. He does not mention Erwin Ackerknecht by name, but attacks his 1943 article in the same book, *Mohave Ethnopsychiatry and Suicide*, regarding what he sees as the erroneous criterion of social adaptation as the basis for differentiating between the normal and the abnormal.[147] The controversy between the two students of Marcel Mauss and Paul Rivet, then both living in the United States, unfortunately was never resolved: neither listened to the other's point of view. But it is important to examine the path of Georges Devereux, who was at the crossroads of several scientific cultures, as was Henri Ellenberger.

HENRI ELLENBERGER AND GEORGES DEVEREUX: PSYCHOTHERAPISTS AT THE MENNINGER FOUNDATION

Georges Devereux was born György Dobó on 13 September 1908 in Lugoj, a Jewish community in the Banat, a region of the Austrian-Hungarian Empire that later became part of Romania. There have been many biographical sketches of him and as well as a feature film (by Arnaud Desplechin: *Jimmy P.: Psychotherapy of a Plains Indian*, 2013). Like Henri Ellenberger, he was multilingual, speaking Romanian, Hungarian, German, and French, in addition to languages he learned for his work as an ethnologist at the École des langues orientales in Paris and while living in America.

According to his biographers, Georges Devereux left Romania in 1926 to study in France. He started out studying chemistry, which he abandoned, then worked as a bookseller in Leipzig, Germany, frequented intellectual circles, tried his hand at fiction and poetry (in German), and struck up a friendship with the writer Klaus Mann (1906–1949). He began studying sociology and anthropology in 1931 at the École pratique des hautes études (EPHE) under the supervision of Marcel Mauss, and conducted his first ethnological fieldwork in Indochina among the Sedang. He then trained at Berkeley and settled down in the United States thanks to a fellowship from the Rockefeller Foundation. It was in this capacity that he studied the Mojave Indians, on whom he wrote his thesis (under the supervision of Alfred Kroeber at the University of California–Berkeley), and published many articles.[148] Fascinated by the attention the Mojave paid to their dreams, he began establishing connections with the psychoanalysis of Sigmund Freud. But to place Georges Devereux's work in a social, political, and cultural context, we should compare it with that of other Americanists.[149]

Georges Devereux and Henri Ellenberger were from very different backgrounds, though many possible parallels can be made: both were exiles, and both had prolonged stays in the United States, and they shared theoretical interests and published on related topics. Both also wrote poetry and fiction. Also, both changed their religious affiliation. Before training in psychoanalysis, Georges Devereux was baptized as a Catholic in 1933; it was at that time that he adopted the name by which we know him. He did his first year of psychoanalysis with Marc Schlumberger (1900–1977) in France, then began training with Robert Jokl at the Menninger Foundation. It was therefore during this period, when he was both a therapist and undergoing analysis, that he published *Reality and Dream*. Henri Ellenberger also did his psychoanalytic training in the 1940s and 1950s. In 1952, Georges Devereux left Topeka for good to work in another private therapeutic institution,[150] this one in Devon, Pennsylvania, where he became engrossed in writing books about ethnopsychiatric theory.[151] In 1956 he settled in New York, where he earned a degree as a psychologist and became a member of the American Psychoanalytic Association. Henri Ellenberger also lived in New York in 1959, before taking up his position at McGill, in Canada.

In 1963, around the time Henri Ellenberger decided to settle permanently in Quebec, having accepted a teaching position at the Université de Montréal, Georges Devereux returned to France. With the support of Claude Lévi-Strauss and Roger Bastide, he obtained a teaching appointment at the École pratique des hautes études the same year. He published *De l'angoisse à la méthode dans les sciences du comportement*[152] in 1967, which had a significant impact in the epistemology of the humanities and social sciences. Other books followed on ethnopsychiatry and ethnopsychoanalysis, which underwent several editions in various languages; most often these were collections of articles. Among them were *Basic Problems of Ethnopsychiatry*[153] and *Ethnopsychanalyse complémentariste*,[154] published in the 1970s but already being drafted during his American years. Henri Ellenberger, for his part, published his important book on *The Discovery of the Unconscious* in 1970. He remained an eclectic doctor, curious about all sociological and psychological theories. Georges Devereux defended a more orthodox psychoanalysis and believed in the universality of the Oedipus complex; he defended a complementary approach between anthropology and psychoanalysis.

It is not possible here to sum up Georges Devereux's entire work, but we will return to it later. The central motif of his ethnopsychiatric work is a conceptual framework for understanding the forms of insanity observed in society, inspired by the framework of social roles developed by the anthropologist Ralph Linton: the insane play roles socially expected of insanity. Indeed, there are patterns in every culture that are provided by its myths and customs, and thus there are normative models of insanity, which lead to a distribution of the role of the insane in society.[155]

In the editorial field, in addition to his methodological works, Georges Devereux founded one of the first French journals of ethnopsychiatry and ethnopsychoanalysis: *Ethnopsychiatrica*.[156] Only five issues of this short-lived venture, launched at the end of his career, were published. Its impact was thus very limited. While Georges Devereux became established posthumously in France in the 1990s and 2000s as the founder of ethnopsychiatry and ethnopsychoanalysis, this was the result of the actions of groups who ran other journals and created university teaching posts in France after his death in 1985. It was in this rather recent context that the influence of Tobie Nathan[157] spread. Nathan defends a relativist point of view[158] radically opposed to the universalism of the man he acknowledged as his master; as a result, we must now take pains to avoid confusing Georges Devereux with his posthumous spokespersons.

Let us return to the sources of the 1950s. Georges Devereux's *Reality and Dream* (1951) is a narrative based on transcriptions of thirty therapy sessions with Native American Jimmy Picard (a pseudonym), a Blackfoot, who was treated at Winter General Hospital in Topeka as a Second World War veteran. Jimmy Picard suffered from mental disorders connected to a series of factors identified as family conflicts, relationship problems, uncontrolled consumption of alcohol, and a head trauma acquired during the war. Georges Devereux exposes his method at the beginning of the book *Reality and Dream* and develops the operative concept of "ethnic personality,"[159] which allows him to link psychology and ethnology. He parses Blackfoot customs and emphasizes the value of dreams in their culture. The account of the treatment is connected to the family saga and the medical history of disorders. Finally, he reproduces the results of psychometric and projective tests administered by a psychologist.

While this book unquestionably influenced the history of cultural psychiatry and psychoanalysis, now, with historical perspective, it must be placed in relation to other similar documents. To do so, I will establish similarities and differences based on documents from the Henri Ellenberger archives. For while Georges Devereux is known for his psychotherapeutic practice with patients of Native origin, it is not well-known that Henri Ellenberger developed a similar practice at the Menninger Foundation.

True to his position as a reserved and eclectic man who tended to look at the overall picture, Henri Ellenberger cites *Reality and Dream* in his articles as a key scientific reference in ethnopsychiatry; however, in the booklets of the EMC, he discusses the various possible psychological interpretations for his Native American patients in Topeka without resorting to Georges Devereux's method, and clearly puts into perspective the value of psychoanalytic interpretation. Henri Ellenberger presented at least two cases of Native patients, from the Potawatomi and Kickapoo groups from reservations in Kansas close to Topeka. Like Jimmy Picard, they were part of the Algonquian linguistic group, Plains Indians, who had once lived by hunting buffalo.

Henri Ellenberger's most developed case study is included in several documents with no great variation. The first known version was published in the EMC in 1965. He used this case, citing new bibliographical references, in 1978 in another booklet of the EMC devoted to drug addiction, an analytical framework important to consider, for it is not central in Georges Devereux's psychoanalytical interpretation. This is therefore an essential difference between the two former Topeka therapists.

Other unpublished documents must be considered: the Henri Ellenberger archives maintain an unpublished version[160] developed for teaching.[161] This is a typed, ten-page document in which he sets out two clinical cases: a brief vignette that serves as an introduction, and a more developed case that he interprets. The document is undated, but in the "Peyote addenda," written by hand, he includes additional bibliographical references found in the 1978 booklet. Thus, the course was most likely given in the social sciences department of the Université de Montréal, where he taught from 1963 to 1977, or at Hôtel-Dieu de Montréal, where he participated in research seminars.

I will briefly sum up the two clinical observations. The meeting with Native American patients at the Topeka State Hospital is dated 1957–58. The first case is that of a Native American from the Mayetta Reservation in Kansas, who was hospitalized at the age of thirty-three. Psychological testing reveals an IQ so low that the result does not seem plausible; indeed, a thorough examination reveals that the results are biased because the patient never attended school. He does not suffer from an intellectual disability but rather from organic brain syndrome. In this case, psychological testing unadapted to the patient's culture has concealed a neurological pathology that went unnoticed until a thorough exam was conducted, one that took into account the Native American patient's socialization on a reserve where he did not receive an education. The second case is that of a man in his sixties, diagnosed as having "alcoholic neurosis." For alcohol neurosis to appear at such a late age seemed unlikely to the psychiatrist:

In 1957, a Kickapoo Indian, aged 65, was admitted to the psychiatric hospital in Topeka, Kansas. Sober until then, he had suddenly begun drinking alcohol to excess following unclear circumstances in which disagreements with his wife appear to have played a role. The case was diagnosed as "alcoholic neurosis." The fact that I knew one of his friends and neighbours well led the patient to tell me his story. Like many of the Indians of his tribe, he had a kind of split personality, an American name and an Indian name, an "official" religion and an "Indian" religion. While nominally Protestant, he belonged to the peyote religion to which he had converted about fifteen years earlier. He practiced his religion sincerely, but had ended up becoming addicted to peyote (a quite rare, though not exceptional, occurrence). His wife, who belonged to another Indian religion, that of the "Drummers," was hostile to the peyote religion. One day there was no peyote to be found: the man suffered deeply, which led him to seek solace in alcohol. That was the real origin of this alcoholism late in life – but the man was loath to speak of peyote or of his religion, which he considered to be purely an Indian matter of no concern to doctors.

Here again, a thorough examination reveals a distinct socialization: the Native patient respected simultaneously the rites of both religions, a surface Protestantism that concealed a private Indian religion, the peyote religion. The latter is founded on the consumption of a toxic product extracted from a cactus that can lead users to experience visions during collective ceremonies. The patient had developed an addiction to peyote and, unable to obtain any, began to consume alcohol to treat the lack experienced, in vain.

We note elements in common with the famous case from Georges Devereux: both times men are involved, who were caught up in profound marital conflict and/or with dominant female figures in their families;[162] psychological tests were conducted in a hospital setting – which emphasizes that psychoanalysis was not the only psychological movement represented in Topeka in the 1950s; and alcoholism was a recurrent pattern, but also an illusory one that hid the real diagnostic issues. There is also of course a common interest in the language, customs, and religion of the patients. Furthermore, far from the stereotype of neutrality in the relationship to the patient, according to the Freudian doxa, the relationships that Georges Devereux and Henri Ellenberger forged with their patients seemed to be combined with friendship. Henri Ellenberger notes in his teaching: "Most fortunately, it turns out that I knew one of his friends and neighbours well; I had visited him on the reservation, and the patient, trusting me, told me his whole story."

But we must also qualify these parallels between Henri Ellenberger and Georges Devereux. Henri Ellenberger minimizes the presence of Native Americans at the Menninger Foundation, which is surrounded by reservations; in fact, Mayetta is less than an hour away by car from Topeka. At the same time, he views drug addiction as a relevant framework for thought – more specifically, the relationship between the toxic and the sacred, between drug addictions and magico-religious rituals, in conflict with Protestant puritanism. From his point of view, this is interesting – a dimension completely absent from Georges Devereux's book. Another difference is that Henri Ellenberger completed his clinical work by observing the religious rituals and practices of the Native Americans he was writing about; such observations are not encountered in the psychoanalysis of Sigmund Freud, who introduced a theoretical parallel between rituals and neurotic symptoms. Similarly, while he draws from the patient's graphic expression in the form of drawings, this is not to depict mental content or interpret Freudian fantasies, but rather to document magic-religious rituals. Finally, Henri Ellenberger is also interested in dreamlike material, yet the psychoanalytic interpretation of dreams is not mobilized; on the contrary, he indicates that the visions were created by the active substance in peyote, as a toxin, and that these were nightmares in the metaphoric sense of the term ("harrowing visions"). He refuses to reduce the addiction-related and religious experiences of the Native Americans to pathological experiences: "The experience is not artificial psychosis," he writes. These are not hallucinations, but "pseudo-hallucinations." The analytical framework of the normal and the pathological is thus not relevant for him. Henri Ellenberger concurs with Erwin Ackerknecht's fundamental criticism of the abusive use of psychopathological notions, and in this way he differs from Georges Devereux.

The knowledge mobilized in Henri Ellenberger's account falls under several rubrics: the social sciences, religious sciences, botany, and psychopharmacology, but also under literature (Aldous Huxley[163] and Henri Michaux[164]), and above all psychology. But which psychology? Straightaway, Henri Ellenberger sets down an analytical framework stemming from classic psychology, that of "double and multiple personalities," which had led to a great deal of scientific controversy in the nineteenth century, and which is not the conceptual framework of psychoanalysis, nor that of Georges Devereux. It takes its explanatory framework from Pierre Janet and Carl G. Jung. Indeed, Pierre Janet authored a summary of nineteenth-century French psychology, notably from the Salpêtrière School (Charcot, Bourneville, and so on) and from the Nancy School (Bernheim), which sustained the controversy around the diagnosis of double and multiple personalities. The origin of this diagnosis goes back a half-century to Freudian psychoanalysis, specifically to the case of Félida, a young woman about whom the Bordeaux doctor Eugène Azam (1822–1899) published remarkable works between 1858 and 1876. Pierre Janet himself was known for his clinical observations of hysteria that featured women plagued by religious turmoil and split personalities. The introduction of this diagnosis at the Menninger Foundation, as an alternative to the psychoanalytical interpretation, is not by chance, for at that time Henri Ellenberger was one of the first serious biographers of Pierre Janet. Furthermore, Henri Ellenberger's interest in the history of double and multiple personalities never flagged; the last article he published at the end of his life dealt with a case history of split personality published by Carl G. Jung.[165]

Having presented the similarities and differences, it is particularly interesting from a historical perspective to note that Henri Ellenberger did not choose to provide a Freudian interpretation of his Native American patients – and I stress this fact once again – although he had just completed training analysis in Switzerland. Clinical observation shows that Henri Ellenberger, as a psychiatrist and therapist, did not prioritize a psychoanalytic explanation in presenting the case of his Native American patient; instead he advanced several psychological interpretations of equal value. His teaching ends with ironic remarks taken from the works of Stanford Unger[166] at the National Institute of Mental Health, noted in a telegraphic style and contained in the booklet he devoted to drug addiction in 1978:[167] the reader may consult the document reproduced in the appendix of this book.

If Henri Ellenberger does not opt for a Freudian interpretation, then how to describe the function he assigns the clinical observations of Native Americans? Above all, it is didactic: it must make it possible to avoid false diagnoses that do not take into account the cultural dimension of psychiatry. The rhetorical style used in this pedagogical exercise is one of demystification: gross errors of interpretation may be avoided through a serious analysis of the sociocultural characteristics as well as a medico-psychological examination.

OTHER ACADEMIC AND INTERNATIONAL NETWORKS:
ROGER BASTIDE VERSUS HENRI AUBIN

Georges Devereux and Henri Ellenberger did not remain isolated from the academic world. To historicize their contributions to a discipline then still being created, it is helpful to see how they related to another contemporary who was well integrated with the academic world: Roger Bastide, a professor at the Sorbonne as well as an ethnologist specializing in the sociology of religion and social psychiatry. Why? The "Georges Devereux" of Henri Ellenberger is above all the author of a corpus of clinical cases about Native people in America or Indochina, from which he excerpts vignettes to illustrate his words, a little like sociologist Erving Goffman (1922–1982).[168] In contrast, Roger Bastide introduced fundamental methodological criticism, repeated by numerous social science researchers in opposition to the statements and clinical vignettes of doctors and psychoanalysts.

Roger Bastide was both similar and dissimilar to Henri Ellenberger, his non-physician and Sorbonne professor colleague. The two men belonged to different generations: Roger Bastide was born in Nîmes in 1898 and was of an age to serve in the Second World War. He passed the competitive teachers' examination (*agrégation*) in 1924, by which time Henri Ellenberger had not yet finished his medical training. They were nevertheless contemporaries, and their interests converged clearly in the 1950s and 1960s, which explains why Roger Bastide spent time as a visiting professor[169] in the department of the Université de Montréal where Henri Ellenberger was working in the early 1960s.

After completing his university education in Bordeaux and Paris, Roger Bastide published some early works in religious sociology. He left for Brazil in 1938, where he remained for close to twenty years, and was there when the Second World War broke out. A sociology professor at the University of São Paolo, he carried on the teaching of Claude Lévi-Strauss between 1935 and 1938. His numerous publications cover a vast range, from Brazilian religious worship, to the cultures and literatures of Brazil, to the epistemological relationships between sociology and psychanalysis, from a perspective close to that of Georges Gurvitch. He defended his thesis at the Sorbonne in 1957 and was appointed director of studies at the École pratique des hautes études (VIth section, which later became EHESS), in the field of social psychiatry. In 1959, he was appointed professor of ethnology and religious sociology at the Sorbonne, a position that had first been held by Marcel Griaule (1898–1956) in 1942; he later shared the chair of ethnology with André Leroi-Gourhan.

Numerous parallels may be established. Like Henri Ellenberger and Maurice Leenhardt, Roger Bastide was Protestant and maintained strong ties with Protestant intellectual and institutional circles throughout his career. He worked with Leenhardt, and both are mentioned in Henri Ellenberger's "Ethnopsychiatry." All three were passionate about the social dimension of mental illness, about the deep links between insanity and religious history – insanity was long considered a sacred illness – and about the systematic and rational study of folklore. Finally, Henri Ellenberger and Roger Bastide had both lived and taught in America and had been to Africa: Henri Ellenberger grew up there as the colonial empires were coming to an end, whereas Roger Bastide went there to work as an ethnologist after decolonization had begun. Both returned there several times to give talks or to participate in scientific meetings.[170]

Besides all this, there are other points of convergence between Roger Bastide and Henri Ellenberger; they also shared a number of collaborators. First, there was the professor of psychiatry Henri Baruk, mentioned earlier, who inspired Henri Ellenberger's thesis topic; a pioneer in social psychiatry,[171] Baruk was a professor at the Faculty of Medicine in Paris. With Roger Bastide he was a founding member of the "Laboratoire de psychiatrie sociale" established in Paris in 1959 at the École pratique des hautes études, along with historian Charles Morazé (who at that time practised a mixture of national history and what was known as characterology), that is, the same year that Henri Ellenberger joined the Department of Transcultural Psychiatry at McGill University. Once again, we see how much this development of the discipline was a transnational phenomenon.

Social psychiatry was defined by an Austrian doctor, Hans Strotzka (1917–1994), as the study of the social and cultural factors that enter into the etiology of mental illnesses as well as the treatment and readaptation of patients through work, care of families, and hospital services.[172] But social psychiatry was above all an American movement dominated by doctors, such as Thomas A.C. Rennie (1904–1956) and Alexander H. Leighton (1908–2007), professors at Cornell University after the war. In France, we note Claude Veil, who collaborated with

Henri Baruk and Roger Bastide and who at the same time held editorial responsibilities at EMC. Claude Veil was then a recognized specialist in hygiene and mental health in occupational medicine and psychology. Finally, Roger Bastide in his works mentions Henri Ellenberger as a participant in social psychiatry,[173] alongside other members of the Évolution psychiatrique group: Georges Daumézon, Henri Duchêne, Henri Ey, and Eugène Minkowski.

The two men corresponded. In 1965, Henri Ellenberger wrote to Roger Bastide to ask him to write a review of his work for the EMC. This letter had a second objective: Henri Ellenberger was also looking for an editor to write a monograph based on booklets devoted to ethnopsychiatry.[174] Roger Bastide himself wrote a very positive review in the university journal that he ran, *L'année sociologique* (1965), but was openly skeptical as to the timeliness of a book. In any event, the exchange had other editorial consequences, for in the months following the review, the editors of the EMC[175] approached Roger Bastide to ask him to write a booklet updating epidemiological methods. That booklet[176] was published with François Raveau in 1971; it deals with a subchapter written in 1965 by Brian Murphy at Henri Ellenberger's request.

The distinctions between the participants in the field are thus subtle, just as their scientific activities are intricate; thus, we cannot treat them as isolated researchers. The renown of Roger Bastide, Georges Devereux, and even Henri Ellenberger in the history of psychiatry acts as a screen. Today, some of their contemporaries are forgotten, notably colonial doctors; people often do not know that they too were very much involved in university networks. In this respect I would mention a francophone and an anglophone: Henri Aubin (1903–1987) and John Colin D. Carothers (1903–1989).

Born in Angoulême, Henri Aubin entered the École du service de santé de la marine et des colonies in 1923 and did his training at the Faculty of Medicine in Bordeaux (internship in 1926). He then entered the École d'application du service de santé des troupes coloniales and obtained his degree in colonial medicine and maritime hygiene at the Faculty of Medicine in Marseille (1928). He began teaching very early on, from 1925 to 1927 as a demonstrator of the nervous system at the Faculty of Medicine in Bordeaux, as a professor of neuropsychiatry at the Faculty of Medicine in Marseille (passing the *agrégation* in 1937), and, in 1931–1932, as a lecturer at the medical school in Pondichéry. His responsibilities as a doctor for colonial troops (1922–38), his teaching, and his numerous publications[177] make him a pioneer of French ethnopsychiatry. He distinguished himself during the interwar years by the rather modern stances he took – for example, he called for an integrated (i.e., combined anthropological and neuropsychiatric) approach to treatment in the colonies.

Henri Aubin specialized in psychiatry and forensic medicine in Paris in the 1930s (at the special infirmary near the prefecture, the Val-de-Grâce hospital, and the Maison nationale de santé de Saint-Maurice). He passed the competition to become a psychiatric hospital doctor in 1936. One year later, he was appointed doctor of colonial troops. After stints as lead doctor of the psychiatric service in Oran (1938–45), then Algiers (1945–48), he returned to mainland France and settled in Clermont-Ferrand as lead doctor of a medical-psychological centre in 1948, then in Pierrefeu (Var, 1956–57). An important collaborator with Professor Antoine Porot (1875–1965) in Algiers, he collaborated in writing the *Manuel alphabétique de psychiatrie Clinique, thérapeutique et medico-légale* (1952), distinguishing himself as the author of particularly racist articles, albeit these were in keeping with theories then being defended at the Faculty of Medicine in Algiers. We note for instance the entries for "Indigenous North Africans," "Magic," "Blacks," and "Primitivism."[178] These articles continued to appear after Algerian independence in the 1965 edition, although they had been revised and updated. Clearly, interest in anthropology and the defence of racist theories are not mutually exclusive in cultural psychiatry; we must consider all the participants in the field.

Let us mention that Antoine Porot was a prominent participant in French colonial psychiatry. A professor of neuropsychiatry at the Faculty of Medicine in Algiers as of 1925, his school was characterized by two elements that at first appear contradictory. The first, unrecognized before the works of American historian Richard Keller,[179] was the trappings of a model medical institution, in that it benefited from health care equipment, modern laboratories, and teaching and research structures, the equivalents of which were hard to find in mainland France in Antoine Porot's time. The second was an openly racist scholarly discourse that associated North African society with primitive psychology. Arabs are described by Antoine Porot and his students as infantile, impulsive, and inferior individuals – and above all, as potential criminals.[180] In fact, Antoine Porot was putting forward ideas that were fashionable at the time: prevailing evolutionism, the cult of progress, anthropological knowledge dealing more with the naturalist narrative than with methods in social sciences, and so on. In taking North Africans' forced submission through colonization for a natural state, the group at the Algiers School was simply legitimizing the colonial order by giving it scientific basis. Not until the 1950s did a courageous minority of French psychiatrists denounce the racism and pseudoscience of colonial psychiatry: the Martinique psychiatrist Frantz Fanon (1925–1961),[181] who joined the National Liberation Front in the midst of the Algerian War of independence, is in some ways the opposite of Henri Aubin.

Frantz Fanon was supported by Jean-Paul Sartre,[182] Simone de Beauvoir, and the intellectual journal *Les Temps modernes,* whereas Henri Aubin was a member of two of the largest French learned societies, the Société medico-psychologique (Medical and Psychological Society) and the Évolution psychiatrique group; he frequently contributed to the Société de médecine et d'hygiène tropicales (Society of Tropical Medicine and Hygiene) and was a member of the editorial committee of several collectives and journals, including the EMC's *Traité de psychiatrie*[183] and *Neuropsychiatrie de l'enfance et de l'adolescence.* We note he was a consulting doctor at WHO, that his list of publications totals more than two hundred titles, and that, with Georges Devereux, he was one of the rare francophone specialists who published in English-language scientific journals in the 1930s.

To complete the picture, on the English-language side, we provide a brief biography of John Colin Carothers, for Henri Ellenberger mentions him on several occasions. Born in 1903 in Simonstown, South Africa, he was the son of an English engineer working for the British navy. He began his medical training in 1921 at St. Thomas's Hospital, University of London. As a young graduate, he accepted to a job offer in Kenya in 1929. He had to travel throughout the entire colony to perform his duties. A turning point in his career occurred in 1938, when the psychiatrist of the Mathari Mental Hospital in Nairobi resigned and he replaced him without having trained in psychiatry. After the Second World War, John Colin Carothers specialized in medical psychology at Maudsley Hospital in London (where Eric Wittkower had completed his specialization a little earlier). In 1948 and 1949 the British Colonial Office ordered him to provide reports on the mental health services in Uganda and Northern Rhodesia.

John Colin Carothers is known for a number of assertions regarding Africans that essentialized and naturalized their radical differences from Westerners. For example, he asserted the rarity, even the non-existence of manic-depressive disorders and depression in Africans, whom he claimed were protected by their culture from this type of morbid reaction.[184] He also attributed Africans' underuse of the frontal lobe to their idleness in an article for which he later was vehemently criticized: "Frontal Lobe Function and the African."[185] Jock McCulloch methodically criticized Carothers in his book *Colonial Psychiatry*,[186] viewing his anthropological and medical conceptions as racist. Certainly Raymond Prince denounced Jock McCulloch's evaluation, as well as McCulloch's simplistic melding of the scientific production of McGill's Department of Transcultural Psychiatry with John Colin Carothers's colonial medicine; the reader may refer to the more recent book by the historian Matthew M. Heaton.[187] That said, the racist prejudice in Carothers's essays is undeniable. In 1951, he left colonial service to take up a position as a psychiatrist in Portsmouth, England. From then on, his scientific output became significant, and he is viewed as a prominent specialist in African psychopathology. Like Henri Aubin, he was named consulting physician at WHO (World Health Organization). His 1953 report published in the "WHO Monograph" collection was translated into French by Henri Aubin himself: *Psychopathologie normale et pathologique de l'African* (1954).

In 1954, Carothers returned to Africa at the request of the colonial government of Kenya, which ordered him to report on the Mau Mau revolutionary movement (1952–59). In 1955, he was assigned another report, this one for Nigeria: readers should refer to the already mentioned historical essay by Matthew M. Heaton to follow Carothers's postwar itinerary in more detail. To sum up, his activity as a consultant cannot be understood outside the context of the Cold War and that of British and American governments using scientists to try to comprehend the burgeoning independence movement. In 1961, he was invited to the first Pan-African Psychiatric Conference in Abeokuta, organized by Thomas Lambo (1923–2004) in Nigeria – proof of his significant place in the psychiatric cultural networks despite his controversial writings – alongside francophones such as Henri Collomb,[188] who took a more progressive stance in favour of reform in Africa.

SOCIAL LAWS, MARXISM, COLLECTIVE
REPRESENTATIONS, AND MEDICAL METAPHORS

The contrast between medical careers like Carothers's and that of an anthropologist like Roger Bastide is striking. The latter sought to arrive at conclusions through social-psychiatric observations that would have the force of sociological method behind them.[189] He did not hide his aversion for psychiatrists' unsystematic collections of case studies.[190] He remained rooted in social theory: the psychic might determine insanity, but only the social could explain how mental disorders were distributed in society:

> Psychotic or neurotic personalities exist naturally everywhere. But in traditional societies, people deny it in a specific way, for the individual exists only through and in the group. One person's illness is considered less ... a personal illness than a *symptom* of an illness found at another level, in the disorganization of the group. Traditional therapy will therefore consist in treating the family group and rebuilding the community by putting a stop to internal tensions, reconciling opponents, and if necessary, by creating around a crisis of possession the communication lost. But the African who comes to France finds himself alone and no longer has these defence mechanisms or community to regain mental health. What emerges from most of our stories of the lives of Africans is that the point of departure of their troubles is by no means the clash of two cultures or two societies inside them – but in their prior life – prior to their arrival in France.[191]

The socialization process offers an explanatory principle of the diversity of mental disorders and is thus seen by Roger Bastide as a sociological law, whereas Henri Ellenberger mainly sees in erroneous diagnoses the key to a medical problem, in the sense that they present the problem of the natural history of illnesses, their expression, their interpretation, and their care. But the misunderstanding goes further: Henri Ellenberger sometimes presents clinical cases in the context of classic social change (industrialization, urbanization, contacts between foreign cultures, migrations, wars, and so on), in such a way that change is always the vehicle of social disorder, conflicts, or pathologies, or the opportunity for a transformation of these symptoms. Yet one of Roger Bastide's major contributions to the sociology of mental illnesses, based on ethnographic fieldwork in Brazil, is to show, on the contrary, that interactions, the phenomena of interbreeding, and rites (which Westerners view as disorder or insanity) are fully socially coded and a source of social stability. Thus, possession may be interpreted as a psychosomatic conversion phenomenon along the lines of hysterical neurosis in the West, but elsewhere it has socializing virtues, with the dance obeying the rules of a symbolic grammar.

Psychiatrists and ethnologists have strongly divergent views, and in that regard, Roger Bastide takes a stand in his publications to specify the forms of a possible, desirable collaboration[192] with doctors. Strangely, the typology of the scenarios outlined by Roger Bastide never mentions the existence of the McGill University group, although it enjoyed high visibility at a top North American university. Should we conclude from this that Roger Bastide's methodological criticisms directly addressed the transcultural psychiatry developed by Eric Wittkower at McGill? The question remains open; institutional relations between Roger Bastide's laboratory in Paris and the McGill team will have to be examined, if the archives permit.

Finally, another major difference between Roger Bastide and Henri Ellenberger resides in the credibility each one gives to Marxist arguments. Setting aside questions of social classes and the relationship between history and economics, for social science researchers the Marxist perspective is also a way of enumerating individual and collective representations, be it in terms of the analysis of superstructures or of ideology.[193] Roger Bastide melds the Marxist perspective with the epistemology of sociology. He had no communist leanings, yet it is clear that he sought to seriously discuss Marxist arguments and that some of his writings and lectures are tinged with Marxist jargon. I disagree on this point with François Laplantine,[194] who ignores the impact of Marxism and who focuses too much on Freudianism in his analysis.[195] Meanwhile, to be clear, Marxism had no influence on Henri Ellenberger. Here his biography is enlightening: his wife was Russian and had fled the persecutions in the early years of the Soviet regime. Moreover, after 1952–53, Henri Ellenberger lived exclusively in North America, where communism was taboo in the academic world. Erwin Ackerknecht may have been an exception: he was a Trotskyist activist until the early 1930s.[196]

But if Marxism served as a path that allowed many thinkers to express individual and collective representations in the twentieth century, there were other approaches that did not draw from economics or sociological models, but rather from psychology. For example, there was the concept of the collective unconscious. Created by Carl G. Jung, the concept is not entirely identifiable with that of the archetype: it is both more vague (archetypes are only one type, alongside instincts and other components) and less identified with its author. For example, for historian Philippe Ariès, the collective unconscious is a useful conceptual tool for coming into closer contact with the "permanence" of a society in the long term, whereas for Henri Ellenberger it offers the possibility of understanding the collective phenomena of insanity – what doctors and psychologists called "collective psychoses." This reminder is useful, for it makes it possible to shed light on the relationship to the "cultural" that ethnopsychiatrists also developed, which may lend itself to a nostalgic taking up of a mythical post or a postcard vision of the Orient, ignoring both the complex realities of the present day. Nostalgia is not perceptible in Henri Ellenberger's articles, yet it is strongly perceptible in the literature he draws from, in which exotic case studies from the past are omnipresent. Indeed, the history of the nineteenth century and accounts of the cultures of Native Americans, Inuit, Africans, and Asians form an implicit corpus. But Henri Ellenberger draws from a second corpus, European and American, that is less known. So we must qualify our observation: certainly we can state that ethnopsychiatry is steeped in exoticism as defined by Edward Said, but at the same time we must point out that Henri Ellenberger innovated by relying on examples and phenomena from recent, Western societies unrelated to the Orient as reconstructed by the West, as analyzed by Edward Said. Let us mention two typically American and contemporary case studies on which Henri Ellenberger relies: the famous panic[197] caused by Orson Welles's (1915–1985) radio broadcast of *The War of the Worlds* in the United States in 1938, and an epidemic of mass hysteria that struck students at an American high school in 1939. These examples serve a didactic purpose, and it is likely that Henri Ellenberger developed them for his teaching in Montreal. Some examples are more difficult to classify, notably the ones involving Japan, which reflect Ellenberger's personal curiosity about the society of that country, which he satisfied by making a research trip there in 1979; we will return to that journey at the end of this presentation.

Other methods connect Roger Bastide and Henri Ellenberger and set them apart from Georges Devereux: for example, the systematic

processing of existing quantitative data about users of psychiatric
hospitals and other mental hygiene services in societies that are mul-
tiethnic (Brazil) or undergoing decolonization, with the objective
of discussing, interpreting, and qualifying the differences between
genres, living standards, and races in the statistics. These data are
rarely acquired using methods of epidemiology or demography;
very often they are arrived at based on empirical data developed by
doctors in the service of those fields. As a general procedure, Roger
Bastide and Henri Ellenberger apply data to show that correlations
between race and illness cannot be explained by simple biological
determinism, which is what people still believed was possible to do
at the end of the nineteenth century. On the contrary, from their
point of view, connections established between skin colour, living
standards, the distribution of mental disorders, and the colonial past
follow *social* logic. To sum up, for both authors the quantitative data
on the cohorts should not be overlooked.

Yet collective phenomena remain a complex problem with their
own particularities. Indeed, Henri Ellenberger's reference work
does not cover just individual illnesses; it also confronts the difficult
problem of mass hysteria. The subject today may appear difficult or
bizarre, but in fact it is a legitimate *topos* in the history of medicine
because it has been known since antiquity and is not easy to dispose
of within the framework of an encyclopedia.

Here again we may create links between issues in the humanities
and the social sciences. We have already recalled the importance
of Maurice Halbwachs, who held a chair in group psychology at
the Collège de France (1944–45). Later on, understanding of certain phenomena such as suicide remained disputed by doctors and
researchers in the social sciences, and mass suicides remained a
controversial problem, whether their significance was religious, sec-
tarian, or heroic, for example in times of war. This topic was the
subject of a report in 1955 by a medical officer[198] during the annual
conference on French psychiatry at a time when the French army was
still very active in the colonial wars. Linking these individual phenomena to collective phenomena introduces the problem of illness
as metaphor, a topic on which American intellectual Susan Sontag
(1933–2004) wrote a famous essay,[199] without being a specialist in
medical history, but in a way pursuing the semiological approach of
Roland Barthes. Medical historian Mirko Grmek also devoted an
analysis to it[200] at the end of his career, in the face of the civil war

ravaging the former Yugoslavia, where he was born and where he witnessed crimes against humanity.

The metaphor of the epidemic is at the centre of Henri Ellenberger's operative concepts, whereas Roger Bastide is wholly opposed to this medical metaphor, explaining his reasons in detail in the example of possession, in which he sets out his transcultural reflections as he developed them during his fieldwork in Brazil: "In Africa, possessions do not constitute an epidemic: they do not spread, they are created, controlled and organized by the cult group."[201] His condemnation is final: psychiatrists therefore err in a most unfortunate confusion, for the analytical framework that would allow us to understand phenomena of possession are to be found not in mass insanity but in the social order.

Even more critical than Roger Bastide, Erwin Ackerknecht[202] does not hide his skepticism of the term "psychic epidemic" (*geistige Epidemie* in German);[203] he prefers to talk about "mass movements" typical of situations of acculturation in terms of situations in which cultures are unbalanced by the introduction of new elements (colonization, a new religion, and so on). He recalls that René Laennec (1781–1826), an important participant in the development of the clinical method in France, wrote a memoir[204] on mental medicine that reiterated the old argument about mass insanity in order to defend his conception of the relationship of the soul to the body. René Laennec, a Catholic and a royalist, upheld the idea that delusions are not organic and that the contagiousness of mass delusions to some extent provides paradigmatic proof, inasmuch as they cannot on any account be organic in origin. His reasoning is relatively simple: mass delusion is not organic in nature, so neither is individual delusion. But this argument has political repercussions. Indeed, Erwin Ackerknecht reminds us that the political and religious instrumentalization of mass delusions served as a means to attack the French Revolution and democracy. In contrast, during the same period, François Joseph Victor Broussais defended an organicist conception of insanity, based on the theory of inflammation, even in cases of mass delusion[205] – thus, his was a secular theory. Clearly, this theme is not politically neutral. Moreover, Erwin Ackerknecht also explains that phenomena caused by suggestion belong to another framework: these are also normal phenomena, such as beliefs and ideologies.

With Henri Ellenberger the metaphor of the epidemic is linked to the notion of "mental contagion," particularly in the classic example of "psychogenic death." This problem became famous in French anthropology after Marcel Mauss[206] attempted to summarize the subject in the early twentieth century. The topic became something of a required *topos*, even if, as the twentieth century advanced, anthropologists and doctors became less familiar with the model of understanding that underlies the explanations of Marcel Mauss, that is, hypnosis and suggestion, as people still may have thought of them in the early twentieth century. This explanatory model, having grown outdated, sank into oblivion after psychoanalysis became established as the explanatory standard for psychological phenomena throughout the world in the mid-twentieth century. But hypnosis and suggestion were not yet anachronistic in the view of Henri Ellenberger, a very erudite man, especially as the problem of psychogenic death had been physically reframed thanks to the works of Walter B. Cannon (1871–1945), a Harvard professor who specialized in psychosomatics and who wrote about the role of endocrine glands and the internal physiological environment in stress phenomena. The state of death attributed to voodoo practices is one of the stereotypes that struck the imagination of scientists such as Cannon;[207] the reader may consult the writings of the Haitian doctor Louis Mars[208] to see how this question was reappropriated from the ethnopsychiatric point of view. Henri Ellenberger appropriated this question very early on, when he was still in Switzerland;[209] in the 1965 booklets, the two explanations (psychological and physiological) coexist, but the cases and observations he reports are included in a specific narrative genre with accounts of magic, possession, and exorcism. In this way, when he gives examples, he tells how, to avoid certain death, the evil spirit is channelled into an object or an animal, and the patient is cured – if not, he dies, with the community as well as the sick person persuaded of the fatal outcome. We would like to know more about what Henri Ellenberger called the phenomenon of "mental contagion"; as we cannot convey his convictions on the problem, it is important here to reintroduce those who promoted transcultural psychiatry in Montreal, concerned with both individual and collective psychopathological phenomena, but who were able to develop new approaches to deal with these issues, notably quantitative methods unrelated to psychological interpretation. I am thinking in particular of psychiatric epidemiology.

THE CONTRIBUTION OF KNOWLEDGE DEVELOPED IN CANADA: PARTICIPANTS AND TEACHING IN THE 1960S

In the 1960s the intellectual landscape was different in Montreal than in Paris, as was the social and political context. Quebec has two linguistic communities, and beyond the frictions between francophones and anglophones, the population of Montreal was highly cosmopolitan after the war, for Quebec's largest city had taken in many refugees from the Second World War and the Cold War. Canadian universities recruited a great many of their teaching staff from abroad to compensate for the lack of qualified personnel at home and also in order to promote new disciplines. In addition, Quebec and the rest of Canada had responsibilities toward the First Nations (still referred to as Indians and Eskimos in France), especially in terms of health policy.

From the time it was founded, the transcultural study group at McGill University brought together psychiatrists and social science researchers, the former in greater number. The group organized its meetings at the university's psychiatry service at the Allan Memorial Institute. The Departments of Anthropology and Sociology were also involved. In 1981 an autonomous research department, the Division of Social and Transcultural Psychiatry, was officially launched. The years that interest us are from 1955 to 1981, when the group was led by "pioneers," to use the term chosen by Raymond Prince,[210] who minimized any ties to colonial medicine.

At first, the section's activities revolved around working meetings and multidisciplinary research seminars, courses that are difficult to describe today, as descriptions based on the archival materials are not available before the 1960s. The department became known largely thanks to a journal, *Transcultural Research in Mental Health Problems*, founded in 1956, which still exists. At first a simple mimeographed newsletter, its function was to centralize and disseminate information on transcultural psychiatry.[211] It contained reviews of books and articles, statistics, and announcements of conferences. The journal as it first existed was a tool for creating social bonds; through it, a questionnaire was distributed around the world to determine the expectations of those who were interested in the field. This was an attempt to develop a new professional specialization and to seek recognition for it. By the end of the 1950s, many of the authors who sent texts to the journal were working in the colonies or former colonies. Among the territories covered (or areas, in the sense of area studies), Asia was strongly represented, even overrepresented, notably by Japan. A former colonial power,[212] Japan was an important Cold War ally of the United States. It also had the most extensive and most modern university network in Asia. This sphere of influence (Southeast Asia) referred more to the British Empire and to the American zone of influence than to Europe. Nevertheless, the newsletter was not a purely Anglo-Saxon journal: Guy Dubreuil, a professor in the Department of Anthropology at the Université de Montréal, quickly took over from Jacob Fried, co-organizing the journal with Eric Wittkower.

Henri Ellenberger joined the editorial committee in 1960, at the same time as Brian Murphy. By then, other francophones were involved with the journal as correspondents, such as Georges Devereux. A little later, in the 1960s, we find reviews of works by Roger Bastide[213] and Henri Collomb,[214] both of whom themselves ran journals: *L'année sociologique* (Bastide) and Henri Collomb headed *Psychopathologie africaine* (Collomb). Collomb was a prominent participant in social psychiatry in West Africa; he stood out by often rejecting the term "ethnopsychiatry,"[215] preferring to integrate practices of traditional care with those of modern psychiatry, with the goal of improving patients' resocialization rather than promoting a form of exoticism. Trained at the École du service de santé de la marine et des colonies, then at the École d'application du service de santé de la France d'outre-mer, a military medical training school, Henri Collomb held positions in Dijbouti, Somalia, Ethiopia, and Indochina before obtaining a chair in neuropsychiatry in Dakar (1958). He then spent twenty years at Fann Hospital in Dakar (the psychiatric service had been created slightly earlier, in 1956), as a medical officer, paid as a lecturer-researcher at the University of Dakar by the French government until his retirement, even after Senegal's independence. He had many colleagues at Fann Hospital: social science researchers, psychologists, and doctors, including René Collignon, Babakar Diop, Moussa Diop, Paul Martino, Marie-Cécile Ortigues, Jacqueline Rabain, Simone Valantin, and András Zempléni. We also note that Collomb underwent psychoanalysis with Angelo Hesnard, a co-founder of the Paris Psychoanalytic Society and the Évolution psychiatrique group, and that he contributed to the *Traité de psychiatrie* edited by Henri Ey for the EMC.

Clearly, the McGill newsletter welcomed francophones. By the early 1960s, Eric Wittkower claimed that it had nine hundred correspondents (a number that cannot be verified) around the world. We excerpt here a circular letter from 1963 that sums up the objectives of the journal, and thus of McGill's Department of Transcultural Psychiatry:

> Recently a section of Transcultural Psychiatric Studies was set up at the McGill University, jointly by the Departments of Psychiatry and Sociology and Anthropology.
>
> The aims of the Section are: (1) to collect and disseminate information regarding the relevance of sociocultural variables to incidence, prevalence and nature of mental disease; (2) to train psychiatrists and social scientists interested in the area of transcultural psychiatry; and (3) to carry out research in this area in Canada and in other countries.
>
> Our program, to date, has succeeded in establishing a communication network of psychiatrists and social scientists in over seventy countries, involving over 900 participants, whose reports on the nature of their research problem, interests and observations are published by us in the form of a Newsletter entitled: *Review and Newsletter: Transcultural Research in Mental Health Problems.*[216]

The use of certain technical terms, such as *incidence* and *prevalence* (utilized by Georges Devereux rarely, if ever), indicate other loans from science at the time, such as epidemiology. Indeed, incidence and prevalence are epidemiological terms, which indicates that transcultural psychiatry and epidemiology were not separate at McGill, or rather that epidemiology was better integrated into the Canadian approach than the French approach. Moreover, the department was involved in training young doctors at the university, which was not the case with Roger Bastide and Georges Devereux in France, who taught students in the humanities and social sciences. A summary document clearly states Eric Wittkower's objective in the mid-1960s:

> The purpose of the program is two-fold:
> a) to train researchers from psychiatry and related disciplines and to supply academic centres with potential teachers in the field;

b) to orient mental health the need to consider the cultural backgrounds of their peoples when planning psychiatric services; and
to assist them in doing so.[217]

To illustrate the circulation of knowledge, note that the Newsletter
was sent to France to the scientific information exchange service of
the Maison des sciences de l'homme (MSH), and to West Germany to
the University of Bremen. The same document indicates five courses,
and their title descriptions:

Social Psychiatry
Application of sociological theory to psychiatry; principles of
social psychiatry; sociopsychiatric research techniques. (20hrs)
H. B. M. Murphy.

Clinical Aspects of Transcultural Psychiatry
Cultural influences on symptomatology; modification of
therapeutic approaches in different cultural settings; indigenous
therapies. (20hrs) E. D. Wittkower et al.

Anthropological Approaches to Psychiatry
Application of anthropological concepts to psychiatry; use of
psychiatric data in anthropology. (20hrs) N. A. Chance & R.
Wintrob.

International Epidemiology of Mental Illness
Cultural variations in incidence and prevalence; survey and
statistical techniques; validity of international comparisons.
(20hrs) H. B. M. Murphy.

*Transcultural Aspects of Administrative and Community
Psychiatry*
Cultural influences on demand for and attitude towards
services; British, French, American and Caribbean models;
incorporation of traditional healers in Africa and India. (20hrs)
M. Lemieux et al.[218]

This teaching was not just theoretical; students had to carry out
supervised fieldwork. Moreover, the program attempted to establish
a balance between students who were doctors and those who were

not; indeed, the intention was to have them work in pairs. To that end, a collaboration with the University of Vermont[219] was developed as a means to achieve an intellectual critical mass and to recruit enough students for the program to produce results.

The department did not grant a specific degree, but courses in transcultural psychiatry were accredited and recognized in the curricula for both medicine and anthropology at McGill. The department was accessible to young psychiatrists in training as well as to psychologists, sociologists, and anthropologists. Its structure was basically open, and it was connected to a network of American universities to which McGill was very close culturally. In fact, many American students and teachers joined McGill, particularly in psychiatry.

The team led by Eric Wittkower was active principally at international meetings. A first meeting was organized during the Second World Congress of Psychiatry (Zurich, 1957), which brought together twenty-four psychiatrists from around twenty countries. Ewen Cameron chaired this meeting, which had been organized by Eric Wittkower.[220] Among those who attended were Tsung-Yi Lin[221] (Taiwan), Thomas A. Lambo (Nigeria), Morris Carstairs[222] (Great Britain), C.S. Seguin (Peru), and Pow-Meng Yap (Hong Kong). At the Third World Congress of Psychiatry (Montreal, 1961), one panel featured a discussion between the teams of Eric Wittkower and Alexander Leighton. The American Psychiatric Association and its Canadian counterpart established transcultural psychiatry committees in 1964 and 1967 respectively. In 1970, Brian Murphy founded the World Psychiatric Association Section on Transcultural Psychiatry.[223] Other international associations could be mentioned, but most of them began after the period we are examining. University study groups also flourished, as did foundations and so on, but they too were not founded before the 1970s.

Brian Murphy became head of the Transcultural Psychiatry Division when Eric Wittkower retired in 1965. At the institutional level, he is remembered for establishing a lasting collaboration with francophone anthropologists at the Université de Montréal and the Université du Québec (UQAM) and for helping to found, in 1974, a bilingual research group, GIRAME (Groupe inter-universitaire de recherche en anthropolgie médicale et en ethnopsychiatrie), which ran for about ten years.[224] At the end of his career he published a reference work titled *Comparative Psychiatry*,[225] in the tradition of Emil Kraepelin and Pow-Meng Yap.[226] This work, the culmination of his career, presented thirty years of quantitative data on several population samples around the world.

Raymond Prince, who witnessed the development of the transcultural psychiatry section from the 1960s to the 2000s (and who headed the section after Brian Murphy), provides a list of the active members at McGill for the initial ten years: Norman Chance, Henri Ellenberger, Brian Murphy, Juan Negrete, Raymond Prince, Jean-François Saucier, Ronald Wintrob, and Eric Wittkower.[227] Oddly, Prince leaves off the list the anthropologists Jacob Fried and Guy Dubreuil. Clearly, that list is unbalanced: doctors are overrepresented in relation to anthropologists, in terms of their contributions.

At the international level, Raymond Prince also points to a number of research centres that were founded after the McGill department: the East-West Centre of Honolulu, the Department of Social Medicine at Harvard Medical School (long chaired by Arthur Kleinman, who also chaired Harvard's Department of Anthropology), the British Culture and Psychiatry Group in London led by Roland Littlewood, and a network called Pacific Rim, which brought together groups from Japan, Hong Kong, Taiwan, and mainland China.[228] Note the absence of francophone research centres on this list, whether in Paris, Dakar, Montreal, or elsewhere. Raymond Prince also ignores the west coast of North America as well as Central and Eastern Europe. However, we must stress that the scientific communities had plenty of intermediaries. It is important at this juncture, before we discuss other ties, to briefly recall the careers of the participants mentioned as the leading pioneers in Montreal: Norman Chance, Juan Negrete, Raymond Prince, Jean-François Saucier, and Ronald Wintrob.

Norman Chance is an American anthropologist, known mainly as a specialist in the Arctic. He studied at the University of Pennsylvania and at Cornell before teaching in Oklahoma and Quebec. He was recruited by Eric Wittkower shortly after Brian Murphy, Henri Ellenberger, and Raymond Prince. In addition to his activities in the Department of Anthropology, he was involved in multidisciplinary teaching in the section and was on the newsletter's editorial committee. He left Canada before the late 1960s to take up a position at the University of Connecticut and at the Department of Psychiatry of the new medical school there. His fieldwork focused on the Far North, Alaska, and northern Scandinavia, on the Cree (one of Canada's First Nations), and on Siberia, China, and so on. At the end of his career, he dedicated himself to environmental studies, in particular at Dartmouth College and at the Institute of Arctic Studies. Besides publishing works arising from his research in the social sciences, he also wrote fiction and ran a website between 1996 and 2009 devoted to the Arctic Circle.

Ronald Wintrob[229] studied medicine in Toronto and New York and had a year's experience in Laos on an international medical team. In 1961 he began a specialization in psychiatry at McGill, under the guidance of Eric Wittkower and Norman Chance. After a year in Paris and another two in Liberia, he returned to Montreal, where he held positions in both anthropology and psychiatry at McGill, and also at the Department of Psychiatry at the Université de Montréal. He trained in psychoanalysis with a francophone. Like Norman Chance, Ronald Wintrob left Canada to take up positions in the Departments of Anthropology and Psychiatry at the University of Connecticut School of Medicine. Ronald Wintrob remained there until 1982, then took a position in Providence, Rhode Island, at Brown University, in the Department of Psychiatry and Human Behaviour. He took part in many international associations and in transdisciplinary groups of specialists, besides chairing the international section of the World Psychiatric Association created by Brian Murphy.

Juan C. Negrete, an Argentinian, did his medical studies at the University of Tucuman before joining McGill in 1963 to specialize in psychiatry (Quebec College of Physicians, 1966; Fellow of the Royal College of Physicians and Surgeons of Canada, 1988). An expert in addictions, he headed a specialized service staring in 1980, the Addictions Unit of the McGill University Health Centre / Montreal General Hospital). He was appointed a professor of psychiatry at McGill in 1985, and then at the University of Toronto in 1995, where he headed a research program on addiction.

Jean-François Saucier, a psychiatrist, developed his first work in transcultural psychiatry at McGill based on the same issue as Henri Ellenberger: the impact of serious illnesses in children of families of different sociocultural backgrounds. He then conducted fieldwork in Africa before starting his academic career at the Department of Psychiatry at the Université de Montréal, where he contributed to anthropological analyses on the health and socialization of children.

Raymond H. Prince (1925–2012) was born Barrie, Ontario, in 1925. He served in the Royal Canadian Air Force at the end of the Second World War and then, as a veteran, studied medicine and social sciences at the University Western Ontario, where he specialized in psychiatry. In 1957, he was appointed by the British Colonial Office to the Aro Hospital (built in 1951 in Abeokuta), just before Nigeria gained its independence (1960). Far from being isolated (unlike John Colin Carothers when he began), Raymond Prince was in contact with Thomas Lambo, the hospital's administrator in charge of consultations at the new University College Hospital in Ibadan, where Africa's first conference on psychiatry was held in 1961. Raymond Prince's earliest published scientific articles were based on his experience in Nigeria. First, he described a syndrome of intellectual exhaustion among Nigerian students, using the term *brain fag*, coined by his patients, who complained that they could no longer read or concentrate and who suffered from hypochondria. Second, Prince established that, for a long time, the traditional healers of West Africa had in their pharmacopoeia an effective anti-psychotic (*Rauwolfia vomitoria*), similar to the one discovered in India (*Rauwolfia serpentina*), and long unknown by Westerners, who had no powerful psychotropic medication before 1952 (Chlorpromazine: trade names Thorazine and Largactil). Wiser for this experience, in 1959 Raymond Prince joined the team assembled by Eric Wittkower at McGill. He returned to Nigeria in 1961–62 through funding from the Human Ecology Fund to study traditional medicine, focusing on soothsayers and Yoruba priests, and participated in the Cornell–Aro Project led by Alexander H. Leighton, a study of mental disorders in western Nigeria; Matthew M. Heaton has demonstrated the project's importance for the globalization of mental health policies.[230] The collaboration with Alexander H. Leighton was long-lasting: Raymond Prince also participated in the Stirling County Study,[231] which Leighton led with Jane Murphy in Nova Scotia, Canada, working on the scientific validation of the study and conducting interviews. His fieldwork abroad also included a study of Rastafarians in Jamaica (1967–69). In 1979, Raymond Prince was appointed a professor of psychiatry at McGill, then director of the transcultural psychiatry section from 1981 to 1991, following Brian Murphy. At the same time, he edited McGill's *Transcultural Psychiatric Research Review*. His numerous medical and administrative responsibilities included working as a consultant with First Nations for the Cree Board of Health from 1978 to 1991. He mainly analyzed the links between religion and mental health (he was the editor of the R.M. Bucke Memorial Society Newsletter[232]) and the use of drugs in traditional medicine. At the end of his life he had become a repository of memory in the university department created by Eric Wittkower in Montreal, publishing his autobiography[233] and commemorative articles. Last but not least, he published fiction (under the pseudonym Rupert de Prenier) and produced documentary films.

These brief biographical notes supplement those of Henri Ellenberger and Eric Wittkower at McGill. Later on, we will be discussing Brian Murphy regarding his collaboration with the EMC. But this small group should not be artificially isolated from other participants in cultural psychiatry around the world, and one day a systematic prosopography of the major contemporaries should be created. As it is not possible to mention them all here, the best solution is to emphasize what made the McGill team stand out: the contribution of epidemiological psychiatric methods to transcultural psychiatry. The research project that most deeply influenced the history of the discipline was the Stirling County Project, which we have already mentioned, a study of epidemiological psychiatry in Nova Scotia from 1952 to present day.[234] Scientific supervision was based at Cornell University, then at Harvard and at Dalhousie (Nova Scotia), led by Alexander H. Leighton[235] and later by his second wife, Jane Murphy (1929–).[236] We will discuss that project later on with regard to Brian Murphy.

THE CULTURALISM IN QUESTION: CONTROVERSY WITH THE PARIS TEAM OF THE EMC

The methods and results of psychiatric epidemiology were undoubtedly among the most important that Henri Ellenberger introduced in France through his actions as an intermediary for his colleagues at McGill. But they in no way created the controversy that would flow from them. Indeed, the archives clearly indicate that the culturalism in which American anthropology was immersed in the twentieth century provoked resistance in France.

The archival materials held at the Fonds Henri Ellenberger and the Fonds Henri Ey[237] demonstrate that Henri Ellenberger had conceived the project of a reference work on ethnopsychiatry independently from his involvement in the EMC run by Henri Ey (he mentions a first order from Basic Books, his publisher in New York). Henri Ellenberger contributed to the *Traité de psychiatrie* from the time it was launched in the early 1950s with more than five hundred contributors. He contacted the EMC when he was seeking a publisher; here is an excerpt of the letter he wrote in early 1962 to Henri Ey, editor of the EMC's *Traité de psychiatrie*, in which he expressed his ideas:

> Another significant part of my time was devoted to ethnopsychiatry, what here is called "transcultural psychiatry." Perhaps you know the Newsletter published twice a year by Drs Wittkower, H.B.M. Murphy, and myself. We have accumulated a great deal of material, probably unique in the world. I have long had the idea of writing an account of all these studies, either in book form or otherwise. Do you think that the Encyclopédie medico-chirurgicale would be interested in publishing in its next supplement an "ethnopsychiatry" booklet? I am aware that there is something on "exotic psychiatry," but ethnopsychiatry is far wider in scope and would contribute a great many new or little-known facts that are also topical.[238]

Henri Ellenberger is here presenting his work as a storehouse of knowledge accumulated by the Montreal team in a university setting, in contrast to the "exotic psychiatry" inherited from colonial medicine and represented at the EMC by Henri Aubin[239] – from whom Henri Ellenberger wished to differentiate himself. Henri Ey[240] replied to this letter that Charles Brisset, another close collaborator, was already in charge of the ethnopsychiatry and anthropology section at the EMC, under the rubric "Social Psychiatry": Henri Ellenberger would have to get in touch with him. Charles Brisset was a psychiatrist and psychoanalyst in charge of a psychosomatic medicine consultation, a close friend of Henri Ey,[241] and a member of the Évolution psychiatrique group.

The editorial projects of Charles Brisset and Henri Ellenberger converged: both wanted all the booklets written for the social psychiatry section to be assembled in a separate volume. There had been at least one precedent at the EMC: a series of booklets devoted to child psychiatry had been assembled in a volume published with the Presses universitaires de France edited by Léon Michaux,[242] in which Charles Brisset had also participated. Contacted through Henri Ey, Brisset enthusiastically welcomed Henri Ellenberger's proposal to collaborate:

An introduction will make it possible to situate this section in the general work and to define methodological points of view. We must show which methods are used and the orientation of modern sociology and ethnology, the concerns of psychiatry compared to these two disciplines, and the development of ideas that allowed their approaches to converge. Then an initial chapter will focus on the study of the first development with the elementary structures of kinship. This involves describing the genesis of creating symbols in the first conflicts posed by primitive social necessities; the second chapter will pursue the same approach, describing the continuation of the relationships of man and his environment up to adulthood. This second chapter will feature the structure of family, school groups, and so on. The third chapter will be devoted to cultures and here I was thinking of using what I wrote, inserting it in the project overall. A fourth chapter will examine the "projected formations," (religion, morality, aesthetics). Finally, a fifth chapter should include basically the practical material that may serve as a tentative conclusion to these studies, that is the concepts that psychiatrists and technicians in various disciplines have drawn from all these works regarding the genesis of mental or psychosomatic illnesses: problems of desocialization, acculturation, and so on, with their pathological consequences.

It seems to me that your assistance may be particularly of value on one hand in terms of working together to lend us your advice and your extensive experience with contacts in North American social anthropology, and to take up again the chapter on cultural anthropology, as well as in writing the final chapter, for which it seems to me the documentation you have assembled with Wittkower is particularly suited, if I can go by my reading of Wittkower. It would of course be easier to discuss all this if you have an opportunity to come to Europe. We would take advantage of that to organize around your visit one of our working sessions.[243]

A first remark: this outline is rather theoretical and quite abstract. He does not mention the fieldwork in social anthropology, nor does he set out the booklets' contents in any detail. It must be stated that this plan would never be applied as such and that the program cannot be compared to the booklets written a few years later by other participants than those that had been contemplated at the start.

A learned doctor, well informed about developments in humanities and the social sciences in the 1950s and 1960s, Charles Brisset wanted to account for the intellectual ferment generated by structuralism, and he quotes Claude Lévi-Strauss's "elementary structures of kinship."[244] But it is difficult to see the connection between this type of concept and psychiatry in his editorial project. Also, Charles Brisset was a French psychoanalyst, and here he was addressing social institutions and the symbolic material handled by anthropologists based on the Freudian notion of projection. It seems that he saw a message to deliver on the cultural aspects of psychopathology in the wake of Sigmund Freud, whose texts included *Totem and Taboo* (1913), "The Moses of Michelangelo" (1914), "Group Psychology and the Analysis of the Ego" (1921), and *Moses and Monotheism* (1939). Charles Brisset worked with three collaborators, all of them doctors and psychoanalysts from the Paris Psychoanalytic Society: Jean-Luc Donnet, Jacques Azoulay, and Michel Neyraut.[245]

Henri Ellenberger was leery of responding to Charles Brisset's program point by point. Instead he emphasized his documentation and his academic experience. In a letter to Brisset dated 13 February 1962 that crossed in the mail with Brisset's letter owing to postal delays between Canada and France, he again explained his approach to ethnopsychiatry, pointing out once more that it no longer belonged to the framework of exotic psychiatry and that he already had a "detailed outline"[246] of his contribution. Charles Brisset then refocused the project in another later dated 1 April, for Henri Ellenberger's proposals overlapped with the "Mental Hygiene" section headed by Georges Daumézon in the same *Traité de psychiatrie* of the EMC, devoted to practical aspects (a section later renamed "Psychiatry and Environment"). For the "Sociopsychiatry" section, Charles Brisset wanted to publish two significant chapters (personality development and epidemiology), and to that end he circulated a detailed outline (dated 8 June 1962).

Late in 1962, after announcing his departure from McGill for a chair at the Université de Montréal, and after meeting Charles Brisset in Paris, Henri Ellenberger suggested that Brian Murphy collaborate. But in France, even if Charles Brisset was not opposed, a lasting misunderstanding occurred, for Brisset intended to support a psychoanalytic conception that aligned with that of his French collaborators and warned that he would oppose culturalist positions,[247] which he believed he would have to face with his North American colleagues.

In his publications,[248] Charles Brisset criticized the theories of Abram Kardiner and especially Karen Horney (1855–1952), an American psychoanalyst of German origin, one of the main representatives of the culturalist movement in psychoanalysis.[249] Although this protest was based on a misunderstanding (Henri Ellenberger and Brian Murphy were not culturalists), it allows us to draw a parallel: Henri Ey's collaborators were forced to enter the debate on structuralism in France, and at the same time, Henri Ellenberger was conveying, inadvertently, fashionable scientific ideas such as culturalism in North America. Here is an excerpt from Charles Brisset's letter:

> Thank you very much for sending me your outline and that of Doctor Murphy. They both seem perfect to me and very complete. My only comment deals with the following. In the spirit of the Encyclopédie, various points of view must be presented and discussed. Yet a difficulty arises for our entire section: European psychoanalysts, especially the French ones, willingly refer to the point of view of the great American school of Margaret Mead, Ruth Benedict, Fromm, and others as "culturalism." As here my colleagues are the young psychoanalysts you have met, I think that, while respecting the rule of the Encyclopédie, they are bound bring to light some of the criticisms leveled by orthodox psychoanalysis against culturalism. You will judge for yourself, as I cannot, whether Dr. Murphy should be informed that the presentation of a sociocultural point of view, while being as complete as he wishes, must be concerned about psychoanalytic purism, which personally I find justified. In the case of this type of article, it is always easy to show the various points of view with reciprocal arguments. I apologize for this perhaps excessive scruple.[250]

Once Brian Murphy was hired as an official contributor to the EMC, Henri Ellenberger suggested reducing his own contribution, allowing more input from Murphy, a specialist in psychiatric epidemiology. We can therefore attribute the introduction of this science in the Encyclopédie médico-chirurgicale to Henri Ellenberger's initiative. Brian Murphy[251] was born in Edinburgh. His father was a teacher with a degree in classics. Brian Murphy was raised as a Scottish Protestant and began his medical studies at the University of Edinburgh before interning in England at Tilbury (Seamen's Hospital) and joining the Royal Army Medical Corps in 1940. An officer during the war, he took part in operations in the Mediterranean zone. In 1945 he started working for the Red Cross and for international refugee organizations, including the United Nations Refugee Resettlement Association (UNRRA) and the International Refugees Organisation (IRO). In 1950 he trained in public health at the London University School of Hygiene, then left for Singapore to study the impact of cultural factors on mental health. He began studying mental disorders, suicide, juvenile delinquency, and psychosomatic disorders. At the same time, he was director of the Student Mental Health Service of the University of Malaya, which gave him the means to develop quantitative data. The data accumulated on the students of Singapore and Malaysia allowed him to develop a longitudinal study that he continued up until the 1980s. Having received a grant from the Milbank Memorial Fund in the United States, he left for New York to complete a doctoral dissertation in sociology at the New School of Social Research dealing with juvenile delinquency (1958). Following this dual training in medicine and the social sciences, he left with his wife and five children to settle in Montreal in 1959, joining Eric Wittkower's team at McGill. Like Henri Ellenberger, his first research project concerned the sociocultural characteristics of patients, specifically how the environment determined the chronicity of mental disorders, and also the effects of placing children in adoptive families. But unlike him, Brian Murphy never left McGill, where he taught from 1961 until his retirement in 1982.

In the end, the result published by the EMC was very different from the plan Charles Brisset had first projected: on one hand, Henri Ellenberger and Brian Murphy rapidly completed their contributions in 1963–64; on the other, all of Charles Brisset's contributors withdrew or did not succeed in writing their articles on time, Therefore, the combined initiatives on each side of the Atlantic resulted in a transfer to France of knowledge developed in Canada in the 1950s and 1960s. In January 1965, Henri Ellenberger's and Brian Murphy's texts were in press. Ellenberger completed them with a subchapter titled "Collective Psychoses" (1967), which he had not been able to finish in time.

Another consequence of the collaborative work was that Henri Ellenberger received other commissions for articles from the EMC, besides acting as an informal editorial adviser on related themes. Texts by Charles Brisset, Henri Ellenberger, and Brian Murphy remained in the EMC's *Traité de psychiatrie* until 1978, at which time they were updated by an extended and younger team that included Raymond Prince and Michel Tousignant (Université du Québec à Montréal, UQAM).[252] These collaborations were obscured due to the way in which Raymond Prince himself wrote the history of his discipline and the McGill department; he does not speak of it in his articles or books. Yet together they give substance to this section, thanks to the ties Henri Ellenberger established with francophone and anglophone academics. Michel Tousignant had an academic career at the crossroads of psychology, anthropology, and epidemiology[253] and participated in the bilingual group GIRAME with McGill's Department of Transcultural Psychiatry. He wrote about his fieldwork in Mexico and Ecuador but also about migrants and adolescents.

The editorial team of the EMC's *Traité de psychiatrie* changed in the late 1960s and early 1970s: Henri Ey parted ways with Charles Brisset; Claude Veil, previously mentioned and a colleague of Roger Bastide, took over running the "Social Psychiatry" section. Interests changed as well: alongside the booklets on neuroses and psychoses, updates now dealt with addictive behaviour, depressive states, and borderline personality disorders. A page in the history of French psychopathology was being turned; the paradigm of structural psychopathology as defined by Georges Lantéri-Laura[254] was coming to an end.

FOR AN INTERSECTING HISTORY OF CULTURAL PSYCHIATRY AND PSYCHIATRIC EPIDEMIOLOGY

Examining the collaboration between Henri Ellenberger and Brian Murphy compels us to wonder about the result of this networking. As we have already stated, the distinctive nature of this collective work was such that socio-cultural and epidemiological questions were not separated and the francophone and anglophone scientific communities of Europe and North America were not pitted against each other. Thus, the booklets published by Henri Ellenberger and Brian Murphy in 1965, updated by an extended team in 1978, provide an observation point for the reception of North American knowledge in France.

The history of epidemiology is still a new field, with only a few specialists in France. Of note are works by Luc Berlivet and Christiane Sinding and, for epidemiological psychiatry, those of anthropologist

Anne Lovell,[255] who heads an ambitious and largely transnational project,[256] following already extensive work in the field of mental health.[257] Works in the philosophy of science, such as that of Anne Fagot-Largeault[258] on morbidity and the scientific approach to the causes of death, and the recent thesis by Élodie Giroux (2006), all touch upon important questions in the history of psychiatric epidemiology. Élodie Giroux's work deals with the emergence of epidemiology as a science and the influence it acquired in medicine in the early 1970s, using the example of cardiovascular disease. Indeed, the epidemiology of cardiovascular patients helped introduce the operative concept of risk factors and a new approach to the illness, involving inferential analysis at the level of both the population and the individual. The author adopts an observation of Luc Berlivet: we "went from epidemiology as a science of epidemics of infectious diseases to epidemiology as a privileged place for a mathematical analysis of complex etiologies."[259] At the international level, there are of course other historical analyses on the history of risk concepts in the history of medicine and related sciences from the 1990s and 2000s, such as those of Robert A. Aronowitz,[260] Patricia Jasen,[261] William Rothstein,[262] Thomas Schlich,[263] and Ulrich Tröhler.[264] But aside from this research program led by Anne Lovell, this work does not take into account the history of transcultural psychiatry.

Epidemiology suffered from the indifference of the medical profession until the 1960s.[265] French psychiatry was slow to introduce methods: one of the main French specialists was Vivian Kovess, a psychiatrist who trained at McGill.[266] A quick glance at the contents pages of the journal *L'évolution psychiatrique* (connected to the EMC for psychiatry) indicates that no entry for "epidemiology" existed until the 1960s. Not until 1966 did the Évolution psychiatrique group devote a workday to this new approach to illness (4 December 1966, with reports presented by Michel Audisio, René Diatkine, Raymond Sadoun,[267] and Claude Veil). In 1968 an issue of the journal brought together a few contributions on the theme.

Epidemiological psychiatry in the United States and Canada was developed earlier than in France, in the postwar years, and was closely linked to scientific communities centred around projects led by Alexander H. Leighton.[268] Again, Henri Ellenberger's correspondence allows us to confirm that ties existed between francophones and anglophones: he met Alexander H. Leighton in January 1966 at Yale University and attested in passing[269] that Leighton was also in contact with Roger Bastide. Alexander H. Leighton[270] trained as a psychiatrist at Johns Hopkins University, where one of his professors was the psychiatrist Adolf Meyer (1866–1950). During this period, he received grants from Columbia University to complete his training in the social sciences and left to do fieldwork with the Inuit and the Navajo (whom he studied again from 1948 to 1953). He was also interested in Japanese American citizens who had been interned and displaced during the war, and in the consequences of the dropping of atomic bombs on Hiroshima and Nagasaki. At Columbia, at the beginning of the global conflict (1939–40), he met internationally renowned anthropologists such as Bronislaw Malinowski, Ralph Linton, Margaret Mead, and Abram Kardiner, as well as researchers who are less well-known today, such as Clyde Kluckhohn (1905–1960), a Navajo specialist at Harvard.[271] Following command experience in the navy during the war, he was appointed professor in the Department of Sociology and Anthropology at Cornell, where he remained from 1946 to 1966. He was appointed professor of social psychiatry at Cornell in 1956 and chaired the Department of Behavioral Sciences at the Harvard School of Public Health from 1966 until 1975. Alexander H. Leighton then held a position in Canada, at the Department of Psychiatry at Dalhousie University in Halifax, Nova Scotia. His research allowed him to build bridges between the United States and English- and French-speaking Canada and to establish lasting working relations thanks, once again, to intermediaries. Among them was Marc-Adélard Tremblay (1922-2014), who collaborated with Alexander H. Leighton and Jane Murphy in the Stirling County Study before becoming a professor of sociology and anthropology at Université Laval in Quebec City.

Aside from the Stirling County Study, Alexander H. Leighton conducted epidemiological studies in New York, Nigeria (1963), and Sweden, as well as with Jane Murphy on the Inuit (Alaska, Bering Sea) in 1955. Jane Murphy arrived in Cornell in 1951 as assistant to the director of the Stirling County Project, quickly becoming his main collaborator.[272] She completed her doctoral dissertation in anthropology there in 1960, and also was affiliated with the Payne Whitney Psychiatric Outpatient Department. Like Brian Murphy, Alexander H. Leighton and Jane Murphy conducted many comparative studies to test and reinforce the validity of their data. Like Raymond Prince, they conducted fieldwork with the Yoruba of Nigeria. Finally, a fact rarely mentioned when speaking of the history of these disciplines (anthropology, psychiatry, and epidemiology) is that Jane Murphy was certainly the first woman to find a place in the centre of the research field (in 1975 she began leading the Stirling County Study at Harvard, and she continues to do so), and is perhaps the only one in her field to have published an article in a scientific review as prestigious as *Science*.[273] She also wrote an article in 1980,[274] when *DSM-III*, the manual of American psychiatry, was published, in which she made positive note of the convergence of methods, thirty years following epidemiological studies, before evidence-based medicine became essential in mental health, which had long been dominated by the dynamic psychiatry approach.

Like other North American researchers not directly affiliated with the McGill group, Alexander H. Leighton and Jane Murphy prefer to speak of cross-cultural psychiatry,[275] rather than transcultural psychiatry, to designate the research field shared by medical anthropology and psychiatric epidemiology. To be more specific, the Cornell and Harvard scientific community has remained distant from that of Montreal, increasingly taking the quantitative approach of epidemiology rather than McGill's hybrid approach, which combines psychiatry, social sciences, and psychology.

Brian Murphy's career path has numerous points in common with that of Alexander H. Leighton, in that their works and fieldwork and investigations demonstrate that it is not possible to separate the history of psychiatric epidemiology from that of cultural psychiatry. Even before settling in North America, Brian Murphy had written a noted collection of studies[276] on refugees in Europe after the Second World War. Published by UNESCO (in a series titled *Population and Culture*), the book focuses on the effects of forced displacement on prospective immigrants to Israel, Australia, and Great Britain. Epidemiology was not part of the book's analytical framework; as was still common at the time, the methodology used by Brian Murphy was based on empirical admission statistics for hospital services, focusing especially on psychoses.

His first major transcultural studies focused on Canada. He conducted a comparative study of fourteen rural communities in Quebec and Ontario with varied cultural backgrounds. This study demonstrated that the high rate of schizophrenia in three francophone communities might be explained by the particularly demeaning social roles for francophone women, who were at the bottom of the social scale in communities that were still deeply rural. His work, like that of Alexander H. Leighton and Jane Murphy, demonstrated that social integration was a determining factor in mental health. His second study focused on the characteristics of psychiatric hospitalizations of immigrants to Canada from various groups. It highlighted the role of family structure and religious factors.

Other noted studies by Brian Murphy dealt with the South Pacific. His editorial role in the journal launched by Eric Wittkower allowed him to maintain a significant information network on schizophrenia and depression; through that network, he collected data from around the world and made comparisons, in particular in developing countries. His work with displaced persons after the war and with various communities in Canada led him to consider the great heterogeneity of populations in Western countries; thus, he was able to avoid sinking into the fascination for exotic peoples and the traditional societies of Asia, America, and Africa. This is why his work, like that of Henri Ellenberger, largely escapes being criticized for orientalism in Edward Said's sense of that term. For example, along with in-depth thinking on *latah*,[277] one of the best-known culture-bound syndromes in transcultural psychiatry, one of his case studies concerns the high rate of schizophrenia in Ireland, which culturally is very close to his native Scotland. Finally, like Emil Kraepelin, he considers that exaggerated feelings of guilt are associated with the severity of emotional disturbances (melancholy) and an unfavourable prognosis.

Ellen Corin and Gilles Bibeau emphasize in their tribute[278] that Brian Murphy was a moderate scientific figure in Montreal, hostile to dogma. He distanced himself from the fashionable schools of thought – something he had in common with Henri Ellenberger, along with a Protestant education and a stubborn tendency throughout his life to perfect one single reference work, which he constantly expanded with new data. Also like Henri Ellenberger, he integrated the results of culturalism though not a culturalist himself.

In his contribution to the EMC, Brian Murphy establishes a list of objectives for social psychiatry based on the operative concept of distribution:

There are a number of goals that research in social psychiatry can pursue. One is the simplest description, either the description of diseases in various populations or in a few unusual conditions in a specific environment.[279]

He also undertakes an inventory of the main social psychiatric approaches:

> 1. Anamnestic studies on the frequency of psychopathological symptoms. 2. Synchronic studies on the comparative frequency of mental illnesses in individuals or in families. 3. Synchronic studies on the frequency of some symptoms in various social groups. 4. Synchronic studies on the frequency of psychopathological demonstrations in various sections of an entire population. 5. Historical studies on the frequency of psychopathological disorders in entire populations. 6. Comparative studies of various populations through psychometric and projective tests. 7. Comparative studies of presumed pathogenic factors. 8. Clinical comparative descriptions of mental patients from different backgrounds. 9. Social studies of groups of individuals subjected to a specific social stress. 10. Diachronic studies. 11. Studies of the phenomenon of interaction in small groups. 12. Opinion surveys and surveys on public attitudes. 13. Experimental manipulation of social change.[280]

He then proposes a typology with three categories: epidemiological, clinical, and interactive approaches. One of the limits cited – one that is important to note, for it is persistent and constitutes a strong horizon of expectations – is the lack of standardization of the categories studied: "Even when we force ourselves to work only with simple social categories, we are likely to find that no standard, uncontested method to verify them exists."[281] For Brian Murphy, the key social variables to consider are age and gender, class and place of birth, marital status, residence, religious affiliation, occupation, and ethnocultural group. Epidemiological methods must help identify what is the significant social variable of an illness. Through these indicators, we must then determine the relevant (i.e., associated) factors affecting the mental health of this population. The incidence rate provides the number of new cases of illness observed in a population over a given period. The prevalence represents the proportion of a population suffering from an illness (it is the product of the incidence in relation to the duration of the illness). These methods make it possible to conduct longitudinal studies, analyze variations in incidence over time, verify hypotheses across vast populations, and so on.[282] The clinic is not cast aside; rather, it is redefined. Epidemiology served to redraw the outlines of the classification categories. In particular, the epidemiological approach applied and promoted categories that were narrower than the broad categories of "neurosis" and "psychosis" in structural psychopathology, or linear graduated scales: as Brian Murphy writes, "in any epidemiological study, the important social variable must encompass limited and precise categories able to apply uniformly to a large population."[283] Here is a rather significant excerpt on schizophrenia:

> Any comparative study on schizophrenia requires the use of rigorous diagnostic criteria and trustworthy statistical reports, conditions that are rarely realized. Recently, the transcultural study group at McGill University in Montreal carried out an international study using questionnaires that contained very specific rules and criteria. Although still incomplete and imperfect, this study showed that the distribution of schizophrenia varies throughout the world in correlation with certain social and cultural factors (Murphy, Wittkower, Fried and Ellenberger, 1963) ... Already we can say that the image of schizophrenic illness as described in our standard textbooks should be seriously revised in light of facts acquired by ethnopsychiatry.[284]

In their contributions, Brian Murphy and Henri Ellenberger readily provide examples on suicide[285] and on the consequences of urbanization[286] to illustrate their statements; yet the phenomena of suicide and the morbidity brought about by urban life are the very basis of sociology in France and the United States. Studies of causes of death and of models of morbidity in medicine are part of the fundamental problematics of epidemiology.[287]

Brian Murphy criticizes the lack of reliable epidemiological data on mental illnesses;[288] quantification, computerization, and statistical tools increasingly determine how concepts of classifications are used. Computers, including personal computers, have become increasingly important professional tools; yet computers are not mentioned in 1965 in the EMC, though they are taken into account in 1978 for interpreting data from tests and for screening. During the same period, academic journals devoted special issues to epidemiology, and works appeared attesting to enthusiasm for computer tools in that discipline.[289] Overall, the 1960s saw the development of standard scales and examination protocols: the Present

State Examination (PSE), the Schedule of Affective Disorders and Schizophrenia (SADS), the Diagnostic Interview Schedule (DIS), the Renard Diagnostic Interview (RDI), the computerized system CATEGO (Norman Sartorius[290] and J.E. Cooper), most of which (the first was British) were the result of two American research teams at the New York State Psychiatric Institute and Washington University in Saint Louis, who were finalizing *DSM-III*, the manual of American psychiatry.[291] Thus a historical analysis of the EMC booklets reveals that in France, psychiatry was becoming more standardized, thanks to text summaries written by a team of researchers established in Canada, before the *DSM* became the world standard: a classic phenomenon of knowledge transfer involving transatlantic communication.

The McGill department played an important role in disseminating and globalizing epidemiological methods in mental health. For example, when Brian Murphy was appointed Emeritus Professor in 1983, he stayed on as head of the transcultural psychiatry section of the World Psychiatric Association. The members of this international network worked closely with WHO and participated in pilot epidemiological surveys, which were used as international indicators. Its website recommends certain reference works, among them Brian Murphy's 1982 work; it also recommends, along with the McGill journal and the section newsletters, transcultural psychiatry textbooks in English[292] that have become standard internationally, demonstrating that this scientific network is connected.

CULTURE-BOUND SYNDROMES AS *TOPOI*: THE EXAMPLE OF JAPAN

As we have already indicated, the term culture-bound syndromes was proposed by the psychiatrist Pow-Meng Yap (Hong Kong) in the 1960s and 1970s. A list of those syndromes was included in an appendix to the American manual of psychiatry, the *DSM-IV* (4th edition, 1994),[293] which also provides a definition: "recurrent, locality-specific patterns of aberrant behaviour and troubling experiences that may or may not be linked to a particular diagnostic *DSM-IV* category." The number of syndromes currently included varies from one work to the next. Here, we note the best-known: *amok, koro, kuru,*[294] *latah, piblokto* (or *pibloktoq*), *susto,* and *windigo.* The most recent edition of the manual, *DSM-V*, includes a

"Glossary of Cultural Concepts of Distress,"[295] which limits itself to nine of these remarkable psychopathological disorders: *ataque de nervios* (Latin America), *dhat nervios* (South Asia), *khyâl cap* (Cambodia), *kufungisisa* (Zimbabwe), *maladi moun* (Haiti), *nervios* (Latin America), *shenjing shuairo* (China), *susto* (Latin America), and *taijin kyofusho* (Japan). It also includes a questionnaire for a structured interview, the Cultural Formulation Interview (CFI), in a revised chapter of the previous version of the manual of psychiatry: this indicates that the problem of cultural specificities is topical in mental health on an international scale. This, however, does not mean that culture-bound syndromes were at the centre of debates in cultural psychiatry from the 1940s to the 1980s: on the contrary, we should be wary of inferring anachronisms and delusions from the DSM, which is why there was no question of addressing this theme at the outset.

Today, essays and descriptive catalogues of culture-bound syndromes (CBSs) abound, from the perspectives of both psychiatrists and medical anthropologists,[296] or those of patients themselves on the Internet. Numerous websites establish inventories of these syndromes or offer assistance to individuals who recognize themselves in a culture-bound syndrome. But one thing is certain from the historical perspective: those syndromes reflect a series of what basically were already established stereotypes classified as exotic since the end of the nineteenth century. From a narrative point of view, we may view them as *topoi* to be consulted each time there is discussion of the relationship between psychiatry and culture, This knowledge, which verges on exoticism, is of course contested; anthropologists have long noted that many categories of Western psychiatry had their hour of glory before being abandoned, disparaged, or marginalized, and that these deserve a place on the same list: chronic fatigue syndrome, multiple personality syndrome, bulimia and anorexia, "type A personalities,"[297] premenstrual syndrome, and so on. The most recent is Gulf War syndrome, which affects American soldiers. Note that the philosopher of science Ian Hacking (University of Toronto and Collège de France, where he was chair of philosophy and history of scientific concepts from 2000 to 2006) has developed an alternative and historical concept: he designates as "transient mental illness"[298] mental disorders that appear in a particular context, which develop in the form of epidemics and then gradually disappear at the same time as the conditions of the context that gave rise to them. He cites as prime examples multiple personality disorder and mad travellers – but this list is not closed-ended, and many other examples on the margins of psychiatric classification provide a great deal to think about in his course at the Collège de France. More recently, the Australian historian Ivan Crozier[299] has borrowed Ian Hacking's analytical framework to reconsider the history of *koro*, a culture-bound syndrome that he analyzes from the point of view of the history of science and gender studies.

Like *latah* and *amok*, *koro* is viewed as an exotic mental pathology: it designates the belief or fear that the penis will retract into the body (this is referred to as genital retraction syndrome in some regions of Southeast Asia populated by the Chinese).[300] It has been known in Western medicine since the late nineteenth century, when a health officer in the Dutch East Indies, J.C. Blonk,[301] published the first article about it (1895). Very quickly, starting in 1908, literature about it appeared in French and in other languages.[302] According to J.C. Blonk, the syndrome was mainly known in people of Chinese origin in Southeast Asia and went back to Chinese Taoist medical tradition. More recently, though, cases have been recorded in individuals not of Chinese origin. Pow-Meng Yap in 1974 proposed characterizing this disorder as an atypical culture-bound reactive syndrome. This type of reactive syndrome is emotional and expresses itself in the form of depersonalization (emotional syndrome, with depersonalization state).[303] Brian Murphy classified it instead among the anxiety orders in his 1982 book. To sum up, it is an old category, but constructed differently by different specialists.

The term culture-bound syndrome is a recent invention, but the discourse is not new. It is not always medical: as we have already pointed out, the oldest observations were provided by travel narratives from the early years of colonial expansion. We also sometimes find on the list of culture-bound syndromes behaviours that were considered pathological, abnormal, or extraordinary in the past but have since been requalified or excluded from current classifications: for example, today homosexuality is no longer associated in the West with mental disorders. The exclusion of homosexuality from American classification dates from the introduction of *DSM-III* in 1980. In 1965, the context was altogether different: leading authors in cultural psychiatry such as Marvin K. Opler (1914–1981) devoted studies to it,[304] and Henri Ellenberger himself chose to present the problematic of culture-bound syndromes, beginning with "Scythian disease." Known since antiquity and mentioned by Hippocrates in his corpus,[305] it refers to those men of the ancient Scythian people who dressed as women and were struck by impotence. This case study is often linked to the *berdache*, who are found in the texts of Georges Devereux and Henri Ellenberger. The *berdache* are a category of cross-dressers, common among the Plains Indians of North America, who are integrated into traditional society in a marginal category. Georges Devereux understands this phenomenon in psychoanalytic terms, as a "complex"[306] resulting from "homosexual urges" and "cultural norms." Note that while Henri Ellenberger cites this example, he never endorses Georges Devereux's psychoanalytic explanation, as in clinical cases of Indian patients treated at the Menninger Foundation.

Specialists have drawn other parallels: for example, with the *sekatra*, a social category of homosexuals or inverts (men dressed as women since childhood) integrated into the traditional society of Madagascar. This transvestism shocked Westerners when they colonized the island. Colonial doctors of the nineteenth century made extremely negative and racist observations about them,[307] disparaging both Malagasy society and the *sekatra*, whose behaviour was reclassified as a mental illness and a moral perversion. However, this type of category is far removed from descriptions of classic mental illness in the West; its medicalization does not draw from the clinical method, but borrows from ethnology and the moral sciences. Here we find ourselves in the framework studied by Edward Said, where science and ethnology were used by colonial administrators to produce stigmatizing knowledge.

In "Ethnopsychiatry" (1965), Henri Ellenberger's position is to consider that there is no specific mental illness; rather, there are specific forms of universal mental disorders. One approach Henri Ellenberger takes when thinking about forms of mental illnesses and their treatment in the world is to consider that the symptoms have a "pathoplastic" aspect in mental medicine[308] – more specifically, the environment (climate, ethnicity, society, culture, social class, rural or urban environment, and so on) has a "pathoplastic" effect. What does this mean? In the *Petit Robert*, plastic has two definitions: 1. "that which has the power to give shape"; and 2. "that which is likely to lose its shape due to an outside force and maintain its new form when the force has stopped operating." What Henri Ellenberger means here is that the environment has a plastic effect on mental disorders (the first meaning of the definition), as these are malleable (the second meaning). To simplify, even the etiology of mental illnesses is biological and universal, the symptoms are not. Of course, many authors have condemned this as too simplistic and as an inadequate approximation: we find criticisms of doctors levelled by social science researchers such as Roger Bastide. Rather than recasting the history of each culture-bound syndrome, going over all the historiography of *amok* and *latah*, or following the evolution of comparative psychiatry since the articles of Emil Kraepelin on the new cross-cultural psychiatry, we propose, finally, to remind readers of the existence of a Japanese culture-bound syndrome that particularly interested Henri Ellenberger: *taijin kyofusho*.[309]

The terminology of course poses translation problems. According to Jean-Claude Jugon,[310] the Japanese term designates more a fear of offending or irritating others than a social phobia in the Western sense. It literally means "an intense fear of others" and is attributed to Dr Morita Masatake (aka Morita Shoma, 1874–1938),[311] who used it in 1932. Morita explains the disorder in his treatise on ereuthrophobia (fear of blushing, which itself brings about the dreaded phenomenon), which he considers to be the typical disorder of anthropophobia (aversion toward men). The term *taijin kyofusho* was not used in the medical treatises of the Edo period (1603–1868), before Japan opened itself to the West (1854), nor is it a loan or adaptation from the Chinese. Apparently it was a common expression in Japanese popular language before migrating to medicine. In the Meiji period (1868–1911), Japanese society was modernizing rapidly; the Japanese translated and quickly adapted Western medical knowledge to Japanese culture, be it German, American, British, French, and so on. German science served as the great model for Japanese academic psychiatry. For example, Morita calls *shinkeishitsu* what the Germans call *Nervosität* (nervousness). We must therefore think of Japanese culture-bound syndrome as a category constructed in relation to Western academic psychiatry within the framework of an imperial culture that has appropriated foreign knowledge since the nineteenth century without every being colonized – not just as an indigenous category.

After Morita, other doctors and psychotherapists stood out in Japanese psychiatry: Doi Takeo (1920–2009), Hawai Hayao (1928–2007), Uchinuma Yukio (1935–), Kasahara Yomishi (1928–), and Fujinawa Akira (1928–2013). Each claimed responsibility for a specific contribution to understanding of the problem and to have been inspired by various schools of thought:

German psychiatry, psychoanalysis, phenomenology, Henri Ey's organo-dynamism theory, and communication theory adapted from the works of Gregory Bateson (1904–1980). We must also consider the American influence following the Second World War, which largely supplanted European knowledge. For example, in the segment of Japanese classification given to the term *taijin kyofusho*, the notion of panic disorders became established, pushing back previous Japanese terminology.

Though articles about Japanese culture-bound syndromes proliferated in the McGill newsletter at the time Henri Ellenberger worked there, it is difficult to know whether this cultural area was the subject of specific discussions or teaching in Eric Wittkower's department. However, even though it falls outside our chronology, note that the current editor of the journal *Transcultural Psychiatry*, Laurence Kirmayer,[312] took a stance against the idea that Japanese psychopathological problems were absolutely and uncompromisingly original to Japan. In fact, he established relationships between *koro* and *taijin kyofusho* in his analysis of social phobia. This emerged from his analytical framework, which posited that excessive social anxiety in a conducive culture may be at the root of implied perceptions in the phobia. Indeed, in *koro*, the phenomenon of body dysmorphic disorder (obsessive or unreasonable fear of being ugly, deformed, or presenting anatomical abnormalities) must be understood in the specific context of social anxiety, similar to the fears in interpersonal relationships in Japan, including the fear of being disagreeable, of offending or hurting others, or of having an imaginary physical deformity.

We await an in-depth historical work that analyzes the construction of the Japanese category based on the analysis that Ivan Crozier produced for *koro*. But what does Henri Ellenberger's interest in Japan signify? Following his contributions to the EMC and his articles on psychologist Pierre Janet in *L'évolution psychiatrique*,[313] we may assume that Japanese culture-bound syndrome reflects the long history of the "social phobia" category in France and the United States; this term of classification is attributed to Pierre Janet and has mostly taken hold in the world through American psychiatry, which borrowed it from the French. To sum up, as with the cases of the Native American patients previously mentioned, Henri Ellenberger often retraced his analysis to Pierre Janet, with ethnopsychiatry and the history of psychiatry being two aspects of his concerns as a learned and encyclopedist doctor.

OPENNESS: CONTINUITY, TRANSITION, AND MISSED
OPPORTUNITY WITH FRANTZ FANON

As we reach the conclusion of this general presentation, we must note that the ways in which ethnopsychiatry was constructed as an academic discipline following the Second World War largely conceal that it was deeply rooted in the colonial period and that it is difficult to link the two periods when attempting to establish the history of this time of transition. Did Henri Ellenberger not warn his colleagues in France at the start of his editorial project? Abandoning exotic psychiatry is the prerequisite for academic knowledge of ethnopsychiatry. The participants who did not understand this – for example, the members of the Algiers School – saw themselves progressively marginalized, and their credibility undermined, or they were even simply ignored by new generations. Yet as we have seen, they contributed to building international academic networks after 1945.

We must emphasize this fact, for it is a specific characteristic of this transitional period: doctors who conveyed openly racist representations collaborated with others who by then had freed themselves from exotic psychiatry. Moreover, the places, participants, and themes we have reviewed have confirmed more than once the continuity between the colonial and postcolonial periods and that scientific networks emerged not only in the academic world. One of the first explanations for this lack of knowledge[314] is that the participants who constructed ethnopsychiatry as an academic discipline and those who criticized colonial psychiatry often ignored each other in the twentieth century. French intellectuals, critical of the colonial system and of the main participants in ethnology,[315] inspired by psychoanalysis, for example Michel Leiris (1901–1990), could have acted as intermediaries, but they did not. Frantz Fanon left his position as a doctor in Algerian psychiatric hospitals before the late 1950s to join the Algerian National Liberation Army, and while his essays inspired many intellectuals, they touched very few doctors. Everything indicates that Henri Ellenberger, Georges Devereux, Roger Bastide, and Henri Collomb did not read Frantz Fanon or explicitly consider his work,[316] for at least three reasons: he was not of their generation, he did not pursue a career in Paris (Frantz Fanon worked in Lyon, Algeria, Tunisia, and Ghana), and he died young of acute leukemia (in 1961). Long after the independence of Algeria, his books remained censored, poorly distributed, and limited to the counterculture. A comparative reading of Henri Ellenberger and Frantz Fanon reveals a missed opportunity.

Henri Ellenberger, born in Africa, caught unawares in mainland France by the beginning of the First World War, then forced to leave the country at the beginning of the German occupation and the Vichy regime during the Second World War, must have had political ideas regarding the colonies and the decolonization process even before making cultural psychiatry his main professional activity at McGill starting in 1959. But this history does not appear in the booklets published in 1965. Similarly, it is also totally concealed in the EMC's reviews of books and articles. Yet this corpus was already a part of postcolonial science. Henri Ellenberger reoriented in particular the perspective of ethnopsychiatry as was practised at the time in Montreal, making possible new reflections on Western culture-bound syndromes. Indeed, he prioritized looking into Western cultural forms of mental illness in countries where he himself had lived, such as the United States and Switzerland, rather than exotic forms. According to Lionel Beauchamp and Raymond Prince, Henri Ellenberger's booklets were widely recognized[317] in the emerging discipline at the time of their publication, and he had the opportunity to present them[318] at the Tenth World Congress of Psychiatry (Madrid, 1966). But outside a circle of specialists, his texts on ethnopsychiatry are rarely cited in France and remain unknown there, which is why it was important to republish them with a scholarly apparatus.

One explanation for the lack of knowledge of this corpus is that it is steeped in the prevailing culturalism typical of the humanities of this era in North America, a paradigm to which France was long resistant. Another explanation is that Henri Ellenberger was not sensitive to French structuralism, even if he had read Claude Lévi-Strauss. But he fully carried out his role as a go-between. Here we must qualify the claim of historian François Dosse, who sees structuralism as a tool that allowed some categories of analysis to be replaced by reflections on minorities that were invisible, silent, alienated, or simply dominant in Western society following the wave of decolonization that saw the return of ethnologists to mainland France: "Ethnologists returned for the most part to mainland France and then discovered colonies inside the Western world, breakwaters resistant to change."[319] Henri Ellenberger was a pioneer in this process: the existence of unrecognized or minor mental disorders in Western cultures is the *basis* of his interest for ethnopsychiatry, not a result.

To conclude, as I have chosen to use Alice Bullard's analytical framework, we can summarize what we have learned at the end of this analysis of ethnopsychiatry as knowledge of and in transition after 1945. *Transition* may be understood as a *period of transition*, resulting from the process of decolonization that ran from the 1940s to the 1960s, that is, from the Fourth Republic until the end of the Algerian War. But I have been careful to not overinterpret the sources of this history and not infer a transition between two periods defined in advance: while the Second World War was indeed experienced by the participants in ethnopsychiatry first-hand, we must be wary of the teleological illusion that sees as obvious what we only now know about the end of the twentieth century. In terms of social, political, and cultural history, no one in 1965 knew how the new independent states liberated from colonial empires would develop in the context of the Cold War that wold divide the world into two blocs until the fall of the Berlin Wall (1989). Also, the DSM-III manual of American psychiatry did not yet exist (1980), and there was no real international standard for classifying mental disorders; the WHO classification had no significant impact. Yet we have seen a series of participants involved at WHO and in the international academic networks of the cultural psychiatry of the 1940s and 1950s. Let us briefly compare the journeys of Henri Aubin and John Colin Carothers on one hand, and those of Alexander H. Leighton and Brian Murphy on the other: while all four were involved in WHO's first international policies of mental hygiene, the first group was marginalized, after the 1960s and 1970s, then later held in contempt for defending or conveying racist portrayals of Africans, while the second pursued careers as pioneers in psychiatric epidemiology, conducting inquiries throughout the world. The global agenda of WHO, which combined prevention policies, scientific inquiries, and more qualitative knowledge on mental health in various cultures, thereafter had an established name, one that was still theoretical in 1965: global mental health.[320] It would be tempting to observe in WHO's large epidemiological studies on schizophrenia, depression, and other major mental disorders (*International Pilot Study on Schizophrenia*: IPSS, 1973 and 1979; *Determinants of Outcome of Severe Mental Disorders*, 1992) the logical outcome of the knowledge Henri Ellenberger summarized in 1965. But that is also an illusion: the statistical methods of these quantitative inquiries, which deal with ten or so countries, are far removed from those used at McGill under Eric Wittkower with the network of correspondents of *Transcultural Research in Mental Health Problems Review* (and later the newsletter).

In short, the corpus assembled and published by Henri Ellenberger teaches us at least two things that usually have been concealed. First, while the construction of an international network like the one at McGill is a condition of possibility for the emergence of transnational knowledge, that does not mean that psychiatric epidemiology was already perceived as an independent and legitimate science in the immediate postwar period, for quantitative methods were still integral to cultural psychiatry, which remained a corpus of knowledge "cobbled together" at the time when Henri Ellenberger was writing for the EMC. Second, none of Henri Ellenberger's chroniclers until now has noted that he taught at a university and published clinical vignettes from his own professional experience at the Menninger Foundation with Native American patients (like George Devereux) but borrowed more from the analytical framework of the psychologist Pierre Janet than from that of Sigmund Freud. Specifically, historians of psychology and psychoanalysis who generally presented him in France as a forerunner of their discipline – the history of psychology or psychoanalysis – overlook that Henri Ellenberger remained an eclectic doctor in North America, and not just a historian. Let us hope that the corpus of "Ethnopsychiatry" will contribute to a more realistic, accurate, and balanced portrait of Henri Ellenberger, the one that Fernando Vidal[321] called for twenty years ago.

This critical edition of Henri Ellenberger's "Ethnopsychiatry" also contributes to renewing the history of dynamic psychiatry of the second half of the twentieth century. Ethnopsychiatry between 1945 and 1965 was not only a hybrid knowledge but also a corpus of knowledge in transition that accompanied decolonization, following on from colonial psychiatry. The history of the first academic networks highlights contrasting positions when we analyze the relationship of participants to exoticism, but scientific communities are still highly polarized by the division of the world imposed by the Cold War. That is why we must avoid speaking too quickly of global mental health, which involves to a greater extent psychiatric epidemiology, the history of which only really started in the 1960s.

Kyoto–Berlin–Montreal, 2015

NOTES

FROM EXOTIC PSYCHIATRY TO THE
UNIVERSITY NETWORKS OF CULTURAL PSYCHIATRY

1 Ey, *Traité de psychiatrie*. On the history of this collection, see Delille, "Réseaux savants"; and Delille, "Une archive."
2 Ackerknecht, "Ethnologische Vorbemerkung," 2. Ackerknecht returned to the topic on several occasions; see his "Transcultural psychiatry."
3 On simplifications and the contested memory of Henri Ellenberger, see Vidal, "À la recherche d'Henri Ellenberger"; and Delille, "Henri Ellenberger et le *Traité de psychiatrie*."
4 Corin and Bibeau, "H.B.M. Murphy."
5 H. Murphy, "In Memoriam Eric D. Wittkower."
6 Prince, "In Memoriam H.B.M. Murphy"; Prince, "John Colin D. Carothers"; Prince and Beauchamp, "Pioneers in Transcultural Psychiatry"; Prince, "Origins and Early Mission."
7 Devereux, "The Works." Note that he used "George" without "s" in the United States and in American publications.
8 Prince, *Why This Ecstasy?*
9 Arnaud, *La folie apprivoisée*.
10 Bloch, "Georges Devereux."
11 Alessandra Cerea (Université de Bologne / EHESS) defended in 2016 a doctoral dissertation based on IMEC's archival holdings for Georges Devereux, which is expected to be noteworthy. Provisional title: *Au-delà de l'ethnopsychiatrie. Georges Devereux entre science et épistémologie* (forthcoming).
12 Becker and Kleinman, "The History."
13 Collignon, "Vingt ans de travaux."
14 Kirmayer, "50 years of Transcultural Psychiatry"; Kirmayer and Minas, "The Future of Cultural Psychiatry."
15 H. Murphy, "The Historical Development."
16 Zempléni, "Henri Collomb." Of Hungarian origin, his name is often Frenchified in journals as Andreas Zempleni.
17 Bains, "Race, Culture, and Psychiatry."
18 Keller, *Colonial Madness*. French historian Jean-Christophe Coffin tried to address the topic, but without making use of the existing critical literature, the issues of which he is unaware. See Coffin, "La psychiatrie postcoloniale."
19 Macey, *Frantz Fanon*.

20 Ernst, *Mad Tales from the Raj*; Ernst, *Colonialism and Transnational Psychiatry*.

21 Coleborne, *Madness in the Family*.

22 Vatin, "Octave Mannoni"; Vatin "Dépendance et emancipation." The second article is a variation on the first.

23 Heaton, *Black Skin, White Coats*.

24 Crozier, "Making Up Koro."

25 Chiang, "Translating Culture and Psychiatry."

26 Fassin and Rechtman, "An Anthropological Hybrid"; Fassin, "Les politiques de l'*ethnopsychiatrie*"; Fassin, "L'ethnopsychiatrie et ses réseaux."

27 Palem, "De l'ethnopsychiatrie à la psychiatrie transculturelle."

28 Bullard, "Imperial Networks and Postcolonial Independence"; Bullard, "The Critical Impact"; Bullard, "L'OEdipe africain, a retrospective."

29 While correcting this manuscript, we noted the publication in Germany of a reference work, both an homage to the German-speaking specialists of ethnopsychoanalysis – Paul Parin (1916–2009), Goldy Parin-Matthèy (1911–1997), and Fritz Morgenthaler (1919–1984) – and an assessment of this movement in various German-speaking countries in the first decade of the twenty-first century. This literature, both professional and memorial, contrasts strongly with French-language publications by a selection of authors with alternative frames of reference following the Second World War. Reichmayr, *Ethnopsychoanalyse Revisited*.

30 There are numerous competing expressions for referring to colonial medicine: exotic medicine, tropical medicine, overseas medicine, medicine in hot countries, and so on. See Monnais, *Médecine et colonisation*.

31 On scientific migrations in contemporary medical science, see Monnais and Wright, *Doctors beyond Borders*. For this research, completed in 2015, I was mainly inspired by the works of British historian Simon Schaffer on the circulation, localization, and spatialization of knowledge. See Schaffer, *La fabrique de sciences modernes*.

32 The history of anthropology is a rapidly growing genre; for a methodological introduction, see Weber, *Brève histoire de l'anthropologie*.

33 See Anderson, Jenson, and Keller, "Introduction."

34 Rechtman, "L'ethnopsychiatrie."

35 Marquer, "L'ethnographie."

36 Bastide, "Psychiatrie sociale et ethnologie."

37 For an analytical framework, see Chakrabarty, *Provincializing Europe*. See also the final chapter and the conclusion of Chakrabarty, *Medicine and Empire*.

38 René Collignon also focuses on mass population movements brought about by the Second World War in his analysis. See Collignon, "Émergence de la psychiatrie transculturelle."

39 See Yanacopoulo, *Henri F. Ellenberger.* This biography presents a more reliable chronological bibliography of Henri Ellenberger than the previous ones.

40 For a stimulating reinterpretation, see Ricard, *Le sable de Babel.*

41 H. Ellenberger, *Essai sur le syndrome psychologique de la catatonie.*

42 She wrote under the pseudonym Vera Hegi in the field of animal psychology with the help of her husband. Henri Ellenberger's first biographers (Mark Micale, Élisabeth Roudinesco, Raymond Prince, and Lionel Beauchamp) agree that Émilie Ellenberger could not join her husband in the United States due to her Russian origins, in the context of the anti-communist postwar witch hunt (McCarthyism).

43 See Van Gennep, *Folklore.*

44 H. Ellenberger, "Les fadets."

45 H. Ellenberger, "Le monde fantastique."

46 For an analysis, see Delille, "Sigmund Freud-Oskar Pfister," 579–82.

47 H. Ellenberger, "Die Putzwut."

48 H. Ellenberger, "La psychothérapie de Janet"; H. Ellenberger, "Un disciple fidèle de P. Janet."

49 See H. Ellenberger, *La psychiatrie suisse.*

50 See Delille, "Le Bouvard et Pécuchet"; Delille, "Le *Traité de psychiatrie.*"

51 See Delille, "Henri Ellenberger"; and Delille, "Un voyage d'observation."

52 Devereux, *Reality and Dream.*

53 Louis Mars studied medicine at the Faculty of Medicine at the Université d'État d'Haïti, then specialized in psychiatry in Illinois, New York, and Paris. A professor at the Faculty of Medicine of Port-au-Prince, then dean and rector at the Université d'Haïti, he was also a member of the Institut d'ethnologie. His book *Crisis in Possession in Voodoo* (1977; original French publication 1946) is prefaced by Georges Devereux, with whom he formed a lasting friendship. Influenced by psychoanalysis, he invented the concept of "ethnodrama" (in the sense of catharsis), along the model of what psychologists call "psychodrama" and Roger Bastide calls "social drama." Louis Mars also had a long political career: he was a member of Parliament by 1946, and later minister of foreign affairs and Haitian ambassador to London, Paris, the Vatican, and Guatemala. A significant part of his of scientific and political career was conducted in the United States. A correspondence exists between Louis Mars and Henri

Ellenberger (Fonds Ellenberger) and between Louis Mars and Georges Devereux (Fonds Devereux, IMEC).

54 See Appendix 3 at the end of the present volume. For more information, see Delille, "On the History of Cultural Psychiatry."

55 Psychiatrist Raymond Prince attributes the English term *transcultural psychiatry* to Eric Wittkower, but Georges Devereux contests this. See Prince, "Origins and Early Mission," 7.

56 H. Ellenberger, *Criminologie du passé et du present.*

57 H. Ellenberger, *The Discovery of the Unconscious.*

58 H. Ellenberger, "L'histoire d'Anna O."

59 H. Ellenberger, "L'histoire d'Emmy von N."

60 H. Ellenberger, "C.G. Jung and the Story of Helene Preiswerk."

61 H. Ellenberger, "La psychiatrie transculturelle."

62 See H. Ellenberger, "Chapitre 50: La maladie créatrice" and "Chapitre 51: La guérison et ses artisans."

63 Fred Elmont (pseudonym of Henri Ellenberger), *Les petits chaperons.* Andrée Yanacopoulo published a very interesting selection of previously unknown autobiographical, light, and literary texts in the appendix of her biography.

64 It is included in the appendix of the present work. It may be compared to the outline of the articles published in the EMC in 1965–67. In her biography, Andrée Yanacopoulo reproduces a teaching brochure from the Hôtel-Dieu de Montréal on ethnopsychiatry, as well as an unpublished "foreword" that Henri Ellenberger either wrote or dictated to his secretary Marguerite Karaïvan, with a view to the book he had imagined at the end of his life, "Études ethnopsychiatriques et ethnocriminologiques." In the end, pressed by illness, he was obliged to resume in one volume the two monographs he had long imagined as separate on ethnopsychiatry and criminology. See Yanacopoulo, *Henri F. Ellenberger,* 301–2.

65 See Micale, "Henri F. Ellenberger"; and H. Ellenberger, *Beyond the Unconscious.*

66 In addition to the scholarly apparatus of the 1994 edition of de *L'histoire de la découverte de l'inconscient,* see Henri Ellenberger, *Médecines de l'âme.*

67 Aside from his father's work, his brother François was an eminent geologist, author of a history of geology, while his other brother Paul, a pastor and paleontologist, continued the work of their father as a missionary and translator.

68 Andrée Yanacopoulo includes an anthology of the unpublished fiction in the appendix of her biography.

69 Many diaries and travel narratives are still unpublished.

70 For broader questioning, see Morrissey and Roger, *L'encyclopédie du réseau au livre*; see also the conference proceedings from 17 and 18 November 2002, organized by the Société Diderot at the Université Paris 7 Denis Diderot, in the form of a special issue of the journal *Recherches sur Diderot et sur l'Encyclopédie*: Collectif, "L'encyclopédie en ses nouveaux atours électroniques." These conference proceedings are largely devoted to the digitalization of the *Encyclopédie*, which updated historiographical thought. Consult also Blanckaert and Porret, *L'encyclopédie méthodique*.

71 Today (2014), three are noteworthy: sciencedirect.com, EM-consulte.com, scopus.com.

72 H. Ellenberger, "Psychothérapie de la schizophrénie."

73 See Delille, "Henri Ellenberger et le *Traité de psychiatrie*"; Delille, "Un voyage d'observation."

74 H. Ellenberger, "Analyse existentielle."

75 See H. Ellenberger, May, and Angel, *Existence*.

76 H. Ellenberger, "Castration des pervers sexuels," 1–2.

77 Dongier and H. Ellenberger, "Criminologie."

78 See Prince, "Transcultural Psychiatry"; and Prince and Beauchamp, "Pioneers in Transcultural Psychiatry."

79 Henri Ellenberger's grandfather, David Frédéric Ellenberger (1835–1919), wrote works about Lesotho: *Histori ea Basotho*; *Catalogue of the Masitise Archives*; and *History of the Basuto*. The father, Victor Ellenberger (1879–1972), continued his scholarly work in the company of one Henri's younger brothers, Paul Ellenberger (who also wrote works as a naturalist), publishing chronicles: see V. Ellenberger, *Sur les hauts plateaux du Lessouto*; *Un siècle de mission au Lessouto*; *La fin tragique des Bushmen*; and *Afrique avec cette peur*. He is also known for translating and publishing traditional narratives, recently republished by éditions Confluences: Mofolo, *L'homme qui marchait vers le soleil levant*; Mofolo, *Chaka*; and Machobane and Motsamaï, *Au temps des cannibals*.

80 A translation of a book by Mofolo.

81 Letter from Henri Ellenberger to Maurice Leenhardt, 27 July 1950; it is part of an exchange of four letters. The end of the letter concerns other requests for documentation, on the same topic.

82 The move coincided with his first article published in Canada: H. Ellenberger, "Aspects culturels de la maladie mentale."

83 H. Ellenberger and Trottier, "The Impact."

84 Prince, "Transcultural Psychiatry"; Prince and Beauchamp, "Pioneers in Transcultural Psychiatry."

85 This argument should be viewed with caution: no archival document indicates that Henri Ellenberger encountered difficulties at McGill as a francophone. The only element to substantiate this hypothesis is recent: the historical work of Alexandre Klein (Université Laval) points out that a McGill psychiatrist was dismissed by Ewen Cameron the year of Henri Ellenberger's departure, against a backdrop of tension between Montreal's two linguistic communities: Charles A. Roberts (1918–1996).

86 A member since 1939 of McGill's Montreal Neurological Institute, in 1946 he founded the Montreal Psychoanalytic Club, bringing together ex-patients, psychiatrists, doctors in training, and other health professionals, though he himself was not trained in psychoanalysis. The club disbanded in 1952, supplanted by the Canadian Psychoanalytic Society. See Naiman, "La psychanalyse au Allan Memorial Institute."

87 See Prince, "The American Central Intelligence Agency." See also Marks, *The Search for the 'Manchurian Candidate'*. Historian Andrea Tone (McGill University) is currently conducting research on the CIA funding from which Ewen Cameron benefited during the Cold War.

88 Canadian historiography is not very helpful in terms of documenting the real relationships between francophones and anglophones in the academic world of psychology and mental medicine, or in terms of the role of intermediaries between the two medical cultures. See Rae-Grant, *Psychiatry in Canada*; Wright and Myers, *History of Academic Psychology in Canada*.

89 H. Ellenberger, *Criminologie du passé et du présent*, 1–50.

90 The term refers mainly to the institute and the journal of Abel Miroglio in postwar France: *Ethno-psychologie : revue de psychologie des peuples*. Doctor Charles Pidoux, close to the Évolution psychiatrique group and active in the journal *Psyché*, was Secretary General of the Société internationale d'ethnopsychologie. But the group did not leave much of a mark on the history of the humanities. See Pidoux, "Freud et l'ethnologie."

91 On the history of the psychology of peoples, see Kail and Vermès, *La psychologie des peuples et ses derives*; and Vermès, "Quelques étapes de la psychologie des peuples."

92 Wundt, *Völkerpsychologie*.

93 Associate professor of philosophy at Le Havre, in 1937 he created the Institut de sociologie économique et de psychologie des peuples, then founded the journal *Psychologie des peuples* in 1946, to which Henri Ellenberger contributed.

94 For a summary of specialized teaching at the Sorbonne following the war, see Gessain, "Ethnologie et psychologie."

95 I refer readers to the correspondence between Georges Devereux and Henri Ellenberger, reproduced in the appendix of the present work.

96 Historian Matthew M. Heaton summarizes clearly the contribution of Arthur Kleinman to cultural psychiatry as of 1977 in the conclusion of his latest book; see *Black Skin, White Coats*, 193–4.

97 Kleinman, "Depression, Somatization and the "New Cross-Cultural Psychiatry"; Kleinman, *Patients and Healers*; Kleinman, "What Is Specific to Western Medicine?"

98 "I use the term transcultural mental health care or transcultural psychiatry to refer to practices in which practitioner and patient are from different cultures, which was the case with the Ortigues' work in Senegal. Ethnopsychiatry refers to local psychiatric systems of knowledge, such as detailed in Zempléni (1968) or Devereux (1961)" (Bullard, "L'OEdipe Africain," 199). This reference is to Zempléni's thesis, *Interprétation de la thérapie traditionnelle*. The couple of Edmond and Marie-Cécile Ortigues is mostly known for a book written based on their experience in the service of Henri Collomb at Fann Hospital: M.-C. Ortigues and E. Ortigues, *Oedipe africain*. See also E. Ortigues et al., "Psychologie clinique et ethnologie (Sénégal)"; and E. Ortigues, "La psychiatrie comparée."

99 "Transcultural psychiatry here is distinguished from 'ethnopsychiatry,' understood as the project launched by Georges Devereux of recuperating entire healing systems from non-Western cultures" (Bullard, "Imperial Networks," 197).

100 Schaffer, "The Eighteenth Brumaire of Bruno Latour."

101 "Colonial psychiatry generally produced knowledge while intentionally ignoring or dismissing local beliefs and practices; postcolonial transcultural psychiatry has reversed this, so that local beliefs and practices including culturally specific healing practices inform and sometimes guide transcultural therapeutic interventions. This transformation is rooted in ways of knowing, in evolving scientific practices and codes of ethics" (Bullard, "Imperial Networks," 198).

102 Lazarus, *The Cambridge Companion to Postcolonial Literary Studies*.

103 Sibeud, "Du postcolonial au questionnement postcolonial," 143. This is an ambitious review essay.

104 Devereux, "Normal et anormal" [1956], in *Essais d'ethnopsychiatrie générale*, 1–83; *Basic Problems of Ethnopsychiatry* [1979], 3–71.

105 Devereux, "L'ethnopsychiatrie comme cadre de reference" [1952], in *Essais d'ethnopsychiatrie générale*, 97.

106 Ibid. Every reader familiar with French anthropology makes the connection between these "meta" categories and the structuralism of Claude

Lévi-Strauss (1908–2009) that Georges Devereux knew well. Yet Devereux does not base his judgment on structuralist episteme; the analogy between the shared scientific concerns of the two ethnologists stops there.

107 Mars, "Nouvelle contribution."

108 I refer the reader to the research of Marianna Scarfone, author of a doctoral dissertation on the history of psychiatry in the Italian colonies. Her sources indicate that terms such as *ethnopsychiatry* and *ethnopsychopathology* were already in use in Italian in the early decades of the twentieth century. This work should help re-establish the chronology. See Scarfone, "La psychiatrie coloniale italienne."

109 Kraepelin, "Vergleichende Psychiatrie." A secondary literature exists in French, English, and German on Kraepelin's contribution, but mainly from a medical point of view. See Huffschmitt, "Kraepelin à Java"; Bendick, "Emil Kraepelin Forschungsreise"; Boroffka, "Emil Kraepelin."

110 Ellis, "The Amok of the Malays"; Ellis, "Latah."

111 The term *amok* has entered the German language; today it is commonly used, and Austrian writer Stefan Zweig published a famous novella in 1922 titled "Der Amokläufer" (in English: "Amok.")

112 Róheim, *Psychanalyse et anthropologie.*

113 The Dutch East India Company established three psychiatric hospitals in the late nineteenth century in Java, at Surabaya (1876), Buitenzorg (1881), and Lawang (1902), and enacted special laws on the insane in 1897. See Collignon, "Some Reflections," 40.

114 Moreau de Tours, "Recherches sur les aliénés en Orient."

115 Micale, "Littérature, médecine, hystérie."

116 For a more historical point of view, in the British context, see Worboys, "The Emergence of Tropical Medicine"; Worboys, "Science and Imperialism."

117 Regarding the codification of these syndromes linked to culture, see Jilek and Jilek-Aali, "The Metamorphosis of Culture-Bound Syndromes."

118 Little information exists regarding the career of this anthropologist, a specialist on Peru, who quickly left McGill for Portland State University in the United States. See Fried, "Acculturation and Mental Health"; and Wittkower and Fried, "Some Problems of Transcultural Psychiatry." The correspondence between Eric Wittkower and Henri Ellenberger reveals that the chair of sociology at McGill in the 1950s, Professor William A. Westley, appears also to have played a role in the early days of transcultural psychiatry.

119 For Eric Wittkower's professional record: Humboldt Universität zu Berlin Archiv, UK W 304.

120 See Hayward, "Germany and the Making of 'English' Psychiatry."

121 Linton, *The Study of Man.*

122 Laplantine, preface to Bastide, *Le rêve*, 14.

123 See Ackerknecht, "On the Collecting of Data," 116–17; Schmuhl, *Kulturrelativismus und Antirassismus.*

124 For a postwar point of view, see Balandier, "La collaboration entre l'ethnologie et la psychiatrie."

125 Berr, *La synthèse en histoire.*

126 Mann, *Lucien Febvre*, 131. See also Dosse, *L'histoire en miettes.*

127 Essays collected in one volume: Mauss, *Sociologie et anthropologie.*

128 Noteworthy is a transitional work between the two sciences, written before medical geography disappeared and modern epidemiology became established: Simmons, *Global Epidemiology.* Not to be confused with "La Géographie psychologique" by Georges Hardy (1884–1972), a colonial public servant: Singaravélou, "De la psychologie coloniale à la géographie psychologique."

129 According to Mirko Grmek, one of the great French-speaking pioneers was Geneva doctor Henri-Clermond Lombard (1805-1895); see Lombard, *Atlas de la distribution géographique des maladies.*

130 Grmek, "Géographie médicale et histoire des civilisations," 1076.

131 Mirko Grmek quotes for example the *Deutsches Archiv für Geschichte der Medicine und medicinischen Geographie*; *Janus, archives internationales pour l'histoire de la médecine et la géographie médicale* (Holland), and so on. This literature is in no way marginal; the last title, for example, is among the literature cited by Erwin Ackerknecht in his essays.

132 The chair in medical geography was awarded in 1878 to Arthur Bordier (1841–1910).

133 Henry E. Sigerist wrote significant articles as of the 1930s. See Sigerist, *Civilization and Disease.*

134 In 1955 they received no less than $80,000 from the Rockefeller Foundation. See Dosse, *L'histoire en miettes*, 123–24.

135 In the French context, see Jean Stoetzel's critical book, *Without the Chrysanthemum and the Sword.*

136 See Chakrabarti, *Provincializing Europe*; Collectif Write Back, *Postcolonial Studies.*

137 Said, *Orientalism.* The book on which he focuses his criticism is Gibb, *Area Studies Reconsidered.*

138 See Friedman, *The Menninger.*

139 Devereux, *Reality and Dream: Psychotherapy of a Plains Indian*: New York, International Univ. Press, 1951.

140 See Ackerknecht, *Malaria in the Upper Mississippi Valley.*

141 Republished as "The Shaman and Primitive Psychopathology in General" in Ackerknecht, *Medicine and Ethnology*, 57–89.

142 Ibid., 82.

143 Ibid., 61. The criticism appears in a footnote: "It is sad to see – but one reason more to take up the problem – that this statement – apparently an 'improvement' of the older slogan that religion is a neurosis – comes from an author who, on the other hand, has done so much to elucidate problems of primitive psychopathology." Erwin Ackerknecht is referring to a 1939 article: Devereux, "A Sociological Theory of Schizophrenia."

144 Ibid., 59.

145 Devereux, "A Sociological Theory of Schizophrenia."

146 Devereux, *Mohave Ethnopsychiatry and Suicide: The Psychiatric Knowledge and the Psychic Disturbances of an Indian tribe* (St Clair Shores, MI: Scholarly Press, 1976).

147 Ibid., 109.

148 Ibid.

149 Works have recently been published in French on the health care practices of Native Americans. See Zaballos, *Le système de santé Navajo.*

150 The school bears his name, but it is just a namesake. The exact name of the institution is "Devereux Schools, Under the Devereux Foundation. Helena T. Devereux Director, J. Clifford Scott, M. D., Executive Director." The headquarters of this network of therapeutic schools was in Santa Barbara, California. Georges Devereux was director of research.

151 This is evidenced in the correspondence between Georges Devereux and Henri Ellenberger.

152 Devereux, *De l'angoisse à la méthode.*

153 Devereux, *Essais d'ethnopsychiatrie générale.*

154 Devereux, *Ethnopsychoanalysis: Psychoanalysis and Anthropology as Complementary Frames of Reference* (Berkeley: University of California Press, 1978).

155 See Linton, *Culture and Mental Disorders.* To be more precise, while Ralph Linton is indeed at the origin of the claim reiterated by Georges Devereux that there are correct ways of being insane in each culture, he is nevertheless a part of American culturalism and of the "culture and personality" movement, an episteme that Georges Devereux always claimed to oppose. See Linton, *The Cultural Background of Personality.*

156 *Ethnopsychiatrica*: 5 issues from 1978 to 1981. Another journal then took the name *Nouvelle revue d'ethnopsychiatrie*: 36 issues from 1983 to 1999.

We cite an older review: *Revue de psychologie des peuples*, 23 volumes from 1946 to 1969 that in 1970 became *Ethno-psychologie: revue de psychologie des peuples* (1970–82).

157 Nathan, "Devereux, un hébreu anarchiste"; Nathan, "Le rôle de Georges Devereux."

158 See Nathan, *La folie des autres.*

159 Devereux returns to this concept in many articles on cultural psychiatry, but also in his essay to obtain the title of psychoanalyst at the Société de psychanalyse de Paris and in his autobiography, where he puts forward a definition inspired by Kroeber: "determined not by child rearing techniques but by the mood of the parents while mediating to him, through such techniques, the culture of his tribe" (Devereux, "The Works," 397). See Kroeber, "Culture Area," 646–7.

160 This version is reproduced in the appendix of the present work. A version is held at the Fonds Henri Ellenberger in Paris, and another at the Fonds Andrée Yanacopoulo in Montreal.

161 On Henri Ellenberger's teaching in the United States, see Delille, "Teaching the History of Psychiatry in the 1950s."

162 This characteristic, which is interesting from the point of view of gender studies, could be an original point of departure for re-examining this corpus from a new perspective.

163 Huxley, *The Doors of Perception.*

164 H. Michaux, *Les grandes épreuves.*

165 H. Ellenberger, "C.G. Jung and the story of Helene Preiswerk."

166 Unger, LSD, *Mescaline, Psilocybin, and Psychotherapy*; Unger, "Mescaline, LSD, Psilocybin and Personality Change."

167 H. Ellenberger, "Les toxicomanies," 5.

168 There was an exchange between Henri Ellenberger and Erving Goffman, with Goffman asking him for a copy of one of his articles.

169 This research study period appears in the calendars of the Université de Montréal. Guy Dubreuil, professor of anthropology there, created the department in 1961, which means that Roger Bastide entered a department that had just been founded, one that sought legitimacy in Quebec. Shortly after this study period, Guy Dubreuil wrote a rather nuanced review of Roger Bastide's book, in which he defended McGill's approach. See Dubreuil, "*Sociologie des maladies mentales* by Roger Bastide."

170 They participated in the conference on African psychiatry and psychopathology held in Dakar, at the invitation of Henri Collomb. An article describes Henri Ellenberger's stay in February and March 1968, at the

time of the second Pan-African Conference on Psychiatry (5–9 March 1968): H. Ellenberger, "Impressions psychiatriques." He also wrote a laudatory review of András Zempléni's doctoral dissertation for the *Transcultural Psychiatry* journal of McGill University in Montreal: *L'interprétation de la thérapie traditionnelle.* András Zempléni collaborated with Henri Collomb; likewise, René Collignon also worked with him in Dakar.

171 See Baruk, *Psychiatrie morale expérimentale*; Braruk, *La psychiatrie sociale.*

172 Strotzka, *Einführung in der Sozialpsychiatrie.*

173 Bastide, "Psychiatrie sociale et ethnologie," 1677.

174 Correspondance Henri Ellenberger–Roger Bastide, 1965–1967, Fonds Henri Ellenberger. Nota bene: there is no call number in the archives for Ellenberger correspondence held in Paris (see bibliography).

175 The publisher's intermediary at this time was Claude Veil, in charge of the "Social Psychiatry" chapter and thus responsible for updates. See, in particular, the letter from Claude Veil to Roger Bastide, on 28 March 1968, Fonds Henri Ey.

176 Bastide and Raveau, "Épidémiologie des maladies mentales."

177 Aubin, "L'assistance psychiatrique indigène aux colonies"; Aubin, "Introduction à l'étude de la psychiatrie chez les Noirs."

178 Aubin, "Indigènes nord-africains," "Magie," "Noirs," and "Primitivisme."

179 Keller, *Colonial Madness.*

180 See Porot and Arrii, "L'impulsivité criminelle chez l'indigène algérien." To place this article in the context of a wider corpus, see Collignon, "Contributions à la psychiatrie coloniale."

181 Fanon, "The "North African Syndrome," in *Toward the African Revolution.*

182 See Jean-Paul Sartre, preface to *The Wretched of the Earth*, in Fanon, *Oeuvres.*

183 Aubin and Alliez, "Socio-psychiatrie exotique."

184 Carothers, "A Study of Mental Derangement in Africans."

185 Carothers, "Frontal Lobe Function and the African."

186 McCulloch, *Colonial Psychiatry.*

187 Heaton, *Black Skin, White Coats.*

188 Collomb and Zwingelstein, "Depressive States in an African Community."

189 Bastide, *Le Rêve*, 280.

190 Ibid., 172.

191 Ibid., 290.

192 Ibid., 152.

193 To situate the problem, see Althusser, "Idéologie et appareils idéologiques d'État."

194 Laplantine, preface to Bastide, *Le rêve*, 15.

195 See Lézé, "Qu'est-ce que l'ethnopsychiatrie?" For the sources, see · Laplantine, *Ethnopsychiatrie psychanalytique*; Laplantine, *L'Ethnopsychiatrie*.

196 In an interview given at the end of his life, Erwin Ackerknecht dates 1933 as the end of his Marxist commitment and the beginning of his interest in sociological and ethnographical methods in France after his emigration. See Ackerknecht, "On the collecting of data," 8.

197 For a contemporary reading of panic, see Dupuy, *La panique*. The book is taken from a report ordered by a department and is characterized by the conception of evil of anthropologist René Girard, author of *La violence et le sacré*.

198 Hamon, "Les psychoses collectives." Professor of child psychiatry Georges Heuyer returned again to the topic in 1973: see Heuyer, *Psychoses collectives et suicides collectifs*.

199 Sontag, *Illness as Metaphor*.

200 See Grmek, *La guerre comme maladie sociale*.

201 Bastide, *Le rêve*, 88–90.

202 Ackerknecht, "On the Collecting of Data," 86–7.

203 Henri Ellenberger cites a rather old source: Hellpach, *Die geistigen Epidemien*.

204 Ackerknecht, "Laennec und die Psychiatrie," 96.

205 Ibid., 97.

206 See Mauss, "Effet physique chez l'individu."

207 See Cannon, "Voodoo Death," 169–81.

208 Mars, *Crisis in Possession in Voodoo*. Robert Alfred Hahn and Arthur Kleinman re-examined this type of problem in the 1980s: see "Voodoo Death" and the "placebo phenomenon."

209 H. Ellenberger, "Der Tod aus Psychischen Ursachen bei Naturvölkern"; and H. Ellenberger, "Der Selbstmord im Lichte der Ethno-Psychiatrie."

210 I refer once again to the series of articles by Raymond Prince titled *Pioneers in Transcultural Psychiatry* (see bibliography).

211 Starting in 1966, the review *Psychopathologie africaine* reproduced excerpts from the McGill Newsletter, with the authorization of Eric Wittkower. Thanks to René Collignon for drawing my attention to the collaboration between the two publications, which remained close over time.

212 Remember that Japan (until 1945: Greater East Asia Co-Prosperity Sphere) and the United States (until 1946: recognition of the sovereignty

of the Philippines) were both former colonial powers. For an analysis, see Singaravélou, *Les empires coloniaux.*

213 Dubreuil, "*Sociologie des maladies mentales* by Roger Bastide."

214 Collomb, "Bouffées délirantes en psychiatrie africaine."

215 See Collomb, "De l'ethnopsychiatrie à la psychiatrie sociale."

216 "Review and Newsletter: Transcultural Research in Mental Health Problems," in "Transcultural Psychiatric Research," 5090B RG: 47 C. 30, McGill University Archives.

217 "Graduate Program in Transcultural Psychiatry," revised version December 1967, p. 1, 5085 RG: 32 C. 2244 Box 2, McGill University Archives.

218 Ibid., 2.

219 This collaboration in the early 1960s with the University of Vermont in Burlington nevertheless remained short-lived, and it is not possible to provide the exact dates. My thanks to the University of Vermont archives for their assistance.

220 Wittkower, "Round-Table Meeting."

221 A pioneer in psychiatric epidemiology after the war. See Lin and Standley, *La place de l'épidémiologie en psychiatrie.*

222 George Morrison Carstairs (1916–1981), also known as Morris Carstairs, was one of the great pioneers in social psychiatry in Great Britain. Scottish like Brian Murphy, but born in India, he studied medicine at the University of Edinburgh before turning to anthropology. President of the World Federation for Mental Health from 1967 to 1971, he returned to India in the 1950s and 1960s and became known for promoting mental health prevention in developing countries. In 1960, Carstheairs founded the Medical Research Council's Unit for Research on Epidemiological Aspects of Psychiatry at the University College Hospital in London, which he set up at the University of Edinburgh the following year when he obtained the chair in medical psychology. He conducted an epidemiological study in the village of Kota (state of Karnataka) in the 1970s, with the help of psychiatrist Ravi L. Kapur (1938–2006).

223 This section's website (consulted in 2011) refers to Emil Kraepelin and Eric Wittkower, from whom he adopts the definition: "Transcultural Psychiatry denotes that the vista of the scientific observer extends beyond the scope of one cultural unit to another." Few sources are cited, but the role of two pilot epidemiological studies is highlighted: (1) *International Pilot Study on Schizophrenia* (1973–79); and (2) *Determinant of Outcome of Severe Mental Illness* (1992). The site explicitly mentions that the cross-cultural approach and the quantitative

approach (scale) of epidemiology enrich each other. As at the time of the founding of the McGill University department, this section of the World Psychiatric Association published a Newsletter to maintain a network internationally.

224 In addition to the journal of GIRAME, see Corin et al., *Regards anthropologiques en psychiatrie.*

225 H. Murphy, *Comparative Psychiatry.* An unsigned review of the work appeared in *L'évolution psychiatrique* 48, no. 1 (1983): 41–2.

226 See Yap, *Comparative Psychiatry.*

227 See Prince, "Transcultural psychiatry at McGill," 180.

228 Ibid., 181.

229 Information partly taken from the site of the World Psychiatric Association.

230 Heaton, *Black Skin, White Coats*, 61–70.

231 For a description of the research project, see A. Leighton, "The Stirling County Study."

232 See Prince, *Conference on Personality Change and Religious Experience.*

233 Prince, *Why This Ecstasy?*

234 A. Leighton, *My Name Is Legion*; D. Leighton et al., "Psychiatric Findings of the Stirling County Study."

235 See *Transcultural Psychiatry*, "Festschrift for Alexander Leighton."

236 Of no relation to Brian Murphy.

237 Correspondence from 1962.

238 Letter from Henri Ellenberger to Henri Ey, 18 January 1962. Fonds Henri Ellenberger.

239 Aubin and Alliez, "Socio-psychiatrie exotique."

240 Letter from Henri Ey to Henri Ellenberger, 25 January 1962. Fonds Henri Ellenberger. Other documents show evidence of a project to create booklets on ethnopsychiatry by François Ravaut in 1960, which was never carried out. Fonds Henri Ey.

241 Together they wrote a textbook of psychiatry: Ey, Bernard, and Brisset, *Manuel de psychiatrie.*

242 L. Michaux, *Psychiatrie infantile.*

243 Letter from Charles Brisset to Henri Ellenberger, 6 February 1962. Fonds Henri Ellenberger. The exchanges between Charles Brisset and Henri Ellenberger extend from 1962 to 1965. The Fonds Henri Ey make it possible to simultaneously read the exchanges between Henri Ey and Henri Ellenberger, and between Henri Ey and Charles Brisset.

244 Lévi-Strauss, *The Elementary Structures of Kinship.*

245 According to the correspondence, Michel Neyraut abandoned the project for health reasons.

246 Letter Henri Ellenberger from Charles Brisset, 13 February 1962. Fonds Henri Ellenberger.

247 Letter from Charles Brisset to Henri Ellenberger, 16 March 1963. Fonds Henri Ellenberger.

248 Brisset, "Le culturalisme en psychiatrie."

249 On the scientific controversy, see Brès, *Freud et la psychanalyse américaine*.

250 Letter from Charles Brisset to Henri Ellenberger, 16 March 1963. Fonds Henri Ellenberger.

251 Corin and Bibeau, "H.B.M. Murphy." See also Prince, "In Memoriam H.B.M. Murphy."

252 H. Ellenberger and H. Murphy, "Les névroses et les états mineurs"; H. Murphy and Tousignant, "Fondements anthropologiques de l'ethnopsychiatrie"; H. Murphy and Tousignant, "Méthodologie de la recherche en ethnopsychiatrie"; H. Murphy and Tousignant, "Les psychoses"; Prince, "Thérapie et culture"; and H. Ellenberger, "Les toxicomanies."

253 See Tousignant, *Les origines sociales et culturelles des troubles psychologiques*.

254 Lantéri-Laura, *Essai sur les paradigmes de la psychiatrie moderne*.

255 Susser, Baumgartner, and Stein, "Sir Arthur Mitchell."

256 For initial results, see Lovell and Susser, "What Might Be a History Psychiatric Epidemiology?"

257 Ehrenberg and Lovell, *La maladie mentale en mutation*.

258 Fagot-Largeault, *Les causes de la mort*.

259 Giroux, "*Épidémiologie des facteurs de risque*," 78.

260 Aronowitz, *Making Sense of Illness*.

261 Jasen, "Breast Cancer and the Language of Risk."

262 Rothstein, *Public Health and the Risk Factor*.

263 I thank Thomas Schlich for answering my questions when I was a visiting scholar at McGill in the Department of Social Studies of Medicine (SSOM), in September 2014.

264 Schlich, "Risk and Medical Innovation."

265 I refer readers to the works of Luc Berlivet and Christiane Sinding.

266 See Kovess, Valla, and Tousignant, "Psychiatric Epidemiology in Quebec."

267 Raymond Sadoun, director of a research unit at INSERM, is a specialist in these matters.

268 Grob, "The Origins of American Psychiatric Epidemiology."

269 Letter from Henri Ellenberger to Roger Bastide, 27 January 1966. Centre de documentation Henri Ellenberger.

270 See Tremblay, "Alexander H. Leighton's and Jane Murphy's Scientific Contributions," 5.

271 Ibid., 6, 7. Clyde Kluckhohn also had psychoanalytic training.

272 J. Murphy and A. Leighton, *Approaches to Cross-Cultural Psychiatry*.

273 J. Murphy, "Psychiatric Labeling in Cross-Cultural Perspective."

274 J. Murphy, "Continuities in Community-Based Psychiatric Epidemiology."

275 See J. Murphy and A. Leighton, *Approaches to Cross-Cultural Psychiatry*.

276 H. Murphy, *Flight and Resettlement*. For a review in a social science journal, see Buettner-Janusch, "Flight and Resettlement."

277 H. Murphy, "Notes for a Theory on Latah." This article discusses various facets of the disorder, the factor of suggestibility associated with it, and its relationship with Tourette syndrome, as well as the epidemiological data. See also H. Murphy, "History and Evolution of Syndromes."

278 Corin and Bibeau, "H.B.M. Murphy," 404.

279 Murphy, "Méthodologie de recherche," 1.

280 Ibid. Anamnesis: account of medical history and the history of a disease.

281 Ibid.

282 See Jenicek, "Les approches épidémiologiques des maladies mentales."

283 H. Murphy, "Méthodologie de recherche," 4.

284 H. Ellenberger, "Ethnopsychiatrie, fasc. no 37725B10," 16.

285 Ibid., 2 ; H. Murphy, "Méthodologie de recherche," 3.

286 H. Murphy, "Méthodologie de recherche," 8.

287 See Fagot-Largeault, *Les causes de la mort*, 34–41.

288 Brian Murphy cites a classic study: the comparison between the rates of mania diagnosed in two regions that are culturally close (London and New York) demonstrated significant gaps and many varied uses of psychiatric nosologies. See Cooper et al., *Psychiatric Diagnosis in New York and London*.

289 See Chanoit and de Verbizier, *Informatique et épidémiologie*.

290 Norman Sartorius headed the team in charge of epidemiology of mental disorders at WHO as of 1963, then headed the Division of Mental Health at WHO as of 1977.

291 American Psychiatric Association, *Diagnostic and Statistical Manual of Mental Disorders*. On this history, see Kirk and Kutchins, *Aimez-vous le DSM?*; in particular the chapter "Contrôler les sources de biais", 88–131. More recently: Demazeux, *Qu'est-ce que le DSM?*

292 For example, two American textbooks: Okpaku, *Clinical Methods in Transcultural Psychiatry*; and Tseng, *Handbook of Cultural Psychiatry*.

293 See Hughes, "The Glossary of 'Culture-Bound Syndromes.'"

294 Kuru has since been reclassified as encephalopathy, transmitted by anthropophagic practices. It is among the diseases caused by prions, such as Creutzfeldt-Jakob disease (mad cow disease). But at the time Henri Ellenberger wrote, the disease remained mysterious and was identified with a cultural specificity, related to the place where it was observed (New Guinea). It disappeared with the end of cannibalism.

295 American Psychiatric Association, "Glossary of Cultural Concepts of Distress."

296 See Simons and Hughes, *The Culture-Bound Syndromes.*

297 Type of personality defined by Meyer Friedman and Ray Rosenman in the 1950s, characterized by hyperactivity and irritability, which increase the risk of cardiovascular disease.

298 For a more in-depth explanation, see Delille and Kirsch, "Le cours de Ian Hacking."

299 Crozier, "Making Up Koro."

300 Doctor and historian of psychiatry German E. Berrios asked about diagnosis among non-Chinese patients: see Berrios and Morley, "Koro-Like Symptom in a Non-Chinese Subject."

301 Blonk, "Koro."

302 Chowdhury, "Hundred Years of Koro." According to Chowdhury, the first known medical description was established in China in 1865.

303 See Chowdhury, "The Definition and Classification of Koro," 42.

304 Opler, "Anthropological and Cross-Cultural Aspects of homosexuality."

305 See Hippocrate, *Airs, eaux, lieux.*

306 See, for example, Devereux, *Essais d'ethnopsychiatrie générale,* 5, 6.

307 As an example, I refer to the observation of Dr Lasnet in "Notes d'ethnologie," 494 and 495.

308 The term *pathoplasticity* is also used in English.

309 The expression is made up of Japanese characters designating a disorder (*shō*), fear (*kyōfu*), and interpersonal relations (*taijin*): thus, *taijin kyofusho,* often abbreviated as TKS.

310 Jugon, *Phobies sociales au Japon,* 79–87.

311 Japanese convention is that the surname precedes the first name.

312 Kirmayer, "The Place of Culture in Psychiatric Nosology." On the same topic, see also Kirmayer, "Culture-Bound Syndromes and International Psychiatric Classification."

313 See H. Ellenberger, "La psychothérapie de Janet"; H. Ellenberger, "Un disciple fidèle de P. Janet."

314 A relative of lack of knowledge, as Anglo-Saxon historiography does not ignore the continuity, despite misinterpretations of the French terminology.

315 Leiris, *L'âge d'homme précédé de L'Afrique fantôme*. For an analysis, see Delille, "Review essay: Holofernes complex."

316 According to René Collignon (personal communication), Henri Collomb read Frantz Fanon.

317 For a selection of reviews, see the unsigned review "Ethno-psychiatrie (Ethnopsychiatry), by H.F. Ellenberger, *Encyclopédie médico-chirurgicale. Psychiatrie.* (18 Rue Séguier, Paris, VI c), (1965), p. 37725C10, 1–14, and p. 37725B10, 1–22 (in French)," *Transcultural Psychiatry* 3, no. 1 (April 1966): 5–8; Bastide, "Ethno-psychiatrie"; and Mathé, "Ethnopsychiatrie in Encyclopédie médico-chirurgicale."

318 H. Ellenberger, "Intérêt et domaines d'application de l'ethnopsychiatrie."

319 Dosse, *L'histoire en miettes*, 163.

320 For a recent historical overview, see Wu, "World Citizenship."

321 Vidal, "À la recherche d'Henri Ellenberger."

BIBLIOGRAPHY

Archives

Archives of the Université de Montréal
Henri Frédérique Ellenberger fonds, 1950–1983. Cote P357.
Andrée Yanacopoulo fonds. Cote P0256.
Henri Ellenberger Fonds from the Centre de documentation Henri
  Ellenberger at the hôpital Sainte-Anne (documents without call numbers)
Henri Ellenberger's professional correspondence

"Un cas de toxicomanie par le peyotl". [Handwritten: "Cours et conférences inédits"], numbered typescript of eight pages, and a manuscript
page titled "Addenda" [and a series of quotes from the poet Henri
Michaux], reproduced in the appendix of the current edition. It deals with
a course on a clinical case of a Native American (Potawatomi), seen at
Topeka (Menninger Foundation) in 1957, although an addendum indicates a bibliographic reference in 1963. Following this document is a five-
page document typewritten in English: a medical report, as well as the
case history of the patient, as well as two drawings that illustrate a vision
dated [to] 1918 (the patient was born in 1891).

The fonds house other files on ethnopsychiatry corresponding to documentation gathered by Henri Ellenberger in the course of his research.
Included is a course synopsis, in English: "Cultural factors in mental
diseases" (no date, paginated from 1 to 66, of which twelve pages are
missing). Without a doubt, this was a lecture delivered at McGill, which
served as outlines for leaflets of the *Encyclopédie médico-chirurgicale*
(EMC), although the structure and content vary.

Humboldt Universität zu Berlin Archiv
UK W 304 (Erich Wittkower's professional record).

Landesamt für Bürger- und Ordnungsangelegenheiten
Abteilung I – Entschädigungsbehörde
Reg.-Nr. 275089.

McGill University Archives
"Graduate program in transcultural psychiatry." Revised Version
  December 1967. Cote 5085, RG 32, c. 2244, box 2.
"Transcultural psychiatric research." 1956–67. Cote 5090, RG 47, c. 30.

*Georges Devereux Fonds at the Institut mémoires de l'édition
   contemporaine (IMEC)*
Correspondence between Georges Devereux and Henri Ellenberger,
   1954–74 (supplied by François Bordes).

Henri Ey Fonds, communal archives of Perpignan
The professional correspondence of Henri Ey and the working documents
of the *Traité de psychiatrie* of *l'Encyclopédie médico-chirurgicale* (EMC)
are held in the fonds and filed under the call number 7s. For a complete
list of Henri Ey's professional correspondence, see the doctoral thesis of
Emmanuel Delille, *Réseaux savants et enjeux classificatoires dans le
« Traité de psychiatrie » de l'Encyclopédie médico-chirurgicale
(1947–1977)*, EHESS, History and Civilizations program, 2 vols., 2008,
365–6. This is the only complete list that matches the numbers on the
archive boxes with the dates of correspondence.

Fonds of journals and specialty notebooks consulted in-library
1) Colonial medicine magazines/journals:
Archives de médecine navale et coloniale (1890–96) was renamed in 1898:
   *Annales d'hygiène et de médecine coloniales. Recueil publié par ordre
   du ministre des Colonies* (1898–1914).
2) Specialized collections and journals in ethno-psychiatry, transcultural
   psychiatry, and medical anthropology:
– *L'autre. Cliniques, cultures et sociétés*, published since 2000.
– *Bastidiana*, published from 1993 to 2006, and eight special issues.
– *Culture, Medicine, and Psychiatry*, published since 1977.
– *Curare Zeitschrift für Ethnomedizin und transkulturelle Psychiatrie*; was
   renamed in 2007: *Curare, Zeitschrift für Medizinethnologie / Curare
   Journal of Medical Anthropology*, published since 1978.
– *Ethnopsy – Les mondes contemporains de la guérison*, 5 issues from
   2000 to 2003.
– *Ethnopsychiatrica*, 5 issues from 1978 to 1981.
– *Nouvelle revue d'ethnopsychiatrie*, 36 issues from 1983 to 1999.
– *Psychopathologie africaine*, published since 1965.
– *Revue de psychologie des peuples*, 23 issues from 1946 to 1969; was
   renamed *Ethno-psychologie: revue de psychologie des peuples* in 1970
   and continued to be published until 1982
– *Transcultural Research in Mental Health Problems*, first series, 9 issues
   from 1956 to 1962; was renamed *Transcultural Psychiatric Research
   Review* for issues 14 and 15 in 1963. The new journal, *Transcultural*

Psychiatric Research Review, vols. 1 to 33, 1963–96, was renamed
Transcultural Psychiatry with vol. 34; has been published since 1997.
– *World Psychiatry: Official Journal of the World Psychiatric Association
(WPA)*, has been published since 2002.
– *Santé, Culture, Health,* journal of Groupe Interuniversitaire de
Recherche en Anthropologie Médicale et en Ethnopsychiatrie
(GIRAME), Montreal, 10 issues from 1983 to 1994.

Interviews with René Collignon, Maurice Dongier, Laurence Kirmayer,
Arthur Kleinman, Anne Lovell, Jane Murphy, Tanya Murphy, André
Normandeau, Andrée Yanacopoulo, Allan Young, and András
Zempléni.

Cited Works by Henri Ellenberger

"Analyse existentielle," fasc. no 37815A10. *Traité de psychiatrie*, 1-4.
Paris: Éditions techniques (Encyclopédie médico-chirurgicale), 1955.
"Aspects culturels de la maladie mentale." *Canadian Psychiatric
Association Journal* 4, no. 1 (1959): 26–37; reproduced in *Médecines de
l'âme. Essais d'histoire de la folie et des guérisons psychiques*, edited by
É. Roudinesco, 431–47. Paris: Fayard, 1995.
"L'autobiographie de C.G. Jung." *Critique* (1964): 207–8.
*Beyond the Unconscious: Essays of Henri Ellenberger in the History of
Psychiatry*, edited by M.S. Micale. Princeton: Princeton University Press,
1993.
"Carl Gustav Jung: His Historical Setting." In *Historical Explorations in
Medicine and Psychiatry*, edited by H. Riese. New York: Springer, 1978.
"Castration des pervers sexuels," fasc. no 37105H10. *Traité de psychiatrie*,
1–2. Paris: Éditions techniques (Encyclopédie médico-chirurgicale),
1955.
"C.G. Jung and the Story of Helene Preiswerk: A Critical Study with New
Documents." *History of Psychiatry* 2, no. 1 (1991): 41–52.
"Chapitre 50: La maladie créatrice" and "Chapitre 51: La guérison et ses
artisans." In *Traité d'anthropologie médicale. L'institution de la santé et
de la maladie*, edited by J. Dufresne, F. Dumont, and Y. Martin,
1015–36. Quebec City and Lyon: Presses de l'Université du Québec /
Presses universitaires de Lyon, 1985.
Criminologie du passé et du present [Inaugural Lecture at the Université
de Montréal, 10 November 1965]. Montreal: Presses de l'Université de
Montréal, 1969.

"Un disciple fidèle de P. Janet: le Dr Léonard Schwartz (1885–1948)."
L'évolution psychiatrique 15, no. 3 (1950): 483–84.

*The Discovery of the Unconscious: The History and Evolution of
Dynamic Psychiatry*. New York: Basic Books, 1970; *À la découverte de
l'inconscient: histoire de la psychiatrie dynamique*, translated by Joseph
Feisthauer. Villeurbanne: SIMEP, 1974; new editions: *L'histoire de la
découverte de l'inconscient*, translated by Joseph Feisthauer, edited by É.
Roudinesco. Paris: Fayard, 1994.

Essai sur le syndrome psychologique de la catatonie [1933], edited by J.
Chazaud. Paris: L'Harmattan, 2004.

"Ethnopsychiatrie," fasc. no 37725A10. *Traité de psychiatrie*, 1–14. Paris:
Éditions techniques (Encyclopédie médico-chirurgicale), 1965.

"Ethnopsychiatrie," fasc. no 37725B10. *Traité de psychiatrie*, 1–22. Paris:
Éditions techniques (Encyclopédie médico-chirurgicale), 1965.

"Les fadets dans le département de la Vienne." *Les cahiers nouveaux de
littérature* 1 (December 1940): 41–3; 2 (January 1941): 89–91.

"L'histoire d'Anna O.: étude critique avec documents nouveaux."
L'évolution psychiatrique 37, no. 4 (1972): 693–717.

"L'histoire d'Emmy von N." *L'évolution psychiatrique* 42, no. 3/1 (1977):
519–40.

"Impressions psychiatriques d'un séjour à Dakar." *Psychopathologie
africaine* 4 (1968): 469–80.

"Intérêt et domaines d'application de l'ethnopsychiatrie." *Actes du IVe
congrès mondial de psychiatrie* (Madrid, 5–11 septembre 1966).
Excerpta Medica Foundation, 1967, 264–8.

"*L'interprétation de la thérapie traditionnelle du désordre mental chez les
Wolof et les Lebou, Senegal (Traditional Interpretation and Therapy of
Mental Disorder among the Wolof and Lebou of Sénégal)* by A.
Zempléni." *Transcultural Psychiatry* 6, no. 1 (1969): 69–74.

*Médecines de l'âme. Essais d'histoire de la folie et des guérisons
psychiques*, edited by É. Roudinesco. Paris: Fayard, 1995.

"Le monde fantastique dans le folklore de la Vienne." *Nouvelle revue des
traditions Populaires* 1 (November–December 1949): 407–35; 2
(January–February 1950): 3–26.

"Les mouvements de libération mythique." *Critique* 190 (1963): 248–67;
reproduced in *Médecines de l'âme. Essais d'histoire de la folie et des
guérisons psychiques*, edited by É. Roudinesco, 449–69. Paris: Fayard,
1995.

Les mouvements de libération mythique. Montreal: Quinze, 1978.

"Pierre Janet philosophe." *Dialogue* 12, no. 2 (1973): 254–87.

La psychiatrie Suisse. Aurillac: Imprimerie Poirier-Bottreau, 1954.
"La psychiatrie Suisse." *L'évolution psychiatrique*: 16, no. 2 (1951):
321–54; 16, no. 4 (1951): 619–44; 17, no. 1 (1952): 139–58; 17, no. 2
(1952): 359–79; 17, no. 3 (1952): 593–606; 18, no. 2 (1953): 299–318;
18, no. 4 (1953): 719–51.
"La psychiatrie transculturelle." In *Précis pratique de psychiatrie*, edited
by H. Ellenberger and R. Duguay, 625–42. Montreal and Paris:
Chenelière et Stanké/Maloine, 1984.
"Psychoses collectives," fasc. no 37725C10. *Traité de psychiatrie*, 1–10.
Paris: Éditions techniques (Encyclopédie médico-chirurgicale), 1967.
"La psychothérapie de Janet." *L'évolution psychiatrique* 15, no. 3 (1950):
465–82.
"Psychothérapie de la schizophrénie," fasc. no 37295C10. *Traité de
psychiatrie*, 1–12. Paris: Éditions techniques (Encyclopédie
médico-chirurgicale), 1955.
"Die Putzwut." *Der Psychologue* 2 (1950): 91–4, 138–47.
"Der Selbstmord im Lichte der Ethno-Psychiatrie." *Monatsschrift für
Psychiatrie und Neurologie* 125 (1953): 347–61.
"Der Tod aus Psychischen Ursachen bei Naturvölkern (*Voodoo Death*)."
Psyche 5 (1951): 333–44.
"Les toxicomanies," fasc. no 37725C10. *Traité de psychiatrie*, 1–5. Paris:
Éditions techniques (Encyclopédie médico-chirurgicale), 1978.

Primary Sources

Ackerknecht, Erwin H. "On the Collecting of Data." In *Medicine and
Ethnology*, edited by H.H. Walser and H.M. Koelbing, 116–17. Berne:
Huber, 1971.
– "Ethnologische Vorbemerkung." In *Kurze Geschichte der Psychiatrie*,
3rd ed. [1967], 1–9. Stuttgart: Thieme, 1985.
– "Laennec und die Psychiatrie." *Gesnerus* 19 (1962): 93–100.
– *Malaria in the Upper Mississippi Valley, 1760–1900*. Baltimore: Johns
Hopkins University Press, 1945.
– *Medicine and Ethnology*. Edited by H.H. Walser and H.M. Koelbing.
Berne: Huber, 1971.
– "Psychopathology, Primitive Medicine, and Primitive Culture." *Bulletin
of the History of Medicine* 14, no. 1 (1943): 30–67.
– "Transcultural Psychiatry." In *Essays in the History of Psychiatry*, edited
by Edwin R. Wallace, 172–83. Columbia: W.M.S. Hall Psychiatric
Institute, 1980.

Althusser, Louis. "Idéologie et appareils idéologiques d'État. Notes pour une recherche [1970]." In *Positions*, 67–125. Paris: Les Éditions sociales, 1976.

American Psychiatric Association. "Glossary of Cultural Concepts of Distress." In *Diagnostic and Statistical Manual of Mental Disorders* [DSM-5], 833–37. Washington, DC, 2013.

Aronowitz, Robert A. DSM: *Manuel diagnostique et statistique des troubles mentaux* [1980 for the 3rd edition]. Edited by Pierre Pichot and Julien Daniel Guelfi. Paris: Masson, 1983.

– *Making Sense of Illness: Science, Society, and Disease.* Cambridge: Cambridge University Press, 1998.

Aubin, Henri. "L'assistance psychiatrique indigène aux colonies." *Congrès des médecins aliénistes et des neurologues de France et de pays de langue française*, Alger, s.n., 1938, 158.

– "Indigènes nord-africains (Psychopathologie des)." "Magie." "Noirs (Psychopathologie des)." "Primitivisme." In *Manuel alphabétique de psychiatrie clinique, thérapeutique et médico-légale*, edited by Antoine Porot, 217, 255, 289–90, 335–6. Paris: Presses universitaires de France, 1952.

– "Introduction à l'étude de la psychiatrie chez les Noirs." *Annales médico-psychologiques* 97, nos. 1–2 (1939): 1–29 and 181–13.

Aubin, Henri, and Joseph Alliez. "Socio-psychiatrie exotique," fasc. no. 37730A10. *Traité de psychiatrie*, 1-8. Paris: Éditions techniques (Encyclopédie médico-chirurgicale), 1955.

Balandier, Georges. "La collaboration entre l'ethnologie et la psychiatrie." *Critique* 21 (1948): 161–74.

Baruk, Henri. *Psychiatrie morale expérimentale, individuelle et sociale. Haines et réactions de culpabilité.* Paris: Presses universitaires de France, 1945.

– *La psychiatrie sociale*, 5th ed. Paris: Presses universitaires de France, 1974.

Bastide, Roger. "*Ethno-psychiatrie.*" *L'année sociologique* 16 (1965): 276.

– "Psychiatrie sociale et ethnologie." In *Ethnologie générale*, edited by J. Poirier, 1655–79. Paris: Gallimard/Encyclopédie de la Pléiade, 1968.

– *Le rêve, la transe et la folie* [1972]. Paris: Éditions du Seuil, 2003.

– *Sociologie des maladies mentales.* Paris: Flammarion, 1965.

– *The Sociology of Mental Disorder.* Translated by Jean McNeil. New York: David McKay, 1972.

Bastide, Roger, and François Raveau. "Épidémiologie des maladies mentales," fasc. no 37878A10. *Traité de psychiatrie*, 1–8. Paris: Éditions techniques (Encyclopédie médico-chirurgicale), 1971.

Berr, Henri. *La synthèse en histoire.* Paris: Alcan, 1911.

Berrios, German E., and S.J. Morley. "Koro-Like Symptom in a
Non-Chinese Subject." *British Journal of Psychiatry* 145 (1984): 331–4.

Blonk, J.C. "Koro." *Geneeskundig Tijdschrift voor Nederlandsch-Indie* 35
(1895): 150–295.

Brisset, Charles. "Anthropologie culturelle et psychiatrie," fasc. no 37715
A 10. *Traité de psychiatrie,* 1–9. Paris: Éditions techniques
(Encyclopédie médico-chirurgicale), 1960.

– "Le culturalisme en psychiatrie. Étude critique." *L'évolution
psychiatrique* 28, no. 3 (1963): 369–485.

Buettner-Janusch, John. "Flight and Resettlement: H.B.M. Murphy and
Others." *American Anthropologist* 38 (1956): 217–18.

Cannon, Walter Bradford. "Voodoo Death." *American Anthropologist* 44
(1924): 169–81.

Carothers, John Colin D. "Frontal Lobe Function and the African."
Journal of Mental Science 97 (1951): 12–48.

– *The Mind of Man in Africa.* London: Tom Stacey, 1972.

– *Psychopathologie normale et pathologique de l'Africain.* Geneva: OMS
Monograph Series, no. 17, 1953.

– "A Study of Mental Derangement in Africans and an Attempt to Explain
Its Peculiarities, More Especially in Relation to the African Attitude to
Life." *Journal of Mental Science* 93 (1947): 548–73.

Chanoit, Pierre-François, and Jean de Verbizier, eds. *Informatique et
épidémiologie.* Toulouse: Érès, 1985.

Collomb, Henri. "Bouffées délirantes en psychiatrie africaine."
Transcultural Psychiatric Research Review 3 (1966): 29–34.

– "De l'ethnopsychiatrie à la psychiatrie sociale." *Canadian Journal of
Psychiatry* 24, no. 5 (1979): 464–5.

Collomb, Henri, and Jacques Zwingelstein. "Depressive States in an
African Community (Dakar)." In *First Pan African Psychiatric
Conference,* edited by T.A. Lambo, 227–34. Ibadan: Government
Printer, 1961.

Cooper, J.E., et al. *Psychiatric Diagnosis in New York and London.*
London: Oxford University Press, 1972.

Corin, Ellen, et al. *Regards anthropologiques en psychiatrie /
Anthropological Perspectives in Psychiatry.* Montreal: Éditions du
GIRAME, 1987.

Devereux, Georges. *De l'angoisse à la méthode dans les sciences du comportement* [1967]. Paris: Flammarion, 2012.

– *Essais d'ethnopsychiatrie générale.* Paris: Gallimard, 1977.

– *Ethnopsychanalyse complémentariste* [1972]. Paris: Flammarion, 1985;

Ethnopsychoanalysis: Psychoanalysis and Anthropology as Complementary Frames of Reference. Berkeley: University of California Press, 1978.

– *Ethnopsychiatrie des Indiens mohaves.* Le Plessis-Robinson: Synthélabo (Les empêcheurs de penser en rond), 1996.

– "Normal et anormal" [1956], in *Essais d'ethnopsychiatrie générale*, 1–83; *Basic Problems of Ethnopsychiatry* [1979], 3–71.

– *Psychothérapie d'un Indien des Plaines* [1951]. Paris: Aubier-Fayard, 1998.

– *Reality and Dream: Psychotherapy of a Plains Indian.* New York, International University Press, 1951.

– "A Sociological Theory of Schizophrenia." *Psychoanaytic Review* 26 (1939): 315–42.

– "The Works of George Devereux." In *The Making of Psychological Anthropology*, edited by G.D. Splinder, 364–406. Berkeley: University of California Press, 1978.

Dongier, Maurice, and Henri Ellenberger. "Criminologie," fasc. nos. 37760A10, 37760A30, 37760A50, 37760A70, and 37760A90. *Traité de psychiatrie.* Paris: Éditions techniques (Encyclopédie médico-chirurgicale), 1958.

Dubreuil, Guy. *Sociologie des maladies mentales (Sociology of Mental Disease)* by Roger Bastide. *Transcultural Psychiatry* 3 (1966): 85–90.

Ellenberger, David F. *Catalogue of the Masitise Archives.* Rome and Morija: Institute of Southern African Studies / Morija Archives, 1987.

– *Histori ea Basotho.* Morija, s.n., 1917.

– *History of the Basuto, Ancient and Modern.* London: Caxton, 1912.

Ellenberger, Henri, Rollo May, and Ernest Angel. *Existence: A New Dimension in Psychiatry and Psychology.* New York: Basic Books, 1958.

Ellenberger, Henri, and H. Brian M. Murphy. "Les névroses et les états mineurs," fasc.no 37725B10. *Traité de psychiatrie*, 1–5. Paris: Éditions techniques (Encyclopédie médico-chirurgicale), 1978.

Ellenberger, Henri, and Jeanne d'Arc Trottier. "The Impact of a Severe, Prolonged Physical Illness of a Child upon the Family." *Proceedings, 3rd World Congress of Psychiatry* 1 (1961): 465–9.

Ellenberger, Victor. *Afrique avec cette peur venue du fond des âges.* Paris: Le livre contemporain, 1956.

– *La fin tragique des Bushmen.* Paris: Amiot-Dumont, 1953.

– *Sur les hauts plateaux du Lessouto, notes et souvenirs de voyage.* Paris: Société des missions, 1930.

– *Un siècle de mission au Lessouto.* Paris: Société des missions, 1933.

Ellis, Gilmore W. "The Amok of the Malays." *Journal of Mental Science* 39 (1893): 325–38.

– "Latah: A Mental Malady of the Malays." *Journal of Mental Sciences* 43 (1897): 33–40.

Elmont, Fred (pseudonym of Henri Ellenberger). *Les petits chaperons de toutes les couleurs.* Montreal: Stanké/Quinze, 1976.

Ernst, Waltraud. *Colonialism and Transnational Psychiatry: The Development of an Indian Mental Hospital in British India, c. 1925–1940.* New York: Anthem Press, 2013.

– *Mad Tales from the Raj: The European Insane in British India, 1800–1858.* London and New York: Routledge, 1991; new edition London and Delhi: Anthem Press, 2010.

Ey, Henri, ed. *Traité de psychiatrie.* 3 vols. Paris: Éditions techniques (Encyclopédie médico-chirurgicale), 1955.

Ey, Henri, Paul Bernard, and Charles Brisset. *Manuel de psychiatrie.* Paris: Masson, 1960.

Fanon, Frantz. *Oeuvres.* Paris: La Découverte, 2011.

– "Le 'syndrome nord-africain'" [1952]. In *Pour la révolution africaine. Écrits politiques* [1964], 16–31. Paris: La Découverte, 2001.

– *Toward the African Revolution.* Translated by Haakon Chevalier. New York: Grove Press, 1967.

Fried, Jacob. "Acculturation and Mental Health among Indian Migrants in Peru." In *Culture and Mental Health*, edited by M.K. Opler, 120–37. New York: Macmillan, 1959.

Gessain, M. [notes taken by André Renard, not reviewed by M. Gessain]. "Ethnologie et Psychologie." *Bulletin de psychologie* 12, no. 162 (1959): 273–81.

Gibb, Hamilton A.R. *Area Studies Reconsidered.* London: School of Oriental and African Studies, 1964.

Giroux, Élodie. "*Épidémiologie des facteurs de risque: genèse d'une nouvelle approche de la maladie.*" PhD diss., Université Paris 1, Panthéon-Sorbonne, 2006.

Hamon, Joseph M.M. "Les psychoses collectives." Report of psychiatry. Congress of alienists and neurologists from France and French-speaking countries. 53rd meeting, Nice, 5–11 September 1955. Cahors: A. Coueslant, 1955

Hellpach, Willy. *Die geistigen Epidemien.* Frankfurt am Main: Rütten & Loening, 1904.

Heuyer, Georges. *Psychoses collectives et suicides collectifs.* Paris: Presses universitaires de France, 1973.

Hippocrate. *Airs, eaux, lieux.* Translated by P. Maréchaux. Paris: Payot et Rivages (Rivages Poche), 1995.

Hughes, Charles C. "The Glossary of 'Culture-Bound Syndromes.'" In "*DSM-IV:* A Critique." *Transcultural Psychiatry* 35, no. 3 (1998): 413–21.

Huxley, Aldous L. *The Doors of Perception.* London: Chatto and Windus, 1954.

Kovess, Viviane, J.-P. Valla, and Michel Tousignant. "Psychiatric Epidemiology in Quebec: An Overview." *Canadian Journal of Psychiatry* 35 (1990): 414–18.

Kraepelin, Emil. "Vergleichende Psychiatrie." *Zentralblatt für Nervenheilkunde und Psychiatrie* 27 (1904): 433–7, 468–9.

Kroeber, A.L. "Culture Area." In *Encyclopedia of the Social Sciences,* edited by E.R.A. Seligman and A.S. Johnson, vol. 3, 646–7. New York: Macmillan, 1930.

Laplantine, François. *L'ethnopsychiatrie.* Paris: Presses universitaires de France, 1988.

– *Ethnopsychiatrie psychanalytique.* Paris: Beauchesne, 2007.

– "Georges Devereux, un savant entre les rives." *La vie des idées,* 19 November 2013. http://www.laviedesidees.fr/Georges-Devereux-un-savant-entre.html.

Lasnet, A. "Notes d'ethnologie et de médecine sur les Sakalaves du nord-ouest." *Annales d'hygiène et de médecine colonials* 2 (1899): 471–97.

Leighton, Alexander H. *My Name Is Legion: Foundations for a Theory of Man in Relation to Culture.* New York: Basic Books, 1959.

– "The Stirling County Study: A Research Program in Social Factors Related to Psychiatric Health." In *Interrelations between the Social Environment and Psychiatric Disorders.* New York: Milbank Memorial Fund, 1953.

Leighton, Dorothea C., et al. "Psychiatric Findings of the Stirling County Study." *The American Journal of Psychiatry* 119 (1963): 1021–6.

Leiris, Michel. *L'âge d'homme* précédé de *L'Afrique fantôme.* Edited by Denis Hollier with Francis Marmande and Catherine Maubon. Paris: Gallimard, 2014.

Lévi-Strauss, Claude. *The Elementary Structures of Kinship.* Translated by James Harle Bell, Rodney Needham, and John Richard Von Sturmer. Boston: Beacon Press, 1969.

– *Les structures élémentaires de la parenté* [1948], 2nd ed. Paris: Mouton de Gruyter, 2002.

Lin, Tsung-Yi, and C.C. Standley. *La place de l'épidémiologie en psychiatrie.* Genève: Organisation mondiale de la santé, 1963.

Linton, Ralph. *The Cultural Background of Personality*. New York: Appleton-Century-Crofts, 1945.

– *Culture and Mental Disorders*, edited by G. Devereux. Springfield: Charles C. Thomas, 1956.

– *The Study of Man: An Introduction*, New York and London: Appleton-Century-Crofts, 1936.

Lombard, Henri-Clermond. *Atlas de la distribution géographique des maladies dans leurs rapports avec les climats*. Paris: J.B. Baillière, 1880.

Machobane, James, and Édouard Motsamaï. *Au temps des cannibales, following Dans les caverns Sombres*. Translated by V. Ellenberger. Bordeaux: Confluences, 1999.

Marquer, Paulette. "L'ethnographie. Ethnographie, psychologie et psychiatrie." In *Histoire de la science*, edited by M. Daumas, 1523–37. Paris: Gallimard (Encyclopédie de la Pléiade), 1957.

Mars, Louis. *La crise de possession dans le vaudou: essais de psychiatrie comparée*. Port-au-Prince: Imprimerie de l'État, 1946 (2nd rev. ed. 1950).

– *Crisis in Possession in Voodoo*. Translated by Kathleen Collins. N.p.: Reed, Cannon and Johnson Co, 1977.

– "De quelques problèmes de psychiatrie comparée en Haïti, psychiatrie et religion." *Annales médico-psychologiques* 11, no. 4 (1948): 99–106.

Mars, Louis P. "Nouvelle contribution à l'étude de la crise de possession." *Psyché* 60 (October 1951): 640–69.

Mathé, A. G. "Ethnopsychiatrie in Encyclopédie médico-chirurgicale par H. F. Ellenberger." *Bulletin de recherches psychothérapiques de langue française* 5, no. 2 (1967): 71–3.

Mauss, Marcel. "Effet physique chez l'individu de l'idée de mort suggéré par la collectivité (Australie, Nouvelle–Zélande) [1926]." In *Sociologie et anthropologie*, 313–30. Paris: Presses universitaires de France, 1968.

– *Sociologie et anthropologie*, 4th ed. With an introduction by C. Lévi-Strauss. Paris: Presses universitaires de France, 1968.

McCulloch, Jock. *Colonial Psychiatry and the "African Mind."* Cambridge: Cambridge University Press, 1995.

Michaux, Henri. *Les grandes épreuves de l'esprit et les innombrables petites*. Paris: Gallimard, 1966.

Michaux, Léon. *Psychiatrie infantile*, 4th ed. Paris: Presses universitaires de France, 1967.

Mofolo, Thomas. *Chaka* [1926]. Paris: Gallimard, 1940.

– *L'homme qui marchait vers le soleil levant* [*Moeti Oa Bochabela*, 1907–1908]. Translated by V. Ellenberger with P. Ellenberger. Bordeaux: Confluences, 2003.

Moreau de Tours, Jacques-Joseph. "Recherches sur les aliénés en Orient." *Annales médico-psychologiques*, vol. 1 (1843): 103–32.

Murphy, H. Brian M. *Comparative Psychiatry*. New York: Springer, 1982.

– "The Historical Development of Transcultural Psychiatry." In *Transcultural Psychiatry*, edited by J.L. Cox, 7–22. London: Croom Helm, 1986.

– "History and Evolution of Syndromes: The Striking Case of *latah* and *amok*." In *Psychopathology*, edited by M. Hammer, K. Salzinger, and S. Sutton, 33–5. New York: Wiley, 1973.

– "In Memoriam Eric D. Wittkower 1899–1983." *Transcultural Psychiatry* 20, no. 2 (1983): 81–6.

– "Méthodologie de recherche en socio-psychiatrie et en ethno-psychiatrie," fasc. no 37720A10. *Traité de psychiatrie*, 1–14. Paris: Éditions techniques (Encyclopédie médico-chirurgicale), 1965.

– "Notes for a Theory on Latah." In *Culture-Bound Syndrome, Ethnopsychiatry, and Alternative Therapies*, edited by W.P. Lebra, 3–21. Honolulu: University of Hawai'i Press, 1976.

Murphy, H. Brian M., ed. *Flight and Resettlement*. Paris: UNESCO, 1955.

– "Méthodologie de la recherche en ethnopsychiatrie," fasc. no 37726A10. *Traité de psychiatrie*, 1–6. Paris: Éditions techniques (Encyclopédie médico-chirurgicale), 1978.

– "Les psychoses," fasc. no 37725A10. *Traité de psychiatrie*, 1–5. Paris: Éditions techniques (Encyclopédie médico-chirurgicale), 1978.

Murphy, H. Brian M., and Michel Tousignant. "Fondements anthropologiques de l'ethnopsychiatrie," fasc. no 37715A10. *Traité de psychiatrie*, 1–4. Paris: Éditions techniques (Encyclopédie médico-chirurgicale), 1978.

Murphy, H. Brian M., Eric Wittkower, and Norman A. Chance. "Crosscultural Inquiry into the Symptomatology of Depression." *Transcultural Psychiatry Research Review* 2 (April 1964): 5–18.

Murphy, Jane. "Continuities in Community-Based Psychiatric Epidemiology." *Archives of General Psychiatry* 37 (1980): 1215–23.

– "Psychiatric Labeling in Cross-Cultural Perspective: Similar Kinds of Disturbed Behavior Appear to Be Labeled Abnormal in Diverse Cultures." *Science* 191 (March 1976): 1019–28.

Murphy, Jane, and Alexander H. Leighton. *Approaches to Cross-Cultural Psychiatry*. Ithaca: Cornell University Press, 1966.

Nathan, Tobie. "Devereux, un Hébreu anarchiste." Preface to Georges Devereux, *Ethnopsychiatrie des Indiens mohaves*, 11–18. Le Plessis-Robinson: Synthélabo (Les empêcheurs de penser en rond), 1996.

– *La folie des autres. Traité d'ethnopsychiatrie.* Paris: Dunod, 1986.

– "Le rôle de Georges Devereux dans la naissance de l'ethnopsychiatrie clinique en France." *Ethnopsy* 1 (2000): 197–226.

Oesterreich, Traugott Konstantin. *Die Besessenheit, Langensalza* [1921]. English translation *Possession: Demoniacal and Other* [1930]. New Hyde Park: University Books, 1966.

Okpaku, Samuel O., ed. *Clinical Methods in Transcultural Psychiatry.* Washington, DC: American Psychiatric Publishing, 1998.

Opler, Marvin K. "Anthropological and Cross-Cultural Aspects of Homosexuality." In *Sexual Inversion,* edited by J. Marmor, 108–23. New York: Basic Books, 1965.

– ed. *Culture and Mental Health.* New York: Macmillan, 1959.

Ortigues, Edmond. "La psychiatrie comparée." In *Encyclopedia Universalis.* 1220–2. Paris, 1980.

Ortigues, Edmond, Marie-Cécile Ortigues, András Zempléni, and Jacqueline Zempléni. "Psychologie clinique et ethnologie (Sénégal)." *Bulletin de psychologie* 21 (15–19), no. 270 (1968): 951–8.

Ortigues, Marie-Cécile, and Edmond Ortigues. *L'OEdipe africain* [1966], 3rd ed. Paris: L'Harmattan, 1984.

Palem, Robert Michel. "De l'ethnopsychiatrie à la psychiatrie transculturelle." *Psychiatries* 140 (2003): 145–62.

Pidoux, Charles. "Freud et l'ethnologie." *Psyché* 107–8 (1955): 477–80.

Porot, Antoine, and Don Côme Arrii. "L'impulsivité criminelle chez l'indigène algérien." *Annales médico-psychologiques* 2 (1932): 588–611.

Prince, Raymond H. "The American Central Intelligence Agency and the Origins of Transcultural Psychiatry at McGill." *Annals of the Royal College of Physicians and Surgeons of Canada* 28 (1995): 407–13.

– *Conference on Personality Change and Religious Experience: Proceedings of the First Annual Conference, January 15–16, 1965, at the Quaker Meeting House, Montreal, Canada.* Montreal: R.M. Bucke Memorial Society, 1965.

– "John Colin D. Carothers (1903–1989) and African Colonial Psychiatry." *Transcultural Psychiatric Research Review* 33 (1996): 226–40.

– "In Memoriam H.B.M. Murphy 1915–1987." *Transcultural Psychiatric Research Review* 24, no. 4 (1987): 247–54.

– "Origins and Early Mission of Transcultural Psychiatry: Some Personal Recollections." *World Cultural Psychiatry Research Review* 6, no. 11 (2006): 6–11.

– "Thérapie et culture." In *Traité de psychiatrie,* 1–6. Paris: Éditions techniques (Encyclopédie médico-chirurgicale), 1978.

– "Transcultural Psychiatry: Personal Experiences and Canadian
  Perspectives." *Canadian Journal of Psychiatry* 45, no. 5 (2000): 431–37.
– "Transcultural Psychiatry at McGill." In *Building on a Proud Past: Fifty
  Years of Psychiatry at McGill,* edited by T.L. Sourkes and G. Pinard,
  177–81. Montreal: McGill Department of Psychiatry, 1995.
– *Why This Ecstasy? Reflections on My Life with Madmen.* Montreal:
  Armor Art and Cultural Foundation, 2010.
Prince, Raymond H., and Lionel Beauchamp. "Pioneers in Transcultural
  Psychiatry: Henri F. Ellenberger (1905–1993)." *Transcultural Psychiatry*
  38, no. 1 (2001): 80–104.
Róheim, Géza. *Psychanalyse et anthropologie* [1950]. Paris: Gallimard,
  1967.
Simmons, James Stevens, et al. *Global Epidemiology: A Geography of
  Disease and Sanitation,* 3 vols. Philadelphia and London: J.B.
  Lippincott, 1944–1954.
Simons, Ronald C., and Charles C. Hughes. *The Culture-Bound
  Syndromes: Folk Illnesses of Psychiatric and Anthropological Interest.*
  Dordrecht: Reidel, 1985.
Stoetzel, Jean. *Jeunesse sans chrysanthème ni sabre.* Paris: Plon, 1954.
– *Without the Chrysanthemum and the Sword: A Study of the Attitudes of
  Youth in Post-War Japan.* New York: Columbia University Press, 1955.
Strotzka, Hans. *Einführung in der Sozialpsychiatrie.* Hamburg: Rowohlt,
  1965.
Tousignant, Michel. *Les origines sociales et culturelles des troubles
  psychologiques.* Paris: Presses universitaires de France, 1992.
Tseng, Weng-Shing. *Handbook of Cultural Psychiatry.* Amsterdam:
  Academic Press, 2001.
Unger, Sanford M. "Mescaline, LSD, Psilocybin, and Personality Change:
  A Review." *Psychiatry: Journal for the Study of Interpersonal Processes*
  26, no. 2 (1963): 111–25.
– *LSD, Mescaline, Psilocybin, and Psychotherapy: An Annotated
  Chronology.* Washington: National Institute of Mental Health,
  1963.
Van Gennep, Arnold. *Folklore. Croyances et coutumes populaires
  françaises.* Paris: Stock, 1924.
Veil, Claude. "Aspects mythiques de la prévention des troubles mentaux."
  L'évolution psychiatrique 31, no. 3 (1966): 493–513.
Wittkower, Eric D. "Round-Table Meeting on Transcultural Psychiatric
  Problems." *Transcultural Research in Mental Health Problems* 4
  (1958): 3.

Wittkower, Eric D., and Jacob Fried. "Some Problems of Transcultural Psychiatry." *International Journal of Social Psychiatry* 3, no. 4 (1958): 245–52.

Wundt, Wilhelm. *Völkerpsychologie*. 10 vols. Leipzig: Engelmann, 1900–20.

Yap, Pow-Meng. *Comparative Psychiatry: A Theoretical Framework*. Toronto: University of Toronto Press, 1974.

Zempléni, András. "Henri Collomb (1913–1979) et l'équipe de Fann." *Social Science and Medicine* 14, no. 2 (1980): 85–90.

– *Interprétation de la thérapie traditionnelle du désordre mental chez les Wolof et les Lebou (Sénégal)*, thèse de 3e cycle, faculté des lettres et des sciences humaines de Paris, 1968.

Secondary Sources

ONLINE

There is a website created by Henri Ellenberger's daughter, Irène Ellenberger, that displays his publications, in particular reprints and translations. Online: www.dizingdesign.com/ellen.htm. The number of blogs and websites about ethnopsychiatry is increasing rapidly, and it would be impossible to list them all here and keep up to date. We would highlight the blogs created by Patrick Fermi (devoted to the history of ethnopsychiatry,) Olivier Douville (about clinical psychology, psychoanalysis, and ethnopsychiatry,) the Centre Georges Devereux (about Tobie Nathan), and Claude Ravelet (about Roger Bastide.)

PUBLISHED WORKS

[Anon.]. "*Ethno-psychiatrie (Ethnopsychiatry)* by H.F. Ellenberger" [Book review]. *Encyclopédie médico-chirurgicale. Psychiatrie*, p. 37725C10, 1–14, and p. 37725B10, 1–22 (in French) [1965]. *Transcultural Psychiatry* 3, no. 1 (April 1966): 5–8.

[Anon.]. "Murphy H.B.M., *Comparative Psychiatry: The International and Intercultural Distribution of Mental Illness*" [Book review]. *L'évolution psychiatrique* 48, no. 1 (1983): 41–2.

Anderson, Warwick, Deborah Jenson, and Richard C. Keller. "Introduction: Globalizing the Unconscious." In *Unconscious Dominions: Psychoanalysis, Colonial Trauma, and Global Sovereignties*, edited by Anderson, Jenson, and Keller, 1–18. Durham: Duke University Press, 2011.

Arnaud, Robert. *La folie apprivoisée. L'approche unique du professeur Collomb pour traiter la folie*. Paris: De Vecchi, 2006.

Bains, Jatinder. "Race, Culture, and Psychiatry: A History of Transcultural Psychiatry." *History of Psychiatry* 16, no. 2 (2005): 139–54.

Becker, Anne E., and Arthur Kleinman. "The History of Cultural Psychiatry in the Last Half-Century." In *Psychiatry: Past, Present, and Prospect*, edited by S. Bloch, S.A. Green, and J. Holmes, 74–95. Oxford: Oxford University Press, 2014.

Bendick, Christoph. "Emil Kraepelin Forschungsreise nach Java im Jahre 1904." PhD diss., University of Cologne. In *Arbeiten der Forschungsstelle des Institutes für Geschichte der Medizin*, vol. 49. Feuchtwangen: C.E. Kohlhauer, 1989.

Blanckaert, Claude, and Michel Porret, eds. *L'Encyclopédie méthodique (1782–1832): des Lumières au positivism.* Geneva: Droz, 2006.

Bullard, Alice. "The Critical Impact of Frantz Fanon and Henri Collomb: Race, Gender, and Personality Testing of North and West Africans." *Journal of the History of the Behavioral Sciences* 41, no. 3 (2005): 225–48.

– "Imperial Networks and Postcolonial Independence: The Transition from Colonial to Transcultural Psychiatry." In *Psychiatry and Empire*, edited by S. Mahone and M. Vaughan, 197–219. London: Palgrave Macmillan, 2007.

– "*L'OEdipe africain*, a Retrospective." *Transcultural Psychiatry* 42, no. 2 (2005): 171–203.

Bloch, Georges. "Georges Devereux, sa vie, son oeuvre, et ses concepts. La naissance de l'ethnopsychiatrie." PhD diss., Université Paris 8. Saarbrücken: Éditions universitaires européennes, 2012.

Boroffka, Alexander. "Emil Kraepelin (1856–1926) and Transcultural Psychiatry: A Historical Note." *Transcultural Psychiatric Research Review* 25 (1988): 236–9.

Brès, Yvon. *Freud et la psychanalyse américaine: Karen Horney.* Paris: Vrin, 1970.

Cerea, Alessandra. "Au-delà de l'ethnopsychiatrie. Georges Devereux entre science et épistémologie." PhD diss., University of Bologne and EHESS, 2016.

Chakrabarti, Pratik. *Medicine and Empire: 1600–1960.* New York: Palgrave Macmillan, 2014.

Chakrabarty, Dipesh. *Provincializing Europe* [2000]. Princeton: Princeton University Press, 2008.

Chiang, Howard. "Translating Culture and Psychiatry across the Pacific: How Koro Became Culture-Bound." *History of Science* 53, no. 1 (2015): 102–19.

Chowdhury, Arabinda N. "The Definition and Classification of Koro."
Culture, Medicine, and Psychiatry 20 (1996): 41–65.
– "Hundred Years of Koro. The History of a Culture-Bound Syndrome."
International Journal of Social Psychiatry 44, no. 3 (1998): 181–8.
Coffin, Jean-Christophe. "La psychiatrie postcoloniale: entre éthique et
tragique." In *L'asile aux fous. Un lieu d'oubli. Photographies de Roger
Camar*, edited by P. Artières et al. Paris: Presses universitaires de
Vincennes, 2009.
Coleborne, Catharine. *Madness in the Family: Insanity and Institutions in
the Australian Colonial World, 1860–1914*. London: Palgrave
Macmillan, 2010.
Collectif. "L'encyclopédie en ses nouveaux atours électroniques: vices et
vertus du virtuel." *Recherches sur Diderot et sur l'Encyclopédie* nos.
31–2. Paris: Les Belles Lettres, 2002.
Collectif Write Back. *Postcolonial Studies*. Lyon: Presses universitaires de
Lyon, 2013.
Collignon, René. "Contributions à la psychiatrie coloniale et à la
psychiatrie comparée parues dans les *Annales médico-psychologiques*.
Essai de bibliographie annotée." *Psychopathologie africaine* 27, nos.
2–3 (1995–96): 265–96, 297–326.
– "Émergence de la psychiatrie transculturelle au lendemain de la Seconde
Guerre mondiale (références africaines)." In *Manuel de psychiatrie
transculturelle*, edited by M.R. Moro, Q. de La Noë, and Y. Mouchenik,
79–107. Grenoble: La Pensée sauvage, 2006.
– "Some Reflections on the History of Psychiatry in French Speaking West
Africa. The Example of Senegal." *Psychopathologie africaine* 27, no. 1
(1995): 37–51.
– "Vingt ans de travaux à la clinique psychiatrique de Fann – Dakar."
Psychopathologie africaine 14 (1978): 133–323.
Corin, Ellen, and Gilles Bibeau. "H.B.M. Murphy (1915–1987): A Key
Figure in Transcultural Psychiatry." *Culture, Medicine, and Psychiatry*
12 (September 1988): 397–415.
Crozier, Ivan. "Making Up Koro: Multiplicity, Psychiatry, Culture, and
Penis-Shrinking Anxieties." *Journal of the History of Medicine and
Allied Sciences* 67, no. 1 (2011): 36–70.
Delille, Emmanuel. "Une archive pour l'histoire des sociabilités savantes
au XXᵉ siècle: Georges Lantéri-Laura (1930–2004) et l'Encyclopédie
Médico-Chirurgicale." *Revue d'Histoire des Sciences* 70, no. 2 (2017):
351–61.
– "Le Bouvard et Pécuchet d'Henri Ey (1955)." *Revue Flaubert*, 2012.

http://flaubert.univ-rouen.fr/article.php?id=24; new edition: *Cahiers Henri Ey* 41-42 (2018): 193–211.

– "Henri Ellenberger et le *Traité de psychiatrie* de l'Encyclopédie médico-chirurgicale: une carrière américaine sous le patronage du groupe de l'Évolution psychiatrique en collaboration avec Henri Ey." *Gesnerus, revue suisse d'histoire de la médecine* 63, nos. 3–4 (2006): 259–79.

– "On the History of Cultural Psychiatry: Georges Devereux, Henri Ellenberger, and the Psychological Treatment of Native Americans in the 1950s." *Transcultural Psychiatry* 53, no. 3 (2016): 292–311.

– "Réseaux savants et enjeux classificatoires dans le 'Traité de psychiatrie' de l'Encyclopédie médico-chirurgicale (1947–1977)." PhD diss. at EHESS, 2 vols. 2008.

– "Review Essay: Holofernes Complex. A new edition of Leiris' *Manhood.*" *History of the Human Sciences*, February 2017. www.histhum.com/?p=322.

– "Sigmund Freud–Oskar Pfister. Briefwechsel 1909–1939 by Isabelle I. Noth, ed. Zurich: TVZ, 2014." *Canadian Bulletin of Medical History* 33, no. 2 (2016): 579–82.

– "Teaching the History of Psychiatry in the 1950s: Henri Ellenberger's Lectures at the Menninger Foundation." *Zinbun* 47 (2016): 109–28.

– "Le *Traité de psychiatrie* de l'Encyclopédie médico-chirurgicale (EMC) sous la direction d'Henri Ey comme lieu d'observation privilégié de la recomposition du champ psychiatrique français (1945–1955)." *Cahiers Henri Ey* 20-1 (2008): 133–48.

– "Un voyage d'observation d'Henri Ellenberger aux États-Unis: Henri Ellenberger entre psychiatrie transculturelle et héritage janétien (1952)." In *Psychiatries dans l'histoire*, edited by J. Arveiller, 85–95. Caen: Presses universitaires de Caen, 2008.

– "Yanacopoulo, Andrée: Henri F. Ellenberger: une vie 1905–1993." *Gesnerus, revue Suisse d'histoire de la médecine* 67 (2010): 295–6.

Delille, Emmanuel, and Marc Kirsch. "Le cours de Ian Hacking au Collège de France: la psychiatrie comme lieu d'observation privilégié de l'histoire des concepts scientifiques (2000–2006)." *Revue de synthèse* 137, nos. 1-2 (2016): 89–117.

Demazeux, Steeves. *Qu'est-ce que le DSM? Genèse et transformations de la bible américaine de la Psychiatrie*. Montreuil: Ithaque, 2013.

Dosse, François. *L'histoire en miettes. Des "Annales" à la "nouvelle histoire"* [1987]. Paris: La Découverte, 2010.

Douville, Olivier. "Quelques remarques historiques et critiques sur

l'ethnopsychiatrie. Questions actuelles à l'ethnopsychiatrie."
Psycho-Ressources, blog d'Olivier Douville, 24 May 2012.

Dupuy, Jean-Pierre. *La panique* [1991]. Paris: Éditions du Seuil, 2003.

Ehrenberg, Alain, and Anne Lovell. *La maladie mentale en mutation.*
Paris: Odile Jacob, 2001.

Fagot-Largeault, Anne. *Les causes de la mort, histoire naturelle et facteurs
de risqué.* Paris: Vrin, 1989.

Fassin, Didier. L'ethnopsychiatrie et ses réseaux. L'influence qui grandit."
Genèse 35 (June 1999): 146–71.

– "Les politiques de l'*ethnopsychiatrie*. La psyché africaine, des colonies
britanniques aux banlieues parisiennes." *L'Homme* 153 (2000): 231–50.

Fassin, Didier, and Richard Rechtman. "An Anthropological Hybrid:
The Pragmatic Arrangement of Universalism and Culturalism in French
Mental Health." *Transcultural Psychiatry* 42, no. 3 (2005): 347–66.

Fermi, Patrick. "Ethnopsychanalyse: esquisse d'un roman familial."
L'autre 3, no. 2 (2002): 329–43.

Friedman, Lawrence J. *The Menninger: The Family and the Clinic.*
Lawrence: University Press of Kansas, 1992.

Friessem, D.H. "Emil Kraepelin und die vergleichende Psychiatrie –
Marginalien zu einer Wiederveröffentlichung." *Curare* 32, nos. 3–4
(2009): 250–5.

Girard, René. *La violence et le sacré* [1972]. Paris: Fayard (Pluriel), 2011.

Grmek, Mirko D. "Géographie médicale et histoire des civilisations."
Annales. Économies, sociétés, Civilisations 18, no. 6 (1963): 1071–97.

– *La guerre comme maladie sociale et autres textes politiques.* Paris:
Éditions du Seuil, 2002.

Grob, Gerald N. "The Origins of American Psychiatric Epidemiology."
American Journal of Public Health 75 (1985): 229–36.

Hahn, Robert, and Arthur Kleinman. "'Voodoo Death' and the 'Placebo
Phenomenon' in Anthropological Perspective." *Medical Anthropology
Quarterly* 14, no. 4 (1983): 16–19.

Hayward, Rhodri. "Germany and the Making of 'English' Psychiatry:
The Maudsley Hospital, 1908–1939." In *International Relations in
Psychiatry: Britain, Germany, and the United States to World War II,*
edited by V. Roelcke, P.J. Weindling, and L. Westwood, 67–90.
Rochester: University of Rochester Press, 2010.

Heaton, Matthew. *Black Skin, White Coats: Nigerian Psychiatrists,
Decolonization, and the Globalization of Psychiatry.* Athens: Ohio
University Press, 2013.

Huffschmitt, Luc. "Kraepelin à Java." *Synapse* 86 (1992): 69–76.

Jasen, Patricia. "Breast Cancer and the Language of Risk 1750–1950." *Social History of Medicine* 15 (2002): 17–43.

Jenicek, Milos. "Les approches épidémiologiques des maladies mentales: priorités, analyses causales, interventions." *Psychologie médicale* 14 (1982): 403–13.

Jilek, Wolfgang G. "Emil Kraepelin and the Comparative Sociocultural Psychiatry." *European Archives of Psychiatry and Clinical Neurosciences* 245 (1995): 231–8.

Jilek, Wolfgang G., and Louise Jilek-Aali. "The Metamorphosis of Culture-Bound Syndromes." *Social Science and Medicine* 21, no. 2 (1985): 205–10.

Jugon, Jean-Claude. *Phobies sociales au Japon. Timidité et angoisse de l'autre.* Paris: ESF éditeur, 1998.

Kail, Michel, and Genevièv Vermès, eds. *La psychologie des peuples et ses derives.* Paris: Centre national de documentation pédagogique, 1999.

Keller, Richard C. *Colonial Madness: Psychiatry in French North Africa.* Chicago: University of Chicago Press, 2007.

– "Taking Science to the Colonies: Psychiatric Innovation in France and North Africa." In *Psychiatry and Empire*, edited by S. Malone and M. Vaughan, 17–40. London: Palgrave Macmillan, 2007.

Kirk, Stuart, and Herb Kutchins. *Aimez-vous le DSM? Le triomphe de la psychiatrie américaine* [1992]. Le Plessis-Robinson, Synthélabo (Les empêcheurs de penser en rond), 1998.

Kirmayer, Laurence J. "50 years of Transcultural Psychiatry" [Editorial]. *Transcultural Psychiatry* 50, no. 1 (2013): 3–5.

– "Culture-Bound Syndromes and International Psychiatric Classification: The Example of Taijin Kyofusho." In *Psychiatry: A World Perspective*, vol. 4, edited by C. Stephanis et al., 195–200. Amsterdam: Elsevier, 1990.

– "The Place of Culture in Psychiatric Nosology: Taijin Kyofusho and *DSM-III-R.*" *The Journal of Nervous and Mental Disease* 179 (1991): 19–28.

Kirmayer, Laurence J., and Harry Minas. "The Future of Cultural Psychiatry: An International Perspective." *Canadian Journal of Psychiatry* 45, no. 5 (2000): 438–46.

Kleinman, Arthur M. "Depression, Somatization, and the 'New Cross-Cultural Psychiatry.'" *Social Science and Medicine* 11, no. 1 (1977): 3–10.

– *Patients and Healers in the Context of Culture: An Exploration of the Borderland between Anthropology, Medicine, and Psychiatry.* Berkeley: University of California Press, 1980.

– "What Is Specific to Western Medicine?" In *Companion Encyclopedia of the History of Medicine*, vol. 1, edited by W.F. Bynum and R. Porter, 15–23. London: Routledge, 1993.

Lantéri-Laura, Georges. *Essai sur les paradigmes de la psychiatrie modern.* Paris: Éditions du temps, 1998.

Lazarus, Niel, ed. *The Cambridge Companion to Postcolonial Literary Studies.* Cambridge: Cambridge University Press, 2004.

– *Penser le postcolonial. Une introduction critique.* Paris: Éditions Amsterdam, 2006.

Lézé, Samuel. "Qu'est-ce que l'ethnopsychiatrie? À propos de *Ethnopsychiatrie psychanalytique* de François Laplantine." *Non-fiction*, 21 April 2009. https://www.nonfiction.fr/article-2424-quest_ce_que_lethnopsychiatrie_.htm.

Lovell, Anne, and Ezra Susser. "What Might Be a History of Psychiatric Epidemiology? Towards a Social History and Conceptual Account." *International Journal of Epidemiology* 43, suppl. 1 (August 2014): i1–i5.

Macey, David, *Frantz Fanon. Une vie* [2000]. Paris: La Découverte, 2011.

Mann, Hans-Dieter. *Lucien Febvre, la pensée vivante d'un historien.* Paris: A. Colin (Cahiers des Annales), 1971.

Marks, John D. *The Search for the "Manchurian candidate": The CIA and Mind Control.* New York: Times Books, 1979.

Micale, Mark S. "Henri F. Ellenberger: The History of Psychiatry as the History of the Unconscious." In *Discovering the History of Psychiatry*, edited by M.S. Micale and R. Porter, 112–34. New York: Oxford University Press, 1994.

– "Introduction." In *Beyond the Unconscious: Essays of Henri Ellenberger in the History of Psychiatry*, edited by M.S. Micale, 3–86. Princeton: Princeton University Press, 1993.

– "Littérature, médecine, hystérie: le cas de Madame Bovary, de Gustave Flaubert." *L'évolution psychiatrique* 60, no. 4 (1995): 901–18.

Monnais, Laurence. *Médecine et colonisation. L'aventure indochinoise (1860–1939).* Paris: CNRS Éditions, 1999.

Monnais, Laurence, and David Wright, eds. *Doctors beyond Borders. The Transnational Migration of Physicians in the Twentieth Century.* Toronto: University of Toronto Press, 2016.

Morrissey, Robert, and Philippe Roger, eds. *L'encyclopédie du réseau au livre et du livre au réseau.* Paris: H. Champion, 2001.

Naiman, James. "La psychanalyse au Allan Memorial Institute." *Filigrane* 10, no. 1 (Spring 2001): 52–60.

Rae-Grant, Quentin, ed. *Psychiatry in Canada: 50 years (1951 to 2001)*. Ottawa: Canadian Psychiatric Association, 2001.

Rechtman, Richard. "L'ethnicisation de la psychiatrie : de l'universel à l'international." *L'information psychiatrique* 79, no. 2 (February 2003): 161–9.

– "L'ethnopsychiatrie." In *Dictionnaire de sciences humaines*, 422–4. Paris: Presses universitaires de France, 2006.

– "De la psychiatrie des migrants au culturalisme des ethnopsychiatries." *Hommes et migrations* 1225 (2000): 46–61.

Rechtman, Richard, and François H.M. Raveau. "Fondements anthropologiques de l'ethnopsychiatrie," fasc. no 37715A10. *Traité de psychiatrie*, 1–8. Paris: Éditions techniques (Encyclopédie médico-chirurgicale), 1993.

Reichmayr, Johannes, ed. *Ethnopsychoanalyse revisited. Gegenübertragung in transkulturellen und postkolonialen Kontexten*. Gießen: Psychosozial-Verlag, 2016.

Ricard, Alain. *Le sable de Babel. Traduction et apartheid: esquisse d'une anthropologie de la textualité*. Paris: CNRS Éditions, 2011.

Roelcke, Volker, Paul J. Weindling, and Louise Westwood, eds. *International Relations in Psychiatry: Britain, Germany, and the United States to World War II*. Rochester: University of Rochester Press, 2010.

Rothstein, William G. *Public Health and the Risk Factor: A History of an Uneven Medical Revolution*. Rochester: University of Rochester Press, 2003.

Roudinesco, Elisabeth. "Présentation." In H. Ellenberger, *Histoire de la découverte de l'inconscient*, edited by Roudinesco, 7–25. Paris: Fayard, 1994.

– "Présentation." In H. Ellenberger, *Médecine de l'âme. Essais d'histoire de la folie et des guérisons psychiques*, edited by Roudinesco, 7–23. Paris: Fayard, 1995.

Said, Edward. *Orientalism*. New York: Vintage Books, 2003.

Scarfone, Marianna. "La psychiatrie coloniale italienne. Théories, pratiques, protagonistes, institutions 1906–1952." PhD diss., Université de Venise Ca' Foscari et Université Lumière Lyon 2, 2014.

Schaffer, Simon. "The Eighteenth Brumaire of Bruno Latour." *Studies in the History and Philosophy of Science* 22 (1991): 174–92.

– *La fabrique de sciences modernes (xviie–xixe siècle)*. Paris: Éditions du Seuil, 2014.

Schlich, Thomas. "Risk and Medical Innovation: A Historical Perspective." In *The Risks of Medical Innovation: Risk Perception and Assessment in*

Historical Context, edited by T. Schlich and U. Tröhler, 1–19. London and New York: Routledge, 2004.

Schmuhl, Hans-Walter, ed. *Kulturrelativismus und Antirassismus. Der Anthropologe Franz Boas (1858–1942)*. Bielefeld: Transcript, 2009.

Sibeud, Emmanuelle. "Du postcolonial au questionnement postcolonial: pour un transfert critique." *Revue d'histoire moderne et contemporaine* 54, no. 4 (2007): 142–55.

Sigerist, Henry E. *Civilization and Disease*. Ithaca: Cornell University Press, 1943.

Singaravélou, Pierre, ed. *Les empires coloniaux xixe–xxe siècle*. Paris: Éditions du Seuil, 2013.

– "De la psychologie coloniale à la géographie psychologique. Itinéraire, entre science et littérature, d'une discipline éphémère dans l'entre-deux-guerres." *L'homme et la société*, nos. 167–9 (2008): 119–48.

Sontag, Susan. *Illness as Metaphor*. New York: Farrar, Straus and Giroux, 1978.

– *La maladie comme métaphore* [1977–78]; *Le sida et ses métaphores* [1988–89]. Paris: Christian Bourgois, 2009.

Sourkes, Theodore L., and Gilbert Pinard, eds. *Building on a Proud Past: Fifty Years of Psychiatry at McGill*. Montreal: McGill Department of Psychiatry, 1995.

Susser, Ezra, Joy Noel Baumgartner, and Zena Stein Zena. "Commentary: Sir Arthur Mitchell – Pioneer of Psychiatric Epidemiology and of Community Care." *International Journal of Epidemiology* 39, no. 1 (2010): 417–25.

Transcultural Psychiatry 43, no. 1 (March 2006).

Transcultural Psychiatry [Special issue]. Festschrift for Alexander Leighton. Edited by J.B. Waldram and G. Bibeau. 43, no. 4 (December 2006).

Transcultural Psychiatry [Special issue]. Festschrift for Raymond H. Prince. 43, no. 4 (December 2006).

Tremblay, Marc-Abélard. "Alexander H. Leighton's and Jane Murphy's Scientific Contributions in Psychiatric Epidemiology." *Les classiques des sciences sociales*, 2003. http://classiques.uqac.ca/contemporains/tremblay_marc_adelard/Leighton/Leighton.html.

Vatin, François. "Dépendance et émancipation: retour sur Mannoni." *Revue du MAUSS* 38, no. 2 (2011): 131–48.

– "Octave Mannoni (1899–1989) et sa psychologie de la colonisation. Contextualisation et décontextualisation." *Revue du MAUSS* 37, no. 1 (2011): 137–78.

Vermès, Geneviève. "Quelques étapes de la psychologie des peuples (de la fin du xixe siècle aux années 1950). Esquisse pour une histoire de la psychologie interculturelle." *L'homme et la société* nos. 167–9 (2008): 149–61.

Vidal, Fernando. "À la recherche d'Henri Ellenberger." *Gesnerus* 51, nos. 3–4 (1994): 88–93.

Weber, Florence. *Brève histoire de l'anthropologie.* Paris: Flammarion, 2015.

Worboys, Michael. "The Emergence of Tropical Medicine: A Study in the Establishment of a Scientific Specialty." In *Perspectives on the Emergence of Scientific Disciplines,* edited by Gérard Lemaine et al., 75–98. The Hague: Mouton, 1976.

– "Science and Imperialism." *Isis* 84, no. 1 (1993): 91–102.

Wright, Mary J., and Roger C. Myers. *History of Academic Psychology in Canada* [1982]. Toronto: Hogrefe and Huber, 1995.

Wu, Harry Y. "World Citizenship and the Emergence of the Social Psychiatry Project of the World Health Organization, 1948–c. 1965." *History of Psychiatry* 25, no. 2 (2015): 166–81.

Yanacopoulo, Andrée. *Henri F. Ellenberger. Une vie.* Montreal: Liber, 2009.

Zaballos, Nausica. *Le système de santé Navajo. Savoirs rituels et scientifiques de 1950 à nos jours.* Paris: L'Harmattan, 2009.

PART TWO

Ethnopsychiatry [1965–1967]

H.F. Ellenberger

DEFINITION

Ethno-psychiatry is the study of mental illness according to the ethnic or cultural groups to which patients belong. This definition delimits ethnopsychiatry in relation:

1. to the *psychology of peoples,* which, as Miroglio (1958) demonstrates, is one of the branches of descriptive sociology;
2. to "*cultural anthropology,*" which may be considered as a branch of ethnology in the broadest sense of the term;
3. to *social psychiatry,* which is the study of mental illness according to the social (but not ethnic) groups to which the patients belong.

HISTORY

Ethnopsychiatry is perhaps as old as medicine itself. Hippocrates, in his treatise *On Airs, Waters, and Places,* provides the famous description of "Scythian Disease": among the nomadic barbarians of the steppes of Scythia (now southern Russia), a number of men became impotent, began speaking in a female voice, and adopted the women's way of life. The old Greek doctor did not content himself with disparaging this anomaly, but sought to explain its origin by the effects of the humid, misty climate of Scythia and by the diet and lifeways of the Scythians.

A multitude of observations of interest to ethnopsychiatry can be found scattered throughout the works of historians, geographers, travellers, and writers from antiquity to the Middle Ages. Starting in the Renaissance, great geographical discoveries aroused curiosity regarding the customs of "savages" and non-European civilizations; by the eighteenth century, forms of pathological disorders such as *amok* were attracting attention. Explorers, missionaries, and historians wrote many precious works in this regard.

With the nineteenth century, more objective and systematic descriptions can be found in writings by colonial and navy doctors, who often speak of "exotic psychiatry." There are a great many such documents, and a German doctor (Obersteiner, 1889) published a general review in a popular magazine in which he describes and compares mental illnesses among primitive Indian tribes and the Blacks of Brazil and of British Guyana, the Egyptians, Turks, Persians, Chinese, gold diggers in Australia, Eskimos,[1] Icelanders, and Laplanders, basing his findings on contemporary medical publications (which unfortunately he omits to cite). But the credit for founding ethnopsychiatry as an independent branch of psychiatry belongs, according to Gregoria Bermann (1958), to Kraepelin, who travelled to Singapore and Java to learn on the spot about disorders such as *amok* and *latah* as well as specific forms that appeared among the Malay such as manic-depressive illness, dementia praecox, and other classic mental illnesses. In 1904 Kraepelin published the first results of his study in an article titled *Vergleichende Psychiatrie* (Comparative Psychiatry), which is the name he gave to this new branch of psychiatry. But Kraepelin was unable to pursue his study in other exotic countries, and his disciples did not really attend to it. After him, it was mainly colonial doctors who continued to develop ethnopsychiatry, adding to it contributions and general reviews (Révész, 1911) that are too forgotten today.

After the First World War, interest in ethnopsychiatry received new impetus from new currents that, had by then renewed interest in ethnology. Around 1930, in Germany, Richard Thurnwald and his school (Wilhelm Mühlmann, Günter Wagner, etc.) launched a systematic study of the effects of contact among races and cultures of different levels. That study, which was later taken up Americans, touches on one of the most controversial problems of ethnopsychiatry: the correlation between clashes of ethnic groups and rapid cultural transformations on one hand, and the frequency of mental illness on the other. The American school of "cultural anthropology" (Abram Kardiner, Ralph Linton, Ruth Benedict, and Margaret

Mead), partly influenced by Freud's theories, sought to establish correlations between techniques of care and the education given to children on the one hand, and, on the other, the collective nature (or "basic personality"), frequency, and forms of neuroses and psychoses in a given population. This brings us back, again, to ethnopsychiatry, albeit by another path.

Today ethnopsychiatry uses extremely varied methods, and there are so many works devoted to it that it is becoming increasingly difficult to develop an overview. A number of general reviews have been published by Róheim (1939), O. Klineberg (1940), Yap (1951), P.K. Benedict and Jacks (1954), and Linton (1956); unfortunately, most of them only address works published in English and provide only a very incomplete idea of current ethnopsychiatric research.

In 1956 a "transcultural study group" was founded at McGill University in Montreal by E.D. Wittkower, to whom we owe a great deal of research in the field (Wittkower, 1958). Wittkower and his collaborators (who included J. Fried, H.M.B. Murphy, H.F. Ellenberger, and N.A. Chance) gathered significant documentation from every country in the world, organized systematic studies, and published a biannual review, (*Transcultural Psychiatric Research*).[2]

GENERALITIES

The usefulness of ethnopsychiatry is both theoretical and practical:

1 As Kraepelin pointed out, the descriptions of mental diseases as contained in our classical works and textbooks are based solely on observation and examination of Western medical patients. However, a given disease often presents different symptoms in different populations. Ethnopsychiatry makes it possible to supplement the descriptions contained in our textbooks so as to uncover a richer and more diversified symptomatology, thus leading to a better knowledge of mental pathology.

2 Through ethnopsychiatry, we become acquainted with some unusual or extreme forms of mental disorders that do not as such really exist in civilized peoples, and this leads to better understanding of the intimate nature of some psychic disturbances observed among Western peoples. For instance, there is the theory of Karl Menninger (1938), who states that suicide is caused by a combination, in variable proportions, of three ten-

dencies: the desire to die, the desire to kill, and the desire to be killed; this theory is confirmed by ethnopsychiatry, which shows that in some populations each one of these three tendencies is clearly manifested in certain forms of suicide (Ellenberger, 1952).

3 In studying pathogenic factors that determine the comparative frequency of mental illnesses in different populations, ethnopsychiatry constitutes a sort of experience instituted by nature, enabling us to analyze the role of ethnic and cultural factors in the genesis of mental disorders.

4 From a practical point of view, knowledge of ethnopsychiatry is necessary for a psychiatrist working among new, different populations (from his own). It will allow him to better understand and treat his patient, and above all to avoid some regrettable errors such as those given as an example by French army medical officer Dr Gustave Martin in 1934:

In a psychiatric hospital in the provinces, a Toucouleur, institutionalized for manic excitement, was only kept there because on nights when the moon was full, he demonstrated his joy and happiness by making an astonishing to-do as was done in his country.

I have seen in a hospital in the capital an Annamite treated for "mental disorders," because the poor wretch, at each of the visits of the ward's head doctor, would prostate himself before him, doing the three big regulation *lais*. Yet this external mark of respect – a sign of great deference and supreme politeness – was conveyed on the observation sheet as "ideas of humility, indignity, and guilt."

The methods employed by ethnopsychiatry are excessively delicate to handle. We will not address the matter, which has been treated elsewhere by H. Brian M. Murphy.[3] We need only to briefly recall the reasons why it is so difficult, in ethnopsychiatry, to avoid causes of error.

The situation of the psychiatrist practising his art in a primitive population in which the customs and language are foreign to him is different from that of the ordinary doctor. When it comes to setting a fracture, a few words translated more or less satisfactorily by an interpreter generally suffice. When it comes to a cross-examination to clarify the origin of an internal disease, the best interpreter will barely be able to overcome the difficulties that arise in obtaining precise information. In the presence of a mental disease, the linguistic difficulties are increased tenfold by the differences in customs and mentality. Nothing is more inaccurate than the idea that the so-called primitive languages are just simple patois and weak vocabulary; quite the contrary, most of these languages are so complex and have such a rich vocabulary that long years of effort are needed to manage to grasp their nuances. It is impossible to understand the experience of a mental disease if we do not have a thorough knowledge of the language in which the patient expresses himself. When these difficulties are overcome, many others arise, which have been described often (Margetts, 1958). There is first the lack of habitual clarity of the patient in the way he describes the disorders he is experiencing, his inability to distinguish their relative importance. It is extremely difficult to obtain satisfactory anamnesis among individuals who are not accustomed to introspection or to looking at their lives in historical continuity. All the more so, it is almost impossible to explore family history. Sometimes the doctor will be led into error because the patient will reply what he thinks the doctor wants to hear. Or it can happen that the patient offers a deliberately incomplete or unilateral anamnesis.

Example: In 1957, a Kickapoo Indian,[4] aged sixty-five, was admitted to the psychiatric hospital in Topeka, Kansas. Sober until then, he had suddenly begun drinking alcohol to excess following unclear circumstances in which disagreements with his wife appear to have played a role. The case was diagnosed as "alcoholic neurosis."

The fact that I knew one of his friends and neighbours well led the patient to tell me his story. Like many of the Indians of his tribe, he had a kind of split personality, an American name and an Indian name, an "official" religion and an "Indian" religion. While nominally Protestant, he belonged to the peyote religion, to which he had converted about fifteen years earlier. He practised his religion sincerely but had ended up becoming addicted to peyote (a quite rare, though not exceptional, occurrence). His wife, who belonged to another Indian religion, that of the "Drummers," was hostile to the peyote religion. One day there was no peyote to be found: the man suffered deeply, which led him to seek solace in alcohol. That was the real origin of this alcoholism late in life – but the man was loath to speak of peyote or of his religion, which he considered to be purely and Indian matter of no concern to doctors.

As for the psychologist, the enormous difficulties he encounters in his new field of activity have been well described by Emerson Douyon (1964), a Haitian psychologist who, after receiving specialized training as a clinical psychologist in the United States and Canada, returned to his country to practise his profession. In an underdeveloped country, he said, the psychologist must constantly question his own role and reinvent his profession. You create a role that is not your own. Your box of testing materials is seen as a magic box, and it just so happens that the usual battery of tests contains many images that are part of the voodoo ritual. Moreover, patients do not allow the psychologist to ask questions; they expect that, like the houngan,[5] he plays, not the role of a listener, but that of an actor. He will be asked to read the lines on the palm of the hand to reveal events foreshadowed by the visit of a big butterfly or by a premonitory dream, or else for help in identifying an enemy, detecting a trap, or in obtaining the love of a girl. In this environment, "the psychologist quickly assesses the inadequacy of his instrument in grasping the new and complex realities of this magico-religious universe," and the majority of subjects prove to be basically "untestable." In such an environment, concepts of psychological stages, mental age, IQ, and of normality, are not applicable. So the psychologist must either continue to apply his ordinary assessment criteria or abandon them to create new ones. Practised according to the Western method, his profession meets no essential need. Should he wish to devote himself to research, he comes up against extreme distrust of the people: recording weight or height, the simplest questions about age and the names of children lead to hostile interpretations that, in our countries, would be considered incredible. "Among the realities of daily existence," concludes Emerson Douyon, "the philosopher Epictetus distinguished necessary things from those that are less so. I am afraid that, among them and in underdeveloped countries, we must place psychology."

Among these "useless things" we must often add most of our methods of psychotherapy, to the extent that they are removed from the most basic suggestive therapy. A psychoanalyst from India, L.C. Bhandari (1960), declared that the majority of his fellow citizens were unamenable to psychoanalytic therapy. Many asked for a powerful drug that would rapidly cure their ills; they could not understand the usefulness of treatment through words. They were loath to lie on the couch and give spontaneous associations. They quarrelled over the fees and the duration of treatment, which they accused the psychoanalyst of unduly prolonging out of dishonesty.

For general and theoretical ethnopsychiatry, the problem is different. The ethnopsychiatrist must have a thorough knowledge of his profession – that is, psychiatry – and in addition should have very sound knowledge of ethnological principles, methods, and theories. This is where major difficulties arise, as have been well indicated by Alfred Bühler (1952) and by other ethnologists. The raw material of ethnology is comprised of on-site observations made by competent researchers who have stayed for an extended period on-site, learned the language, and won the confidence of the locals. Unfortunately, very few observers fulfil these wishes! (Often, they are administrators, doctors, or missionaries with no ethnological training). Yet these privileged observers are likely to commit serious errors, resulting from their preconceived ideas or personal theories. An ethnologist who wishes to confirm his favourite theories may more or less unintentionally suggest them to his local informants, who will later repeat them to him or to others. Radin (1951) convincingly showed that the imprecise notions of *wakanda, orenda*, and *manito*, respectively described by A. Fletcher, J.W.B. Hewitt, and W. Jones, hold no credence; their promoters let themselves be influenced by preconceived ideas, which did not prevent many ethnologists from accepting them without criticism, assimilating them with Polynesian *mana*[6] and constructing many adventurous theories based on them. Bühler tells the story of ethnologist G. Peekel, who was so sure that the worship of the sun and the moon used to exist on an island in the Bismarck Archipelago that he persuaded the locals to modify some of their ceremonies in order to align them with what they must have been in the past according to his personal theories. Today, most ethnologists only stay briefly on-site; they arrive there with well-prepared questionnaires; they question the administrators, doctors, teachers, or missionaries, as well as a number of more or less Westernized locals. This method is easier, but cannot give results comparable to those obtained by the experience of a man such as Codrington (to cite but one name), who spent almost his entire life in close contact with a native tribe. Then comes the ethnologist theorist, who, based on material gathered by field researchers, develops theoretical constructions. Nothing is more beneficial than if this man combines a keen critical sense with great caution in terms of generalizations (Durkheim, Mauss); but

often the theorist will develop a construction that is more remarkable for its scope than for its soundness (Bachofen, Tylor, Frazer).
Unfortunately, it is on this fragile foundation that psychiatrists and
psychologists construct highly speculative systems. Bühler notes
that the conception of a period of matriarchy inevitably experienced by all nations at one point in their history, as well as the
notion of a universal worship of the sun and the moon, have no
serious foundation, which does not stop them from being claimed
to be indisputable truths by some disciples of Jung, who think they
see in them confirmation of their master's theories. Nor should
we be amazed if theories presented by Freud in *Totem and Taboo*
proved more successful with psychoanalysts than with ethnologists.
To conclude, we cannot be too cautious in ethnopsychiatry regarding the [...] ethnological data chosen to try to explain the facts, and
especially in terms of major theoretical systems.

DIVISIONS OF ETHNOPSYCHIATRY

Ethnopsychiatry is divided into a theoretical and general part that
analyzes the various general problems of this science, and a descriptive and clinical part that classifies, defines, and describes the various
mental diseases as they are presented in various peoples.

Theoretical and General Ethnopsychiatry

The main problems that arise in theoretical and general ethnopsychiatry are those of cultural relativism, cultural specificity, cultural nuances of mental illnesses, differentiations within the same cultural group, pathogenic cultural factors, and biocultural interactions.[1]

THE PROBLEM OF CULTURAL RELATIVISM

Is the concept of mental illness universal, or is it relative to specific cultures? In other words, are certain psychological manifestations considered normal in one ethnic group and abnormal in another, and vice versa? The theory of cultural relativism asserts that this is so. It is generally presented as follows:

> Let us imagine that a man, barely covered with a loincloth, frightfully emaciated, his face painted in red and blue, scratching his vermin, should squat in the corner of a town hall in Paris and remain there for hours and days, chewing a few grains of millet, sometimes humming, but most of the time not moving or speaking. If at least he were begging, his behaviour could be understood, but he is not ... It is most likely that he will soon go through the gates of the Sainte-Anne mental hospital ... But this man, I have seen him a hundred times in India! The faithful were gathered in front of him, staring at him in the hope of receiving some emanation of his wisdom. *A man is insane relative to a given culture.* (Albert Béguin, 1952)

Among ethnologists, it is mainly Ruth Benedict who systematically expounds the theory of cultural relativism in her book *Patterns of Culture* (1934), supporting it with facts and arguments that have become classic. She points out, for instance, that megalomaniac behaviour, which elsewhere would be called delusions of grandeur, was considered normal among the Kwakiutl[2] of British Columbia, and that an attitude of morbid distrust and hostility, which elsewhere would be called "paranoiac," is quite usual among the natives of Dobu Island.[3]

There is no doubt about these highly interesting facts. Nevertheless, cultural relativism also has its limitations, which sometimes have been overlooked. A critical survey of dependable data shows that a few basic forms of mental disturbance – idiocy, senile dementia, and acute delirium with agitation and fury – are considered abnormal all over the world. Or at least there is no known instance of a population where these troubles would not be considered pathological.

In fact, the question is more complex, because to our two categories (normal and pathological), many populations add a third: the supernatural. Certain kinds of delusions may thus be considered by the patient's relatives as phenomena of supernatural inspiration, or as possession by good or evil spirits. Such beliefs existed in civilized countries up to comparatively recently, along with the belief in changelings (children of fairies or goblins who were substituted for human children at their birth); thus, when children were born idiotic or malformed, they could be abandoned without remorse, since they allegedly did not belong to the human race (Piachewsky, 1935).

What makes the question more intricate still is the existence of an intermediate state between the "normal" belief in mythical and supernatural entities, and delusional ideas of undoubtedly pathological nature. Tanzi (1890) expounded this idea in a famous paper in which he pointed to striking parallels between superstitious beliefs or customs of certain primitive populations and the delusional ideas of Western mental patients (mainly those who today are called paranoid schizophrenics). This idea was later taken up and further developed by C.G. Jung in his theory of archetypes, that is, specific types of powerful images commonly known to all mankind. These archetypes may have a destructive effect upon a schizophrenic, whereas normally they exist as myths, folklore, or dreams.

It is noteworthy that those mental disturbances considered everywhere as pathological – idiocy, severe dementia, acute agitated delirium – all manifest what ancient psychiatrists called "total insanity." Divergences of opinion start as soon as one has to deal with "partly insane" individuals, for instance, those who have delusional ideas but are able to express themselves clearly and can carry on a logical discussion: the "folies raisonnantes" (reasoning madmen) of classic French psychiatrists. Here, depending on whether the emphasis is on the "sound" or the "sick" facet of an individual, a given culture will consider him normal or mentally disturbed. But in fact, these cultural divergences in the evaluation of mental illness do not differ very much from the individual divergences of our psychiatrists, notably the conflicting diagnoses of forensic psychiatric experts during a judicial trial.

Cultural relativism, in a broader sense, covers not only the question of mental disease, but also the question of differences between populations in their attitudes toward mental patients, and toward the social status given to certain groups of psychically abnormal people.

John Koty's *Die Behandlung der Alten und Kranken bei den Naturvölkern* (1934) contains a vast amount of data on attitudes toward the aged, invalids, and the sick (including mentally ill people) in primitive societies. Surprising differences are found between various populations: some are kind and friendly, others cruel and insensitive toward "useless mouths." Such facts have not received enough attention from ethnopsychiatry and deserve more extensive study. Koty only writes about the most primitive societies and says nothing about the more civilized, which certainly also merit investigation. There also we would find noteworthy differences from one region to another, or from one era to another. To give but one example: up to a century and a half ago, cretinism was endemic in the upper valleys of the Alps. In spite of their poverty, mountain dwellers in these villages took care of their cretins[4] in the most touching way. (Balzac gives a remarkable description of one of these villages in his novel *Le médecin de campagne, The Country Doctor*). Here is an example that must be exceptional in our Western countries, which are dominated by a hedonistic-utilitarian philosophy.

An instance of this is found in a memoir by Pearl S. Buck, *The Child Who Never Grew* (1950). The celebrated American novelist, born and educated in China, returned there after her marriage, where she gave birth to her daughter, whose true story is told in the memoir. The child, a mongoloid idiot,[5] lived in China until the age of three, when her mother brought her back to the United States. The contrast she draws between Chinese and American attitudes toward mentally retarded children[6] casts the Chinese in a good light.

The respective attitudes of various ethnic groups toward their mentally sick has another consequence, which seems to have escaped the attention of researchers in terms of the methodology of ethnopsychiatric research. It is obvious that among ethnic groups hostile to the aged, chronically sick, or crippled, these unfortunate people have a tendency to disappear more rapidly than elsewhere, dying from misery or in mysterious circumstances. In a population where the incidence of mental illness is very low, this point – usually difficult to clarify – should be carefully examined before any conclusions are drawn.

THE PROBLEM OF SPECIFICITY OF MENTAL DISEASES

Our second problem is the following: Are mental diseases the same all over the world, or do certain mental diseases exist only in one country or cultural setting so that they are therefore the specific product of that given culture?

The problem is not new. Hippocrates wrote a treatise describing Scythian disease, mentioned earlier. In past centuries, a great number of diseases were described as being specific to the population of a given country.

In the Middle Ages, a strange disease was observed sometimes among Scandinavian warriors: "the fury of the berserk." A very strong man, called a "berserk," was suddenly seized with such fury that he developed supernatural energy and killed a great number of people in a very short time. The *berserks* disappeared when Scandinavian countries became Christian (Güntert, 1912).

In the seventeenth century, a supposedly new disease appeared in England, the "English disease," first described by George Cheyne (1735) as a mixture of true organic symptoms and hypochondria. To those symptoms, later authors cited, as additional features, disgust with life and a propensity to suicide. The density and humidity of the air in England was believed to be one of its main causes.

About the same time, a "Swiss disease" – known as *Heimweh*, or nostalgia – became conspicuous among Swiss soldiers in the service of foreign princes. A Swiss soldier would become indifferent to everything while constantly dreaming about his native country. His condition would gradually worsen and end with death unless the soldier was discharged and sent back home, in which case he would rapidly be cured. That "Swiss disease" resulted, it was believed, from climatic factors, that is, from the contrast between the thin, pure air of the Swiss mountains and the heavy, thick air of other countries (Ernst, 1949).

Gradually, it became known that quite a few other supposedly specific conditions existed in other parts of the world – running *amok* and *latah* in the Malay countries, *kayaksvimmel* among the Eskimos "Arctic hysteria," "Pacific hysteria," and so on – to which we shall refer again later.

Thus it would seem that the proponents of the theory of "cultural specificity" are right when they claim that a number of mental diseases exist specific to certain cultures, and therefore resulting from unknown cultural factors.

Closer investigation, however, shows that none of these conditions are really as limited, geographically and culturally, as has been contended. Occasionally, they can be found in Western culture, although in less conspicuous forms.

"Scythian's disease," for example, the case of men dressing and living as women, is none other than what we call "transvestism." The difference is that generally we do not accept transvestism, while in the past among the Scythians and still today among certain primitive nations, it is (or recently was) not only permitted, but even institutionalized. An example is the *berdache* among American Indians, the *sekatra* and the *sarimbavy* in Madagascar, and so on.

The fury of the *berserk* and the running *amok* of the Malay are two manifestations of an identical phenomenon: a sudden impulse to commit multiple murders. But a phenomenon of this type may occur in any country in the world. Recently, American newspapers told the story of a nineteen-year-old man who, during a car ride, killed eleven people. If that young man had lived in Iceland in the tenth century, he would have been called a "berserk"; if he had lived in present-day Java, he would have been said to be "running *amok*." The difference is that, living today in the United States, this young man became an object of horror and was called a criminal, whereas if he had lived in medieval Scandinavia or contemporary Malaysia, he would have been called a hero and honoured as such (though perhaps he would have been killed during his killing spree).

In terms of the fury of the *berserk*, and running *amok*, the influence of culture manifests itself in two ways:

1 By *cermemonialization*, that is, the socio-psychological model to which the manifestation conforms. It unfolds as a drama written in advance where the lead actor has learned his role well, or as a ceremony, the details of which are dictated by tradition.

2 By the element of *tolerance* conferred by the culture in question. It is characteristic that the *berserk* disappeared in the eleventh century of our era, immediately after the church declared they would no longer be tolerated. However, running *amok* continues to exist in Malaysia and Indonesia.

It would be easy to demonstrate that the "English disease" had nothing to do with the London fog, and that it was a condition that, to this day, occurs in any part of the world, and has been called "spleen" (Le Savoureux, 1913). As for nostalgia, it has nothing to do with climatic factors either: it can be encountered in several parts of the world, in any location where an individual who has integrated into a closed cultural environment is suddenly placed in another cultural environment in which he does not manage to integrate.

We may therefore conclude that the so-called specific mental diseases – those of the Scythians, Malay, Eskimos, Swiss, and English – are only specific forms of common mental diseases, although the symptoms are shaped by cultural factors.

It is obvious that the more a disease is psychogenic in nature, the more it will be marked by cultural factors, and this may give the disease the false appearance of having a specific cultural component. When we consider the meaning of words such as *spleen, cafard, Koller,* and so on, we realize that although there are some slight psychological differentiations, depending on English, French, or German national characters, they all indicate an identical or very similar depressive or neurotic syndrome.

A more difficult problem is presented by the case of *shinkeishitu,* a condition often considered to be a typical Japanese neurosis. According to Takeo Doi (1958, 1959, 1962), it would appear that the word *shinkeishitu* is a translation of the German word *Nervostät,* but it seems to have rapidly acquired a particular meaning in Japanese. The psychiatrist Shoma Morita (1928), author of a therapeutic method well-known in Japan under the name "Morita Method," has given an extensive clinical description of this disease as well as a theory on this neurosis. *Shinkeishitu* includes those neurasthenia conditions that in our countries are termed anxiety neuroses and obsessions. Morita claims that these disorders derive from a common hypochondriacal constitution, *toraware*, which is a kind of constant preoccupation of the patient, not only about his health but also about the activities of those around him and other men. Doi thinks that *toraware* derives from the frustration of a basic psychological tendency, called *amae*, an untranslatable word meaning the need to be loved, protected, and guided. *Amae* seems to be a fundamental feature of the Japanese character, to which *shinkeishitu* is therefore closely related, and this explains the success of the Morita Method in the treatment of this neurosis. The Morita therapy is said to be based on the principles of Zen Buddhism. We hope that Morita's work will soon be translated into Western languages, because the data at our disposal are not sufficient for a profitable discussion of the problem. It would seem, however, that Morita's clinical synthesis agrees with Janet's psychasthenia and that the *amae* is somewhat similar to the "besoin de direction" (need for guidance), to which Janet attributes a major role in the psychology and treatment of neuroses.

If we shift from Japan to some more primitive types of cultures, we encounter concepts that differ even more from ours. Hans Koritschoner (1936) briefly described the concepts of native physicians in eastern Africa regarding mental diseases and their classification. *Shaitani*, as he calls them, are attributed to the influence of evil spirits and occur mainly in women. The native medicine classifies *shaitani* into two groups, respectively the *shaitani ya pwani* and the *shaitani ya bara*; they all agree on the group to which each *shaitani* belongs, but Koritschoner admits that he does not understand the principle of this classification (if there is one). Each *shaitani* has well-defined symptoms, but almost none of them fit into our nosological categories, as is shown in this table:

I. *Shaitani ya pwani*:
Ruhani: pain throughout the body, restless dreams, hallucinations.
Subiani: a pregnant woman complains of unbearable pain and shouts that she is going to give birth to an animal.
Kibwengo: starts with headaches, nighttime restlessness, shouting, and amnesia the following morning, but the headaches persist.
Makata: sudden fall.

Maimon: anxiety, then nighttime restlessness, inarticulate cries, rhythmic body movements; the attacks are repeated every evening; in the intervals, sexual desire is heightened.

Sherifu: agitation, the patient begins speaking in a language supposed to be Arabic, but with only intonations of it.

Tari: rhythmic movements of the head, without exclamations.

Bedui: fits of nighttime stupor interspersed with shouting and agitation.

Mahaba: exceptionally, this is a disease of men: impotence.

II. *Shaitani ya bara*:

Kinyamkera: the patient leaves her bed at night and wants to climb trees.

Kirima: patient is restless, feverish, noisy, but immobile.

Simba: patient is aggressive, bites and scratches, wants to escape into the bush.

Ngombe: the patient complains each day of a pain in a different place and then begins to walk on all fours and swallow inedible things.

Masai: the patient suddenly begins imitating the attitude, gait, voice, and the dance of a Masai person.

Gobegobe: the patient falls, rolls on the ground, and puts everything she can find into her mouth.

Songosongo: the patient, seated, is troubled by rhythmic movements of the head and thorax and utters monotone cries.

Kokorai: the patient is cold and goes so close to the fire that she burns herself.

Mluguru or kivugo: paralysis of the lower limbs and stomach pains.

Mafite: as with Masai, the difference being that the group imitated is the Mafites (or Ngoni).

Kukwaire: the patient catches spiders or lizards and swallows them.

Kidiri: breathing is rapid, shallow, and laboured, without interruption.

Ndungumaro: patient is immobile and unconscious.

What are we to think of this strange nosology? Are these really mental disorders specific to a particular African culture? In some cases, they appear to be symptoms of a physical illness. Moreover, Koritschoner reports that these *shaitani* occur mainly in women who have left the interior of the country to live on the coast, and who are influenced by suggestion while they are watching treatments administered publicly by native doctors – that is, these *shaitani* are victims of other women. It is thus likely that most often these are specific forms of hysteria, protean neuroses *par excellence.* The classification of the *shaitani* of East Africa is no more absurd than some classifications of neuroses in the classic treatises of the eighteenth century, in which various forms of hysterical troubles were classified every which way alongside tetanus, rabies, and epilepsy.

A study similar to that of Koritschoner, but a good deal more comprehensive, is the one Devereux devoted to the Mojaves, an Indian tribe of the American southwest (1961). Devereux systematically studied their psychoses and neuroses, as well as their ideas about these mental illnesses. He described these one by one and classified them. Unlike the native doctors of eastern Africa, the Mojaves did not imagine a psychiatric classification of their mental disorders.

Devereux thinks these Mojave disorders can be divided into three groups. The first encompasses instinct disorders, which include – under names in the Mojave language that we will spare the reader – attacks of homicidal fury, hunter's neurosis, scalper's psychosis, witch-killer's psychosis, a disease of people who are too active, the psychosis of the god Mastambo, neuroses of singers and shamans, and so on. In a second group, Devereux places "heart neuroses" such as *Hi: wa itck* or the sorrow of an older husband abandoned by his young wife. The third group includes disorders attributed to the subject who encounters various supernatural beings: a dream vision of a divinity, suffering from a mental disease, meeting a supernatural snake, a Mojave ghost, a ghost from a foreign tribe, a witch, and so on; within this group, Devereux connects the effects of magic with those of toxic substances, including alcohol.

As Devereux clearly demonstrates, all Mojave mental illnesses are subject to a dual diagnosis, one according to native psychiatric conceptions, and the other according to our usual nosology. We must hope that Koritschoner's article and Devereux's work will inspire ethnopsychiatrists to express more interest in the psychiatric conceptions of different nations. But we should not expect native nosologies to reveal the existence of mental diseases specific to their respective cultures. All the data currently known seem to indicate that the general processes of mental diseases are basically the same throughout the world, even if their symptoms are modelled and infinitely diversified by cultural factors.

CLINICAL ASPECTS AND NUANCES
OF MENTAL DISEASES

Ethnopsychiatry introduces us to numerous aspects and nuances of mental diseases in the many populations of the world. This variety results from two major factors:

1 *The influence of mores, customs, beliefs, and superstitions*, in which the patient participates as a member of his group.
2 *Culturally determined attitudes of the surrounding society toward the disease*, and the patient's reaction toward this attitude.

The influence of mores, customs, and beliefs on the clinical aspects of phobias, obsessions, delusional ideas, and hallucinations was demonstrated long ago by traditional psychiatry in civilized countries, and applies all the more so when the cultural environment is steeped in magic or animistic concepts. Some examples will suffice to illustrate this influence. Dr G. Martin (1935), a surgeon in the French colonial army, published some instructive observations gathered in French West Africa,[7] illustrating how differently delusions of grandeur can manifest themselves in African natives, whether they are "savages" of the bush or more "civilized" or "acculturated" individuals. I borrow from Martin's publications a few instances of delusions of grandeur among Bush Negroes:[8]

1 A native of the Congo, a megalomaniac, enumerated his wealth: "I have three bottles of Cologne, two canteens, and a cupboard filled with food."
2 Another megalomaniac Bush Negro: "I possess a loincloth that is expensive, and also a mat. Nobody has such a beautiful one."
3 A third one, a paddler: "I am a chief, and the son of a chief. I have as much authority as a white man. The White is my equal, but does not give me orders. I am a great warrior. I went up the river, leading many soldiers and many canoes. I killed everybody and conquered the whole country ... I am not a dirty Negro."
4 A fourth one is a Yakoma; his tribe is probably not yet quite rid of cannibalism: "My fellow patients are lowly slaves. I have the right to kill them. I will cut their heads off and eat them

because I am hungry. I am a great chief, the most handsome, the most powerful. I do not want a corpse, or a sick man. I want a man, but I want him alive. I want to kill him myself."

In contrast to these four Bush Negroes, here are now two of their compatriots who belong to tribes that have been more exposed to the influence of civilization:

1 A merchant from the African coast speaks of his "large fortune," his "vast plantations," his "numerous trips to France," and of his "many expenditures."
2 A native of Madagascar declares: "I have lots of cars, thousands of herds of cattle. I have visited all the capitals of Europe. The palace of the Governor-General belongs to me. I have donated millions of francs to military aviation. I own airplanes, railroads," etc.

Such instances enable us to measure the influence of civilization on the content of delusional ideas. We see that the extent of these patients' megalomaniac delusions can be evaluated only through an accurate knowledge of their respective ways of life. Thus, for a Bush Negro, the idea of possessing "two canteens," "an expensive loincloth," and so on may be a symptom of delusion of grandeur whereas in our Western civilization it would express a sense of dire poverty. On the other hand, the delusions of grandeur of the two latter patients, the acculturated ones, are not very different from similar delusions observed in European or American patients.

In regard to the Yakoma patient, it is obvious that the same clinical importance could not be ascribed to his declarations as for a patient in our culture. A patient in our culture who expressed cannibalistic wishes of that kind would no doubt be considered a "serious case," whereas for a man of this tribe these would simply indicate aggressive tendencies on the border between normal and abnormal. In this patient, evidence of mental illness rests perhaps less on the patient's cannibalistic feelings than on his uninhibited way of expressing them openly in the presence of a white doctor!

Let us now consider the cases of two young men of the French Congo, both of them Roman Catholics and former pupils of a mission school. They are described in the same article by Dr Gustave Martin:

A former student of a Catholic mission in Brazzaville assures us that he [had] ascended to Heaven. There he was greeted by the angel Gabriel and by Saint Peter who held a large cross in his hand. These messengers of the Lord placed a rosary around his neck, saying: You will be Christian and your name will be Joseph.

What are we to think of this subject's declaration? Was it simply a dream? (According to the missionaries, many conversions immediately followed this type of dream). Or was it a vision similar to those of certain mystics or saints of the Catholic Church? Or was it a delusional, schizophrenic idea?

Another explains to us that one of his friends, a bad Christian, is sending him the demons with which he is possessed. He sees and hears these devils. He spends his time chasing them, but at night they climb on the roof. They enter his room. They pursue him. Recently they tied him up. It is they who have caused his weight loss, headaches, the pain from which he suffers, and so on.

Imagine that a patient living among us, in our Western civilization, brought us the same complaints. Few psychiatrists would hesitate to call them "delusional ideas." But for a Black man in America, or even a Christian studying in a missionary school, things are not that simple. In a culture where everyone from time immemorial has ascribed disease to the influence of evil spirits and witchcraft, one must be very cautious before assuming that complaints of that order are delusions. Maybe the patient really was afflicted with severe mental illness. Maybe it was only a mild type of neurotic depression whose symptoms were coloured with ancestral beliefs and other cultural elements.

It would be superfluous to cite more clinical instances. They would only confirm our assertion that in many instances only a close knowledge of the cultural background will enable the psychiatrist to distinguish whether an individual is normal or mentally ill and, if he is ill, to what extent.

The attitude of the surrounding society and the reaction of the patient are strong, culturally determined factors that modify the symptomatology of mental diseases depending on the ethnic or cultural group. Any illness may be considered to comprise a nucleus[9] of symptoms directly created by the morbid process, around which gather the reactions of the patient toward his ailment, toward his doctor, and mainly toward the attitude of the surrounding society toward himself.

W. Schulte, in a paper titled *Die gesunde Umwelt in ihrer Reaktion auf Psychosen und Psychopathien* (1958), tried to briefly define the specific formula that, in our countries, expresses the attitude of the immediate society toward ordinary mental diseases. The mentally retarded provoke a reaction of aversion, and feelings of superiority, and sometimes (especially with idiots) hostility or disgust. Maniacs provoke an attitude of amusement, very different from that produced by schizophrenic pseudo-maniacs. The depressed patient irritates and tires; he gives the impression that he could "shake himself out of it" if he tried. When his condition worsens, he may be better tolerated, or provoke anxiety; when he commits suicide, the members of his family show feelings of guilt, and so on.

It is unfortunate that this particular aspect of psychiatry has not been investigated more closely. Ethnopsychiatry could make a significant contribution to it. It would confirm that the influence of the attitude of the surrounding society is often more important than the illness itself and is even likely to create a serious pathology.[10]

An unusual example of this is given in a study by Johann Frick: *Körpergeruch als Krankheit* (1963).

This is a bizarre illness that is quite frequent in the two provinces of Kansu and Tsinghai,[11] in the northwest of China, where it is designated as *sao ping* or *ch'ou ping*: the patient is perfectly healthy and normal, except for body odour that affects the Chinese sense of smell very unpleasantly, whereas Europeans do not notice it or notice only a vague odour which has no special association for them. The Chinese distinguish three varieties of it, the worst of which is comparable to that of rancid butter. They find it so nauseating that they sometimes feel ill just smelling it. The Chinese claim it is a hereditary illness but that it may be contracted through too-close contact with one of the subjects. Individuals suffering from *sao ping* are victims of social ostracism, which makes their lives excessively unpleasant. They cannot, for example, marry outside the families in which this infirmity exists. It contains an element of shame so that it is never mentioned (saying to someone that he has it would be a way to provoke inexpiable hatred).

If society's reactions may create a pathological syndrome from a simple physiological anomaly, it is even more likely to have the same effect on a physical or mental illness, already painful in itself.

Epilepsy is a classic example. In many countries, in past centuries, it has been considered an illness different from others, the result of supernatural and awe-inspiring causes. It has been told how Romans interrupted their public assemblies if an individual had an attack of epilepsy. A Norwegian physician, Dr Louise Aall, who worked in Tanganyika, gave a remarkable description of epilepsy and the reactions to it among the Wapogoro[12] (Aall, 1962).

This agricultural tribe is poor and undernourished and has many infectious and parasitic diseases. The Wapogoro show a peculiar indifference toward illness and only accept treatment when it becomes unbearable. The only illness they really dread is epilepsy, and when a formerly sane individual experiences his first epileptic attack it is a catastrophe for the family; they call in a witch-doctor and are prepared to sacrifice anything to stop the plague. The Wapogoro have no idea that epilepsy is a natural illness; they blame it on the action of evil spirits, as punishment for some sin committed by either the patient or a member of his family, or as the result of an evil curse. They also believe that the disease is contagious. That is why, when an epileptic has an attack, all bystanders frantically run away, with the result that the patient is often injured in his fall and receives no help. In the intervals between attacks, he is feared and despised; he is obliged to live in a separate hut, eat alone, and get water for himself. It is difficult for him to find a job, and he lives in abject poverty and filth. Exceptionally, an epileptic whose attacks are not frequent may become a witch doctor. But the majority have a pitiful existence and often die during attacks, or die prematurely of some physical or infectious illness.

Mrs Louise Aall assures us that with a little experience, one can instantly recognize an epileptic in a group of natives: he has a swollen face, a miserable expression, and a dull look. Before a European doctor, his attitude is characteristic: he is a repulsively dirty individual who comes in, does not dare sit on a chair, crouches on the floor, and stares humbly, at first unable to talk, while his family does it for him, nagging him at the same time. Then he starts talking in a monotonous voice, harsh and grating, inarticulate and hardly intelligible. Curiously enough, there is a type of dream called a "Wapogoro dream," which comes only to epileptics (who, according to Mrs Aall, never fail to experience it): the patient dreams he is washing his hands in a basin of water and enjoys it. Suddenly, he notices that the water is red like blood and he awakens, terrified.

The treatment of epilepsy with modern anti-convulsives not only makes the attacks disappear but also brings about an extraordinary change in the personality of the patient: his eyes and his expression light up, his voice changes, he becomes clean, hardly recognizable as the individual who was once in such a deplorable state. But often at this point he becomes quarrelsome and dangerous, complaining of bad treatment suffered during his illness, and it becomes all the more necessary to take care of him. The treatment then consists of social readjustment of the patient, working on him as well as his family and all the people surrounding him.

Social reactions toward mental disease vary infinitely depending on the disease, the accepted views on this disease, and local superstitions. An extreme example was published by a Haitian ethnopsychiatrist, Dr Louis Mars (1947).

In 1936, a woman who appeared to be about forty years old was found wandering in a field, naked, silent, and completely amnesic. The people could not identify her but took her for a zombie. The Haitians believe that a dead person can rise from his tomb a few hours after he is buried and continue to live, mechanically working as a slave for a master who will take him in; however, if a zombie eats salt, he will be delivered from slavery, though he will also lose his memory. It was believed that the unknown woman was a zombie to whom that had happened, and a family came to claim her as a dead relative, buried in 1907 (thus twenty-nine years earlier); their declaration was supported by neighbours, who claimed to recognize her as well. It is unfortunate that Louis Mars did not tell us the rest of this story or share how the patient played her role of ex-zombie.

The more an ethnic mentality differs from ours, the more the clinical aspect of mental illnesses will differ, under the double influence of native beliefs and people's attitude toward mental patients. A Swiss doctor, Erna Hoch, in a series of publications (1957, 1959, 1961), gave precise details on the mental diseases of Hindus in the Lucknow region.[13] Among this population accustomed to a fatalistic attitude, many cases of mental depression may go unnoticed. Refusal of nourishment by a depressed or schizophrenic individual may be easily mistaken for a pious performance of some duty imposed by religious belief. Obsessions, as long as they have not reached considerable proportions, will not strike in a population accustomed to taboos and rites. As for schizophrenia simplex,[14] it will not be easy to distinguish from the idle way of life of certain individuals under the shelter of a large patriarchal family. That an individual starts neglecting duties and responsibilities will not provoke social stigma (it is more or less the life designated in Russian by the word *oblomovchtchina,* from the name Oblomov, who is the hero of a novel by Goncharov.)[15] Paranoiac delusions of persecution would not be surprising either in a setting rife with religious, racial, and political hatreds. And most of all, delusional ideas that are religious in nature may be misjudged. If a Christian announces that he is Christ, or a Moslem proclaims that he is Mahomet, their delusion will immediately be detected; but if a Hindu pretends to be the reincarnation of Vishnu, or if a mother says that Krishna is reincarnate in her newborn, or if a melancholic displays deep sorrow and remorse for sins committed in a previous life, such ideas may be accepted, or at least tolerated. Severe schizophrenia may also be socially accepted when the ailing person leaves his family and becomes a hermit or a wandering fakir. It is highly improbable that such patients will ever consult a European psychiatrist, and this, according to Mrs Erna Hoch, explains why the usual statistics inform us of the kinds of patients hospitalized in India, but not of the actual frequency of mental ailments. Another important remark: Hindu schizophrenics do not show the "lack of emotional contact" that, according to European authors, is an essential feature of this illness, and this leads Mrs Erna Hoch (1959) to suspect that "loss of emotional contact" is not a basic symptom of schizophrenia, but a consequence of the forbidding, humiliating, and hostile attitude of the European society, and of the social stigma attached to this ailment in Western nations.

Observations similar to those of Mrs Hoch in India were made in many other countries. Bruno Lewin (1957) described how the practice of psychiatry in Egypt requires that the doctor have a close knowledge of mores and customs, economic and social conditions, and the local language, failing which he may commit serious mistakes in his diagnosis. The Egyptian is naturally inclined to gesticulate, to take theatrical attitudes; he believes in spirits (particularly in evil spirits, the "djinns"), so that a simple psychic reaction may easily appear to be a serious psychosis. Lewin relates the case of a young woman who, under a spell cast by another woman, became possessed by the spirit of Karina, supposedly her husband's woman-*djinn,* until a stronger counter-spell made all the symptoms instantly disappear. Hearing voices, or believing one is possessed or persecuted by evil spirits, is not necessarily symptomatic of schizophrenia. However, genuine schizophrenia may be hidden under the clinical appearance of hysteria.

Rather than provide multiple examples of this type, we indicate another situation that may be the source of serious misunderstandings and conflicts – that in which *two or more ethnic groups live side by side and have very different ideas and attitudes about certain illnesses*. This is the case in Israel, where Mrs Phyllis Palgi (1960) described difficulties encountered by social assistance services in terms of rehabilitation of the disabled. These services are made up of European-trained doctors, nurses, and social workers, to whom it appears obvious that any disabled person necessarily wants to begin functioning normally again as soon as possible and become again a useful member of the community. With this "Western" way of seeing things, disabilities are approached with a "scientific" mindset; they are attributed to natural causes, though often people cannot help but experience a degree of disgust for them. This attitude differs entirely from that of some groups of immigrants. Among Iraqi Jews, the cripple is initially considered to be unable to ever become a normal member of the community, and as necessarily becoming dependent on his family and his social group, for whom he is a painful burden, and whom he discredits. Among Yemeni Jews, the element of social shame is absent; however, the group's behaviour toward the cripple is inspired by a fatalistic mentality. Moroccan Jews show even more kindness toward cripples, but no effort is made to rehabilitate them. It is easy to imagine the difficulties that may result from conflicts between such different points of view.

Conclusion. Ethnopsychiatry has started to give us numerous and precise data on the behaviour of mental patients and their families, and on the clinical differentiations of various mental ailments, but considerable work is still ahead before we have a "psychiatric geography" covering the whole world and all peoples. When this tremendous work is completed, we shall probably have to revise many current concepts regarding the frequency and respective value of symptoms of mental illnesses such as they are presently described in our usual textbooks.

DIFFERENTIATION OF MENTAL DISEASES
WITHIN THE SAME ETHNIC GROUP

It is not enough to establish the frequency and the clinical aspects of mental illnesses in a specific ethnic group: further study is needed to ascertain how these diseases are clinically distributed and differentiated within that group. The frequency and clinical differentiations of mental ailments vary according to sex, the urban/rural profile of the population, caste, the marginalization or isolation of groups, and social class, it being understood that we consider here only differentiations within one ethnic group.

Variations according to sex. Doctors have always observed that physical and mental illnesses differ in frequency and in clinical aspects according to the sex of the patient. These differences were traditionally attributed to biological factors inherent in the sex, or sometimes to the social roles of men and women.

It was J.J. Bachofen who introduced a new point of view. In his fundamental work, *Das Mutterrecht* (1861), he expresses the assumption that mankind has lived through three important stages: primitive promiscuity, matriarchy, and patriarchy. In each of the three stages, the roles of men and women have been very different, though precisely determined in every detail as well as in all aspects of social, economic, religious, and cultural life. The transition from one stage to another has been lengthy and arduous. Many apparently paradoxical manifestations, such as sacred prostitution, hetaerism, amazonism, and collective psychoses associated with the cult of Dionysus were explained as accidents attributable to this cultural evolution.

Bachofen's theories are no longer accepted in their original form, but they had considerable influence on ethnology, sociology, and psychology. These theories, for instance, inspired the notion of *Kulturkreis*, or the "cultural circle" (Wilhelm Schmidt, W. Koppers, Gräbner, and so on). M. and M. Vaerting (1921–23)[16] tried to distinguish two types of society, one dominated by men and the other by women; they concluded that what we call the "masculine character" and the "feminine character" are but the character of the dominating sex and that of the dominated sex, so that in a society dominated by women, the latter would have the "masculine" character, and vice versa. Such theories have been popularized by various authors, and similar views may be found in some works by Margaret Mead.

Another major concept is that of *gonochorism* (Winge 1918–19). Winge defined gonochorism as the "the distance or difference between sexual types." This distance and difference may concern the primary sexual characteristicss (sexual organs), the secondary (other anatomical differences), and the tertiary (the field of instincts and character). Winge contends that in mammals and birds there is a correlation between gonochorism of primary characters and sexual behaviour: a strong gonochorism is characterized by polygamy and a slight gonochorism by monogamy (comparing the ways of a rooster with those of a pigeon). As for mankind, Winge only looks at the gonochorism of tertiary characters, which changes according to age (reaching its maximum between the ages of twenty and twenty-five and declining after age fifty), and according to social and cultural factors. Certain influences increase or maintain gonochorism, while others decrease it, resulting in what Winge calls *applanation*, that is, psychological equalization of the sexes. Teaching little boys to play with tin soldiers and weapons and little girls to play with dolls increases gonochorism, whereas coeducational schools and playing together decrease it; gonochorism increases in the same proportion as the differentiation in clothing, occupations in men and women, and so on. According to Winge, matriarchy reduced gonochorism, whereas patriarchy increased it tremendously, until it reached its peak in the large states of patriarchal structure; its decrease characterizes the processes of urbanization and of political and cultural decline. According to Winge, the increase and decrease of gonochorism are among the causes of the greatness and the decadence of nations.

The problem of *correlations between gonochorism and variations of mental illness* according to sex does not seem to have been systematically studied. However, a superficial investigation shows some irrefutable facts. In Europe, there has traditionally been a dominant masculine disease and a dominant feminine one. In the eighteenth century, hypochondriasis was a definitely masculine disease; its feminine counterpart was the "vapours." In the nineteenth century, these were replaced respectively by neurasthenia as masculine neurosis and hysteria as feminine neurosis. Was it a coincidence that at the end of the nineteenth century, when gonochorism began to decrease in Europe, a masculine hysteria appeared, whereas feminine hysteria almost completely disappeared? In some ways, alcoholism was traditionally a masculine disease, but due to the contemporary equalization, it has become more and more frequent in women, mainly in countries where the socialization of sexes is more advanced, as it is in the United States. By contrast, in Switzerland, where gonochorism is more solidly maintained, there is a typically feminine neurosis, the "house-cleaning compulsion of Swiss housewives" (see further down).

Enzo Agresti (1959), who studied delusional ideas in three groups of patients hospitalized in an Italian mental hospital, the first from 1857 to 1866, the second from 1920 to 1922, and the third from 1957 to 1958, noted a remarkable fact: the difference in the content of delusional ideas in men and women, previously very marked, has almost complexly disappeared over the course of that century.

Similar differences are found in other peoples. Among the Malay, traditionally there exist two very specific conditions, *amok* and *latah*. *Amok* is exclusively masculine – Malay men are accustomed from early childhood to handle weapons and exercise violence; whereas *latah* affects mostly women, who are often accustomed to the most servile submission.

The correlations between gonochorism and sexual psychopathology are still very obscure. According to Winge, the increase in gonochorism tends to produce sadism in men and masochism in women. But what are its effects on male and female homosexuality, and on transsexuality? Probably similar situations have been resolved differently from one people to another. But we must wait until special studies are devoted to this issue.

Cities, countryside, and suburbs. The differences between mental illnesses in cities and those in the countryside has long been noted, and interesting observations have been gathered by isolated authors.

M. Terrien (1893, 1897), who practised rural medicine in the Vendée, noted extremely frequent hysteria among the peasants of this region; he blamed it on the alcoholism of the parents, religious fanaticism, and superstitions (ghosts and sorcery).

During the same period, Baderot (1897) described in his thesis the clinical particulars of Breton patients hospitalized in an asylum in Rennes. The most striking fact, according to him, was the high frequency of religious delusions. "These delusions," he wrote, "are generally sad ones and ideas of damnation predominate." He found it in 28 percent of the patients in the Rennes asylum, compared to 7 percent of 757 observations throughout other French provinces and other countries. Baderot explained this frequent religious delusion as the result of the education and way of life of Breton peasants:

their first book was the catechism; they regularly go to church, hear many stories about ghosts and sorcerers, get drunk on Sunday, but only after attending Mass, and so on. Note that Terrien and Baderot show us the same factors existing in peasants of Vendée as in those of Brittany (intensity of religious faith, attachment to the Catholic faith, superstition, alcoholism), yet one of them notes, as an essential clinical characteristic, hysteria among the inhabitants of the Vendée, while the other notes mystical delusion among the Bretons. It would be interesting to compare their data on rural psychiatry with those available in other provinces in France and in other countries.

Among more recent works, we note that of Garbe (1960). The author first distinguishes three types of rural regions: those that are gradually being deserted (Massif Central, Aquitaine Basin); those where large farm operations prosper and where rich land industrialists contrast with an impoverished farming proletariat (the north of France); and regions of traditional polyculture where growers are very much attached to their land and their traditions. Garbe describes the last category. The mentality of peasants consists primarily of a deep feeling of insecurity, the result of centuries of natural catastrophes, political turmoil, and feudal exploitation, which explains the attitude of distrust, caution, and cunning. To this must be added a fundamental belief in the supernatural, but also a strong attachment to a combination of traditional, domestic, moral, and religious values. The peasant has little emotivity and is slow to react, but beneath his somewhat coarse appearance, he conceals cold, critical judgment. The peasant social group is characterized by its stability and cohesion and by the strength of family bonds and traditions, sometimes resulting in bitter family conflicts, but also in great tolerance toward the mentally retarded and the mentally ill. In such an environment, Garbe says, the practice of psychiatry is very different from what it is in the city, and mental illnesses do not resemble the classical descriptions given in textbooks; they are often disguised as psychosomatic ailments. The psychiatrist needs much discretion and patience.

This picture of French rural psychiatry is, on the whole, confirmed by Borgoltz (1960), who adds a few details. Rural society is tolerant toward mental retardation, chronic schizophrenia, exhibitionism, and alcoholism; delusions of persecution or jealousy are often unrecognized until they lead to violence. Superstitions and belief in sorcerers often produce anxiety. In cases of acute mental disturbances, the family tries to keep the patient at home as long as possible; they consult the psychiatrist only as a last resort. There is a general belief that some normal individuals are being confined to jail-asylums following a plot arranged by heirs apparent and doctors for personal gain. Disorders in a child's character often go unrecognized, or else the teacher is blamed for them. Hysteria is frequent and often takes the form of "Charcot's hysteria." Fear of impotence and frigidity is frequent. The practice of psychiatry is difficult; information given by the family is surprisingly inaccurate. The same words are used by the parent and by the doctor but are assigned different meanings. The majority of patients report physical rather than emotional complaints; they and their families do not easily accept a diagnosis of mental illness.

Particulars of rural psychiatry. In a country like France, these particulars are mainly expressed therefore by the atypical form of the disturbances, which readily take on a psychosomatic disguise; by frequent anxious conditions and hysteria; and in certain regions by frequent religious delusions. A large part of this psychopathology can easily elude the attention of the psychiatrist unless he makes a special effort to understand rural populations. Moreover, a strong attachment to tradition explains that some psychopathological conditions that have supposedly disappeared may unexpectedly be shown to exist. In the early nineteenth century, Esquirol sometimes saw a werewolf, who had been brought to him from some remote place in the countryside; in the years 1880 to 1830, cases of demoniacal possession were sometimes brought to Salpêtrière (such as the famous "Achille," a patient examined and cured by Janet); today, a tragedy sometimes reveals that sorcery still has a dangerous hold in certain regions. Here is a recent example, published by L. Israël and Mrs E. North (1961).

In a little village in Alsace, a five-year-old boy, Jacques Z., died under suspicious circumstances, his body covered with signs of beating. The child was known to have poor health and a difficult character, and perhaps was mentally ill. The father, a poor weaver, was arrested and admitted to having beaten the child to death; but anonymous letters arrived, accusing the mother. She was also arrested and proved to be retarded and illiterate and once to have been a victim of her father's incestuous behaviour. As for Jacques's father, he was himself the son of an alcoholic father and a schizophrenic mother. Jacques's mother was convinced that her husband was possessed by evil sprits sent by "bad women" (i.e., witches). She saw herself as the true victim, because these witches wanted to take her husband; it was to drive away these evil spirits that she beat Jacques into unconsciousness. The husband protested but did not have the strength or courage to stop her; he admitted to killing the child because he wanted to protect his wife from arrest. The court decided to commit the mother to a mental hospital, and the father was sentenced to two years in prison. The authors point out the role of the villagers: they knew what was going on, but no one intervened, for it satisfied their need for tragedy and mystery. When the child died, anonymous letters were sent, and the miserable couple, vehemently accused by the population, served as scapegoats.

To what extent can we apply rural psychiatric observations in France to rural societies in other countries? To answer this question, we would need precise documentation covering numerous regions and be able to compare the data. Garbe indicated the existence in France of three kinds of regions: industrialized, disorganized, and traditional/stable. One can assume that each of these types has its distinct rural psychopathology. Certain countries, such as the United States, have predominantly "land industrialists," for whom the word "peasant" is an insult; their special psychopathology is not well-known. Other countries, by contrast, have an underdeveloped type of peasantry whose special psychopathology is the object of rather numerous studies. We may get an idea of this from the work of a rural psychiatrist in Guadeloupe (Pineau, 1960).

The setting in which this Guadeloupe population lives is conditioned by some constant geographic and climatic factors. The climate is hot and humid. The population is constantly threatened by tornadoes, earthquakes, and volcanic eruptions. They have an insular mentality, while being politically and culturally attached to France. The majority of inhabitants have a poor, unbalanced diet. The rural population is extremely mobile and moves to other parts of the island, sometimes every year, which leads to a constant feeling of instability and insecurity. In most families, the mother constantly changes husbands or companions, and consequently children change "fathers"; 45 percent of births are illegitimate. At each new birth, the food ration of the children decreases, as does the space, so that they have to leave the house as soon as possible, knowing they will not easily find work. The inhabitants suffer not only from food shortages but also from hemoglobinopathies, hepatic ailments, and intestinal parasitoses such as amoebiasis, bilharziasis, and ancylostomiasis, as well as paludism; add to these intoxications due to anti-malarial medicine. This population is therefore miserable, starving, unstable, illiterate, and superstitious. Their belief in ghosts, in mythical beings, and in sorcery is a constant source of fear, depression, and anxiety attacks. Unfortunately, Pineau does not give precise details on rural psychopathology as it compares to that of the island's urban population. He only indicates differences regarding criminality. Among the urban population there are cases of swindling and organized crime. Rural delinquency includes murder caused by political quarrels or jealousy, thefts often inspired by hunger and misery, and sexual offences. Superstitious beliefs, intolerance, and religious fanaticism often play a part in all of these.

Some rural populations are even more underdeveloped than those described by Pineau in Guadeloupe. Such are the miserable peasants of northeastern Brazil and the slopes of the Andes and of several countries of Latin America, of whom Pacheco e Silva (1960), among other authors, provided a striking picture. Mental diseases in these populations are one ingredient in an amalgam of extremely complex economic, social, and political problems. These peasants live in abject destitution, suffering from food shortages and imbalances, endemic diseases (parasites, trachoma, anemia), and epidemics (malaria, yellow fever, and others, depending on the region), not to mention natural catastrophes such as droughts in the Brazilian northeast that lead to acute dehydration in the inhabitants. Puerperal infections are frequent, and the high incidence of imbecility and epilepsy is probably due to acute encephalitis in small children. Low vitality among the peasants diminishes their resistance to physical and mental diseases. Pacheco e Silva points out the frequency in these regions of acute confusional syndromes such as Korsakoff's psychosis. Misery and hunger induce alcoholism in many individuals and also (among the Indians of the Andes) chewing of the coca leaf. To complete this picture, it is precisely among the most miserable of these people, in the Brazilian northeast, that a number of epidemics of collective psychoses have occurred.

The study of such rural societies, aside from its present interest, can help us understand the mentality that, in Europe during the fifteenth and sixteenth centuries was the background against which certain psychic epidemics, such as the witch hunt, took place.

Urban psychopathology is as complicated as rural psychopathology, and notwithstanding the great number of investigations on the topic, it is still difficult to obtain an overview of it. To start, we should distinguish between the traditional city, which contains a small proportion of the total population of a region, and the modern city, which includes a huge proportion and whose inhabitants have a very different way of life. We should also distinguish between actual urban psychopathology (that of the stable urban population) and the psychopathology of "urbanization," which involves an influx of rural people undergoing social and economic disintegration and proletarianization. We should also bear in mind the intermediate formations between the city and the countryside: where we previously referred to the "outskirts" of a city, we now hear in America the word "suburbia" to designate large new districts in which the population is comprised mainly of young adults living in mass-produced housing developments or in large apartment buildings far from the city centre, and the word "exurbia" to designate more remote neighbourhoods, including fragments of rural elements that they gradually absorb.

Once these distinctions are established, several questions arise, which mainly belong in the field of social psychiatry and which we can only mention briefly:

(1) *Is there a difference in the occurrence of mental diseases between urban and rural populations?* Most studies conclude that mental diseases are more likely to occur in cities. Gartly Jaco (1960), in Texas, finds that the average occurrence is two and a half times higher in cities, with some variation related to the different types of mental diseases. But his work simply shows that mental patients in cities are more likely to be hospitalized and to consult a psychiatrist than those in the countryside. So far there is no indisputable evidence in true morbidity.

(2) *Is there a particular distribution of mental diseases among different areas of the same city?* Faris and Dunham (1939), in their classic work based on an extensive investigation in Chicago, state that rates of mental disease are higher in slums that in other residential districts. Mental illnesses, according to Faris and Dunham, decrease steadily from the city centre to the periphery, thus showing the same pattern that other authors have found in the distribution of juvenile and adult delinquency. Faris and Dunham find, moreover, that each type of mental disease has a maximum frequency in certain types of districts:

paranoid schizophrenics dominate in districts with furnished lodgings, catatonics in areas inhabited by recent immigrants and Negroes, manic-depressives[17] in districts with higher rents, alcoholics in "transition" areas, general paralytics in "areas of vice," senile dementia in neighbourhoods with a high proportion of renters. Schroeder (1942–43), who conducted investigations in five cities – Kansas City, Milwaukee, Omaha, St Louis, and Peoria – found that the total frequency of mental illness followed the same general tendency as in Chicago – that is, a maximum amount of it was centred in the slums. However, the differential distribution of the various mental diseases found by this author was not as precise as that indicated for Chicago by Faris and Dunham. Data obtained since that time do not seem to have clarified matters.

(3) *Are there specifically urban forms of psychopathology?* Many authors have described the evils caused by large modern cities. Hygienists have denounced air pollution from fumes, dust, and toxic gases; poisoning as a result of spoiled food; nervous strain caused by noise; neon signs; nervous fatigue resulting from commuting; cramped living quarters lacking air, soundproofing, and privacy; and the combined effects of social pressure and existential emptiness. Setting aside the purely physical effects of "urbanitis" (Zivy), what are the psychopathological effects? The problem has been studied mainly from the point of view of juvenile delinquency (Chombart de Lauwe) and of diffused demoralization, already well described by earlier novelists.

In the United States, many studies have been devoted to the psychopathology of suburbia – that is, newly built districts that provide neither the pleasures of the city nor those of the countryside, where the husband comes home late, fatigued from work and a tiring commute, and his wife is bored to death, her life limited to "four walls and a baby," all of which leads to anxiety, irritability, quarrels, and neurosis. Other studies have focused on the plight of bachelors, the aged, and the lonely, all of whom suffer the *vae victis* of modern life. In France, Courchet (1963) described a specific syndrome characterized by brutal fits of aggressiveness, sometimes suicidal, and attacks of acute mental confusion that spontaneously disappear after forty-eight hours; he attributes these disorders to overexertion, combined with living in inadequate housing, and above all to a lack of social ties. Therefore, it seems to be a syndrome of being worn down and to be social in origin.

In conclusion, we may say that the most precise fact detected so far in the comparison between towns and countryside is that more ancient forms of disorders are found mostly in the countryside, while more recent ones are more often found in cities. The countryside is inclined toward the psychopathology of the past, while the city tends towards that of the future.

Castes. Castes are a phenomenon almost exclusive to India and can only be understood within the framework of the large conglomeration of philosophies, mythologies, rites, and economic and social rules that is called Hinduism. From a sociological point of view, caste has been defined as a system of segmented and hierarchical divisions of society. In India there are a multitude of castes, many of which are subdivided into subcastes. At the top is the sacred caste of Brahmans; at the bottom are the inferior castes and outcasts (or pariahs) and the savage tribes. Each individual is born into a caste and remains there until he dies, unless expelled for a serious offence. For the individual, belonging to a certain caste determines his way of life, profession, marriage, friendships, attitudes, and social behaviour, both within his caste and in his relations with individuals of other castes. It is highly probable that each caste has its own psychopathology and that there are correlations between the frequency and variety of mental disorders and the castes to which the patients belong. This vast field of study is still unexplored, open to generations of explorers. Let us hope that India, which has given the world so many great philosophers, will also produce psychiatrists at the level of Sankara Acharya who will some day examine these problems. To date, very little information is available on these topics.

Sreenivasan and Hoenig (1960) have analyzed the admission figures for the psychiatric hospital in Mysore, starting with the four highest castes: Brahmans, Kshatriyas (warriors), Vysyas (merchants), and Sudras (agriculturalists). They found a very high percentage of admission for the first three categories and a much lower one for the Sudras as well as for the inferior castes. The percentage of admissions is even higher for Christians. These figures show a positive correlation between the degree of education of the members of these castes and their urban character; they only indicate which castes have been hospitalized more often.

More interesting is the work of Carstairs (1954) on a limited but precise subject: the attitudes of castes toward Indian hemp. The Brahmans have a tolerant attitude toward it and use it often; the Kshatriyas (warriors) usually abstain.

A subject that has attracted more investigators is that of criminal castes or tribes. It is well-known that they exist in great numbers in India. Their origins remain mysterious. The total number of these individuals is estimated at one million. Each province of India has its criminal castes or tribes, most of them nomadic, whose members embrace unique morals and customs, religious practices, and criminal activities. Abundant literature exists on this subject, but it is not easily available. Some official publications and works of criminologists (Pillai, 1924) or ethnologists (MacMunn, 1934) give information that is too often vague or contradictory, with no indication of the psychopathology of these castes or groups (apart from their criminality).

MacMunn (1934) mentions among the main criminal groups the Ramoosies (thieves, middlemen, and night watchmen); Brindijaras (male cattle thieves, women prostitutes); Bhamptas (train robbers, travelling in respectable disguise); Kaikadis (exhibitors of trained monkeys and armed robbers); Kolis (robbers who are particularly dangerous, disguised as policemen); Harnis (bandits disguised as begging monks; their women become wives or mistresses of rich men and one day disappear after robbing the house); and so on. The present government in India is making a tremendous effort to resocialize these tribes, building on past attempts by the British colonial government (Gillin, 1931, 105–64).

The most famous criminal tribes was the Thugs, or Phansigars, who terrorized the entire country for centuries. They travelled disguised as merchants or pilgrims, carefully choosing their victims, strangling them quickly with a piece of string, then burying them rapidly and fleeing with their belongings, thus honouring Kali, the goddess of death, and making a profit at the same time. They were exterminated in the early nineteenth century by the British colonial government, thanks to Captain W.H. Sleeman, whose works (1826, 1839), along that of Edward Thornton (1837), are the main source of information on the Thugs (see also James Sleeman, 1933). W.H. Sleeman provided interesting details about the careful training of young boy Thugs, who were progressively initiated into the criminal practices of their tribe. One Thug, named Feringea, told Sleeman (1836, 148–9) how a young boy inadvertently witnessed for the first time such practices and was so shocked by them that he died before the end of the day. Such facts, incidentally, are difficult to reconcile with the psychoanalytic concept of superego and agree more with the traditional concept of an autonomous moral instinct.

Marginal groups and isolated communities. Hindu castes are organically differentiated within the general community. But there are other types of differentiated social groups. Some of them isolated themselves of their own will; others have been excluded from the general community by the community's will. Others were separated of their own will as well as by the will of the general community.

Over the course of history, many groups have separated and differentiated themselves from other men, often for religious reasons. Psychiatrists have focused more on those that are considered antisocial or eccentric. A famous example is a Russian sect, the Skoptsy, founded in the mid-nineteenth century by Selivanov, who taught his disciples a combination of beliefs, rites, and ceremonies, as well as the principle of voluntary castration. Despite being persecuted, the sect flourished, growing to several thousand followers by the early nineteenth century. We know about it thanks to the work of a Russian forensic expert, Pelikan (1876), who was appointed by the Russian government to conduct an extensive scientific study of the sect, in the course of which he had the opportunity to examine several thousand Skoptsy. Pelikan was surprised by the low incidence of mental illness among them, apart from the collective diagnosis: "fanatic infatuation, without religious delusion" (121). Eugène Pittard (1934) conducted an anthropological investigation of a group of one hundred Romanian Skoptsky. Half of them had been castrated before puberty, the other half after. Pittard mentioned that he knew of only one or two of them who could have been called neurotic. These two studies found a low incidence of mental disorders in a community of fanatic sectarians whose members were strongly integrated into their social group. However, studies conducted later among the Hutterites show that one must be very careful when drawing conclusions, because the real frequency of mental disorders within a sect may prove to be greater than previously assumed.

The Hutterites, an Anabaptist sect,[18] were the subject of a thorough psychiatric study that produced significant results. The sect was founded in Bohemia in the sixteenth century and, after numerous and often tragic vicissitudes, immigrated to North America, where today it numbers nine thousand people scattered throughout nearly one hundred colonies in parts of the United States and Canada. Hutterites have preserved their religion, traditions, and German dialect, as well as their social and economic system based on common property. The faithful are tightly integrated into their community, within which they enjoy complete economic and emotional security. They are said to have perfect mental health. The results of an exhaustive psychiatric investigation conducted by a team between 1950 and 1953 were published in a book by Eaton and Weil (1955) and another by Kaplan and Plaut (1956). These authors found that the mental health of the Hutterites was not as perfect as previously stated, though their rate of mental diseases was still less than that of the general population. Criminality, sexual deviation, and alcoholism were almost non-existent among them. The prevailing mental ailment was depression, in a particular form, *Anfechtung*,[19] which constituted roughly 70 percent of the total figure of mental illness (see Kaplan and Plaut, 65–77). A patient afflicted with *Anfechtung* has deep feelings of guilt and firmly believes he has done something wrong or has had bad thoughts. This disease is viewed as a temptation by the devil. A patient suffering from *Anfechtung* can find relief by confessing to his preacher; he enjoys the sympathy of the community but is not exempt from his work and his obligations. In short, Hutterites show a lower rate of emotional disorder than the average population, and their ailments tend to take a particular form. This conclusion, of course, cannot be extended to other isolated communities, but so far no extensive investigation of the same kind has been performed elsewhere.

It is important to note that similar studies have been conducted on *marginal groups that have been set aside or are despised by the general community.* In times past, there existed in all civilized countries "accursed races" – for example, inhabitants of villages where there had once been leprosy, or that were home to descendants of foreign settlers. A few such communities still exist, such as the Eta in Japan,[20] who are said to have a high rate of criminality; it would be interesting to find out their percentage of mental diseases.

Still other *groups separated themselves from the general community and were also excluded from it.* This seems to be the case with gypsies, descendants of an ancient "criminal tribe" [a stereotype that was long ago abandoned – *Ed.*] that migrated to Europe from India at the end of the tenth century and lived as nomads in small groups scattered across all civilized countries. Their high rate of criminality is noted everywhere, but the frequency and form of their mental disorders have never been studied. The Yenish are among the best-known of the nomadic groups;[21] they wander through the canton of Graubünden in Switzerland, where they have been studied mainly by Jörger (1919) and Bertogg (1946). It is generally assumed that they are descendants of the German population of villages devastated during the Thirty Years' War, compelled to lead a nomadic life in order to survive. They earn their living as itinerant workers, tinsmiths, basket weavers, and so on, and have preserved very specific customs and superstitions (for instance, the use of dog fat as medicine). Dr Oskar Pfister (1951) (son of the famous psychoanalyst of the same name),[22] superintendent of the Beverin psychiatric hospital in Graubünden, examined their delusional ideas, which are in marked contrast to those of other patients in Graubünden. Those suffering from delusions of persecution do not talk about material devices, radios, spies, and detectives, instead referring to the sale of human beings, people being mutilated, beheaded, and buried, magic spells, conspiracies, and quite a number of horrifying sadistic or magical things. Such ideas are precisely the same as those that folklorists have noted among the beliefs and superstitions of normal Yenish individuals.

Here we broach the much more extensive problem of mental disorders among Jews in various countries, and among black minorities in the United States as well as Brazil. Many works have been written about this subject, many of which contradict one another, and we cannot examine all of them here. Let us just mention that it has often been alleged that young immigrants to Israel are spontaneously cured of their neuroses, for instead of living as an ethnic minority in other nations, they are now buoyed up by the feeling that they have acquired national independence. Such facts deserve thorough and well-conducted research.[23]

Social classes. It has long been recognized that the rich and the poor face different pathologies, and not only for nutritional diseases. In 1905, Niceforo published a work about diseases among the working class titled *Les Classes pauvres : Recherches anthropologiques et sociales*. It has often been said that psychoses are more frequent among the poorer classes and neuroses more frequent among the wealthier. But is this really a matter of incidence of illness? We remember Janet's adage: When a patient is poor, he is institutionalized with a diagnosis of psychosis; when he is rich, he is sent to a private sanatorium with a diagnosis of neurosis; if he is extremely wealthy, he is called an "eccentric"[24] and cared for at home by private nurses. A methodical study of this problem was started in New Haven by Hollingshead and Redlich (1958), who conducted an exhaustive investigation into all psychiatric cases, from serious psychosis to mild neurosis, treated in 1950 in hospitals, clinics, and doctors' offices in that city. Patients were categorized into five socio-economic classes. The authors found that the higher the social class, the greater the number of neuroses treated. Patients from the upper classes were more often treated by prolonged psychotherapy, those from lower classes by shock therapy or drugs. The percentage of schizophrenia increased as one descended the social scale; the highest proportion of chronic schizophrenics kept in psychiatric hospitals were from the poorest population.

The studies of Hollingshead and Redlich, conducted in a city with a stable and homogeneous population, give the impression that from one class to another we encounter various subcultures. So it is easy to foresee that differences will be even greater among populations in which social classes also contain various ethnic groups. In Peru, for instance, the upper class consists of the descendants of the Spanish conquistadors, and the lower class of Indians of almost pure descent; in the middle are the mestizos (a mixture of Indians and Spaniards who have preserved many Indian customs) and the cholos (people of mixed race who have adopted the Spanish way of life. Louis Mars (1958) emphasized that in Haiti, the three main social classes have distinct psychopathologies, and each of these classes is comprised of a different proportion of white and African elements.

PATHOGENIC CULTURAL FACTORS

We now come to the most difficult and most contentious part of ethnopsychiatry. In a given culture, what are the pathoplastic factors,[25] and what are the properly pathogenic factors? The numerous studies conducted in this field are far from producing definitive results.

(A) Let us start by eliminating non-cultural factors that intervene in most of the observations:

(1) Some research has dramatically underestimated *genetic factors* as well as consanguinity. In a group like the Hutterites, who for four centuries have led life on their own and among whom only fifteen surnames exist (three of which comprise half the population), consanguinity is obviously strong, and it has played a significant role in the frequency of depression in this population.

(2) *Climate* has a well-known pathogenic effect on white people who go to tropical or polar countries, but what role does it play in indigenous psychopathology? Sal y Rosas (1958) showed that in Peru the rate of epilepsy in the population changes with the climate and the altitude.

(3) *Dietary factors* are no less important. Windigo psychosis would not exist among the Indians of Canada's northeast without the famines they endure. Undernutrition, nutritional imbalance, and avitaminosis contribute to mental disturbances and are sometimes themselves the result of superstitions and dietary taboos (Heun, 1963).

(4) *Infectious and parasitic diseases* may also play a role. We know that malaria has been indicated as a cause in Malay *amok*.

(5) *Demographic factors* are not negligible. The structure of a population by age group plays a part in the distribution of mental disturbances. For example, in places where life expectancy is short, there is less senile dementia.

(6) As for the *sociological factors*, it is excessively difficult to distinguish them from cultural factors, as we have seen regarding social class.

Having left these various elements aside, we can try to analyze cultural pathogenic factors. But many authors do not appear to have noticed that there also exist inhibiting cultural factors in mental illness. As for the pathogenic cultural factors, some authors have tried to establish a list (Leighton, 1961). We could, following the concept of Auguste Comte, classify these factors as static or dynamic, the former in relation to a stable social order, the latter in relation to changes in society.

(B) In the first group, which relates to "static sociology," we need to begin by examining civilization itself. There is a tendency, going back to the Greek cynics and later taken up by Rousseau and Diderot, and then by Paul Rée, Nietzsche, and Freud, to accuse civilization of being the cause of all evils, or at least of psychic disturbances and neuroses. Others merely incriminate urban or technological civilization, or the division of society into classes. These problems are too extensive for us to respond precisely to them; it is preferable to tackle factors that are more limited and also well-defined.

(1) The theory that calls into question *primary education* embraces two hypotheses simultaneously: on the one hand, a correlation is postulated between national character and methods of care and education

(use of swaddling clothes, form of crib, method of breast-feeding, corporal punishment, toilet training, repression of sexual curiosity, and so on); on the other, a correlation is postulated between national character and predisposition to certain neuroses or psychoses. The school of cultural anthropology has published many studies of this type. Some are hypothetically adventurous, such as the theory that seeks to explain the Russian national character by the practice of swaddling infants up to the age of nine to twelve months (Gorer and Rickman, 1949). Other seem more plausible, such as the study by Spiro (1959) of the people of Ifaluk, in Micronesia, a small atoll of 250 inhabitants who enjoy a good climate and abundant food produced without much labour; they are kind and sociable. In three cases of mental diseases among these people, features of restrained aggressiveness were noted. Spiro explains the latent aggressiveness and anxiety of the inhabitants of Ifaluk by the fact that, on the island, mothers dip their young children every morning into the icy waters of a lagoon; apart from this, they are treated with the greatest indulgence and can direct their hostility toward evil spirits, of whom the children have been told stories. Regarding the problem of the relationship between cultural anthropology and psychiatry, we refer to the article by Charles Brisset (1960), previously mentioned.[26] The future of this research will depend on comparative studies, objective and very precise, such as that of Madame Faladé (1960), who compared the development of one hundred infants from Dakar, Senegal, to the development of one hundred French children from Paris. The development of these two groups of children, measured by psychomotor tests, showed very different curves, which were explained by the differences in primary education.

(2) Another pathogenic cultural factor is the psycho-social pressure directed against certain categories of individuals, either against deviants where they are not tolerated by the community, or against others in some critical situations. Specific neuroses and psychoses have been described in Egypt by Lewin (1958) and in Algeria by Sutter and colleagues (1959) among young women forced to marry a man they hate; after the marriage, these women have periods of mental confusion and agitation. There also seems to be a specific psychopathological gerontology in cultures in which there is a hostile attitude toward the aged, but the research on this is not yet sufficient. An extreme example of a social pathogenesis is present in Malay *latah*, which, as we will see further on, mainly occurs in women after a certain age following an accumulation of ill treatment.

(3) A third pathogenic cultural factor is the encouragement given to certain pathological behaviours, be it openly or implicitly. This is why the *berserks* or *amok* runners could continue to exist – in their own countries, they were seen as heroes. Any hysterical manifestation follows trends that are encouraged by the general attitude of society. Each time a particular form of neurosis becomes "fashionable," its frequency increases; this was the case with the "vapours" in the late eighteenth century and with "hysteria" until 1900.

(4) A fourth factor is the collective attitude toward human relations. The studies of Bateson and Mead (1942) on the inhabitants of Bali are instructive. There, the child is continually stimulated by his mother, but as soon as he starts to express an emotional response, she turns away from him, so that by age three or four, the child acquires a kind of emotional indifference. The entire population of Bali presents very strong schizoid features; it has even been stated that this collective schizoid disorder has lent its characteristics to the culture of Bali, including its art and religion. In an essay on mental health in Thailand, Stoller (1959) points out that the culture in that country preaches contentment and self-indulgence, with the exception of aggressiveness. It appears that Thai children are very much inhibited, and that crimes of violence are frequent and the number of mentally ill is high. Stoller thinks that Thai culture is responsible for this, because it preaches abstention rather than an active resolution of difficulties and because it offers no outlet for the release of aggressive instincts. A picture almost diametrically opposed is the one in the United States, where, according to David Landy (1958), the culture is dominated by five fundamental values: work, success, prestige, money, and leisure. Hence the isolation of the individual and the married couple, a loss of personal identity, and strong constraints imposed by the social group to which the individual belongs, all of which lead to a proliferation of emotional disorders resulting from isolation and social conflicts.

(5) In general terms, there are two main types of culture: verbal and literary (Varagnac, 1959), and people have wondered whether a correlation exists between these and the frequency or form of mental diseases. Carothers (1959), who studied this problem among the black population of Africa, shows that they live in a world dominated by sound; it lacks the written word, which is the intermediate element between thought and action and therefore the prerequisite of abstract individual thought. Hence the power of collective

representations and magic among these people. No doubt these conditions determine the form of mental disorders, but it has not yet been proven that they increase their frequency.

(C) The second group of pathogenic cultural factors relate to "dynamic sociology" (in Auguste Comte's terminology). Here as well, several factors have been blamed:

(1) *Geographic mobility*: population displacement (refugees and the like) and migration from the countryside to cities are both factors pertaining to socio-psychiatry rather than to ethnopsychiatry. This has been examined elsewhere (Gillon, Duchêne, and Champion, 1958).

(2) *Cultural changes* have often been blamed, but many forms and degrees of these exist. They range from slow and imperceptible adjustments to rapid changes arising from massive social disruption. Leighton (1959) stated that rapid and sweeping cultural change has a disastrous effect on mental health, and his opinion was shared by Wittkower and many others. Leighton analyzed how rapid socio-cultural transformations could become pathogenic: during childhood, the formation of personality is influenced by the lack of organization of family life and by the contradictions between the family's values and those of the outside world. The efforts of the adult, who is struggling in life, exceed the resources of his personality. At a later age, emotional disorders are unleashed by a harmful environment. Moreover, preventative measures formerly offered by religious authorities, professional healers, and wisemen gradually disappear when these men become unable to exercise their former influence. However, A.M. Rapoport (1959) claims that the correlation between sociocultural changes and increased frequency of mental diseases is true only in capitalistic countries, not in Soviet Russia where the frequency of mental diseases has decreased since the establishment of a socialist regime.[27]

(3) *Cultural conflicts* are probably an important cause of emotional disorders, but so far this role has only been studied in terms of collective psychoses, among which the most significant are movements of mythic liberation (Ellenberger, 1963).[28]

(4) *The isolation of the individual within the community* may be viewed as resulting from the factors of "dynamic sociology" that we listed earlier. In 1879, F.N. Manning noted in Australia the high frequency of mental diseases among unstable immigrants – that is, homeless people without family or permanent friends,

who often changed locations and jobs. After years of this existence, they developed delusions of persecution, accompanied by auditory hallucinations, and spent their later years in mental hospitals. It is interesting that seventy-seven years later, Listwan (1956) also described the frequency of ideas of persecution among immigrants to Australia. Many other observations confirm that social isolation is a mechanism through which sociocultural transformation leads to mental illness. Long ago, Halbwachs (1930) and von Andics (1940) noted that suicides occur more often in places where people are isolated socially.

(D) In addition to cultural factors that produce or stimulate mental diseases, there are factors that may inhibit or repress them. Clinical experience provides clear instances of repression of mental illness. In some neurotic individuals, all symptoms disappeared completely when they entered concentration camps and reappeared as soon as they had been liberated.[29] Sometimes the repression of illness may be incomplete. This is what happened with the hysterical disturbances that were so frequent during the First World War (1914–18). During the Spanish Civil War, as pointed out by López Ibor (1942), but mainly during the Second World War, these hysterical symptoms were considerably less frequent, but at the same time, there was a notable increase in peptic ulcers and other psychosomatic ailments. It is as if the soldiers' neurotic suffering had been repressed, but not completely; repression remained midway, as it were, on the psychosomatic level. Inhibition of mental diseases also manifests itself as a reduced number of mental diseases during wars and other times of great political and social upheaval; perhaps this is due to a temporary tightening of social ties. Attention must also be paid to the systematic catharsis of incipient mental disorders such as observed in certain cultures. Kilton Stewart (1961) describes how the Negritos of the Philippines tell one another their dreams every morning, and by discussing them aloud, expunge their anxiety and resentment. Among the Navajos, any state of depression and anxiety is referred to the shaman for his kindly intervention.

This brief account has shown that the study of cultural factors that stimulate or inhibit the production of mental ailments has only begun. However, we can state that fewer mental diseases will be found where there is strong social cohesion accompanied by positive collective values, and that the highest incidence of mental diseases will be found where, in the wake of socio-cultural disintegration, the individual is isolated and deprived of positive collective values.

BIOCULTURAL INTERACTIONS
AND MENTAL DISEASES

The intermingling of biological and cultural elements is another insufficiently studied aspect of mental illness. Civilization leads man to discoveries; these discoveries change the patterns of human life, bringing cultural and social upheaval, which in turn modifies the biological constitution of man, with far-reaching consequences in regard to mental illness, and so on.

In this wide and as yet unexplored field, we shall only mention here facts that are comparatively recent in human history but of great importance.

(1) The first fact is *the prolongation of the average length of human life*. Two or three centuries ago, a forty-year-old was called an "old man" or an "old woman"; today – as the saying goes – "life begins at forty."[30] A natural consequence has been the increase in diseases of old age, including senile dementia and cerebral arteriosclerosis. But many people fail to recognize another – probably more important – consequence of the prolongation of life. It is obvious that the framework of an individual biography and the general fabric of society must necessarily both be very different in a population according to whether the average human life is very short or very long. In a population in which the average human lifespan is generally short, an individual must choose his profession, complete his education, earn his living, and marry and start a family at an early age. In other words, he must become an adult at a point in his life when today's young people are still big babies. Those who wonder that Napoleon was already a great general at the age of twenty-five forget that such precocity was the rule at that time. The Great Condé was twenty-two when he won the Battle of Rocroi that broke Spanish domination. Lafayette married at fifteen; at twenty-one he was commander-in-chief of the French expeditionary forces in America. In short, everyone was expected to be an adult soon after the advent of puberty.

The prolongation of the average human life completely changed the framework of human biography, to the point of creating "a new human species" (Bouthoul). Adolescence in Europe today is now several years longer than it was two centuries ago, and it appears to be even longer in the United States. We enjoy a much more pleasant childhood and adolescence than our ancestors did, but at the same time, this long, protracted period of artificially maintained immaturity and irresponsibility may well be a principal cause of the extraordinary increase in juvenile delinquency. In any comparison between the psychopathology of a developed Western country and that of an underdeveloped country, one wonders to what extent the clinical differences observed are caused by a difference in the average lifespan.

(2) A second fact is the psycho-biological revolution determined in man by the *discovery of general anaesthesia* and the dissemination of analgesic medication. Today we take for granted that the simplest surgical operation must be performed under general or local anaesthesic. From the moment of our birth we are accustomed to take a sedative or analgesic as soon as we feel the slightest pain. Men have always tried to protect themselves from pain, but up to a century ago they had little success. Certainly they suffered much more than we do, but their tolerance for pain was far superior to ours. We can scarcely imagine how Napoleon's soldiers could undergo amputations outdoors, sitting on a drum and smoking a pipe. Even Louis XIV lived under conditions which would seem incredibly uncomfortable to us; he continued his work despite toothaches we would call excruciating. Our ancestors were very tough; they would call us ridiculously soft. This was probably not – as Leriche (1936) has pointed out – because they had more moral fortitude, but simply because their nervous systems were conditioned to pain in different way. For us, life is much more pleasant, and the prospect of severe pain is much more frightening to us than it was to our ancestors. Pain has been excluded from our daily lives, but it plays perhaps a more important role in our inner lives as a source of existential anxiety, hence of a certain form of neurosis.

(3) A third fact is the enormous *increase in stimulation* to which we are subjected. Over the last century or two, our Western culture has gradually increased the sources of sensory and psychological stimulation to which we are exposed, to a point that would have seemed unthinkable to our ancestors. Our children have been subjected to

obligatory schooling with broader and longer programs of study; they have children's books and magazines, toys, movies, radio, television, frequent travel, and a quantity of stimulation often amounting to psychic aggression against them. Because of the resulting neuroglandular stimulation and the different types of brain conditioning, our psycho-biological constitution is different from that of our ancestors. This is easy to recognize when one considers how people lived less than two centuries ago. Take, for instance, a novel such as Goethe's *Elective Affinities (Die Wahlverwandschaftern)* and try to visualize living like its protagonist. We would have found that life terribly boring. Conversely, our ancestors would have found our present way of life dangerously frenetic. Though we cannot be certain, it may be that our way of life has a traumatic effect on many individuals, especially in populations where this increase in stimulation has occurred rapidly in the course of one generation. There are reasons to suspect a direct correlation between the enormous increase in the quantity of mental stimulation and the increase in schizophrenia, which seems to be another characteristic of our culture.

Clearly, our Western culture has made discoveries that have changed the psycho-biological nature of Man, making him a modified species with a different psychopathology.

Descriptive and Clinical Part

The mental disorders studied in ethnopsychiatry may be divided into three groups:
(1) Mental diseases that have an organic cause.
(2) Mental diseases that have no known organic cause.
(3) Collective psychoses.[1]

MENTAL DISEASES OF ORGANIC CAUSE

Mental diseases of organic origin may be of interest to ethnopsychiatrists in that their frequency is influenced by certain mental attitudes of populations.

Example: In Guatemala, Cakchiquel children often suffer from diseases caused by malnutrition, but their parents refuse to believe that these diseases are caused by poor nutritional and blame them on evil spirits. This belief allows the disease to continue and at the same time relieves parents from any feelings of responsibility. (Dr Gustavo Castaneda,[2] Guatemala City, personal communication.)

Moreover, symptoms of organic diseases may be moulded or coloured by psychological factors or other cultural causes of unknown nature. This is sometimes the case for infectious diseases and even more so for intoxication.

(1) *Infectious and parasitic diseases.* We are not going to describe here diseases such as malaria, trypanosomiasis, leprosy, and so on. We shall only mention that in West Africa, according to Tooth (1950), many cases of trypanosomiasis among bush natives resemble schizophrenic syndromes. This is all the more surprising given

that the clinical aspects of schizophrenia in bush natives are rather undifferentiated, whereas schizophrenia among Blacks in cities has the same aspects as in Europeans.

(2) *Poisons deemed magic.* Poisons have played a considerable role in the history of mankind, as shown by Lewin in his well-known book *Die Gifte in der Weltgeschichte* (1920). For many centuries, the making and using of poisons was a secret knowledge held by a small number of initiates, and was also a branch of magic. The advent of the science of toxicology in the nineteenth century delivered humanity from its obsession with poisons and from the ancient fear of magic. Along with their very real empirical knowledge of the nature, preparation, and effectiveness of certain poisons, many sorcerers applied the secondary psychological effects of these drugs; it is highly likely that these effects could even cause death by pure psychic action, in other words, individuals died because they merely *believed* they had been poisoned. A veil of legends, some more fantastic than others, was wrapped around the main poisons, which ethnopsychiatry cannot separate from the study of their purely pharmacological effects.

In Mexico in the sixteenth century, the conquistadors were shocked to learn that Aztec sorcerers possessed powerful magic drugs that could produce all kinds of extraordinary effects. This mysterious knowledge was suppressed, along with magic itself, and driven into remote areas. The German pharmacologist Victor Reko, a professor at the School of Medicine in Mexico City, conducted long and difficult study of these magic poisons; he managed to find, isolate, and identify a number of them, and described them in his book *Magische Gifte* (1936).

Ololiuqui is said to produce a particular kind of intoxication, accompanied by a clear-sightedness, hence its use as an "oracle beverage" by the Zapotecs, or as a "truth-drug," given that while under its effects an individual is considered unable to keep a secret.

Ayahuasca, or the "beverage of weird dreams," is supposed to create a state of intoxication with intense visual and auditory hallucinations, with visions of spirits and ghosts.

Prolonged use of *sinicuichi*, the "drug of oblivion," produces a loss of memory of recent facts, together with a hypermnesia for experiences far in the past. Remote memories are vividly revived as if they were being experienced for the first time.

Colorines paralyze the muscles and destroy willpower while producing a distinctive psychic excitement accompanied by dizziness and cutaneous hypersensitivity. Blood pressure rises tremendously so that a cerebral hemorrhage may easily occur in individuals who are predisposed, and the victim, who has been poisoned for revenge, may thus die with every appearance of a natural death.

Xomil-xihuite, or "crystal coffin," is the name given to a drug that is said to paralyze an individual while leaving him conscious, so that he lucidly witnesses his own death without being able to give any sign to his family and friends.

Camotillo is said to be the most dreaded of all poisons because of its delayed action. An individual who absorbs it remains in perfect health for several weeks, then gradually plunges into a twilight state, showing complete indifference. After some weeks of slowly worsening, the individual suddenly dies of paralysis and suffocation. Indians maintain that the sorcerer can regulate the administration of this drug in such a way that he determines the exact day the victim will die.

But all magic poisons are not so dismal, and some are even useful, such as *cohombrillo* and *eyosod*, both of which rapidly counteract the effects of intoxication due to alcohol or other narcotics.

The Mexican Indians called a group of drugs that produce the appearance of insanity, at least temporarily, *toloache*; intoxicated by these, an individual behaved ridiculously and was scoffed at by those who had offered him the drug.

Other magic poisons described by Reko include *marijuana*, a product made from Indian hemp, which is widely known in Mexico and the United States, and *peyote* (or *peyotl*), which has also become renowned for the ever-changing and coloured hallucinations it produces, and which Mexican sorcerers knew how to use. Recall that among North American Indians, a religion of peyote has been founded, whose adherents take this drug ritually in order to produce visions that are believed to be revelations of divinity.

Let us finally mention the mushroom that Reko calls *nanácatl* or *Amanita mexicana*. It is perhaps the same mushroom that, under the name of *Psilocybe Mexicana*, has been the subject of recent studies and has entered experimental pharmacology. However, *nanácatl* is not used only for religious or magic purposes, as proved by the strange anecdote told by Reko (1936, 127). A young Indian woman was admitted to a Mexican psychiatric hospital following a state of

manic excitement that rapidly subsided. However, it was observed
that each visit from her family was followed by an unusual state of
aggression. It was eventually discovered that the patient had a little
box containing a dried vegetable product; the Biological Institute
declared it to be fragments of *Amanita mexicana*, and the mystery
was solved.

Reko has been criticized for describing his "magic poisons" in
insufficiently scientific, indeed rather journalistic ways. He did in
fact dwell quite deliberately on the exaggerated or even absurd
properties attributed to certain drugs. He did so because those properties, even when imaginary from a purely pharmacological point
of view, were part of the myths[3] surrounding these drugs and thus
contributed to their clinical effects to a degree that should be neither
exaggerated nor underestimated.

(3) *Habituation poisons.* This huge field, on which a great deal of
medical literature exists, cannot be entered into here. We will merely
indicate in what respects this subject concerns ethnopsychiatry.

The first aspect concerns the *cause of the impulse that drives one
to take the poison,* and the effect expected by those who take it.
As shown by Félice (1936), who compiled the works of previous
authors, most of today's addictions are ancient in origin and, in the
beginning, were means to obtain "religious intoxication" in primitive populations (*kava,* hashish, peyote, tobacco, alcoholic drinks),
or "divine intoxication" in Indo-European populations (the *soma* of
the Hindus, Dionysiac intoxications, and so on). To this day, peyote is used as a sacred substance in the peyote religion of North
American Indians and tobacco is smoked ritually during certain
Indian ceremonies and in some Brazilian sects. As for hashish, it
is well-known how it was used by the "Order of Assassins" in the
Middle East in the eleventh century (Lewin, 1920, 207–14). Around
1880, Kalamba, king of the Baluba in the Congo, established in his
kingdom the Religion of Hashish. Other examples could be mentioned. For a long time, the majority of poisons have been available
to the layman; they have become a part of social habits and individual ways and customs. Often as well, a drug is meant to alleviate
misery and make life a little less intolerable. Sometimes it is more or
less imposed upon individuals who use it.

Such is the case, for instance, among Indians in the mountainous
provinces of Peru. Most of them are *mestizos,* in whom Indian blood

predominates. Also, most of them speak the language of their ancestors, *Quechua*, but heavily infiltrated with Spanish words; they are ashamed of this language and in the presence of strangers pretend not to understand it, thus revealing the deep feelings of inferiority prevailing in these populations since the loss of their national independence. These peasants live poorly on infertile land, which they cultivate with outdated methods. Water is scarce, and sources of water are fought over in numerous lawsuits. Housing and clothing are miserable, and food is insufficient – low in protein and consisting mainly of starches. Working conditions are such that these Indians are paid partly in coca, tobacco, and alcohol. In order to understand the tremendous importance of coca for Indians, one has to keep in mind this social, economic, and cultural background. The coca leaf, chewed by the workman, eases his fatigue and his hunger, breaks the monotony of the endless work, and helps him to establish human contact, despite his sadness – in short, it makes life a little less unbearable (Aliaga-Lindo, 1959).

The second aspect concerns the *description of religious or social rites and ceremonies, and the ways and customs associated with the use of addictive poisons,* as well as the multitude of beliefs related to these drugs. This topic has been treated in a great number of detailed studies, but there have been very few general surveys for substances such as opium and alcohol. The ethnological literature offers a number of general surveys on the diffusion of certain varieties of alcoholic drinks and on customs associated with their consumption (Crawley, 1931), and there are some very incomplete psychiatric studies on the clinical forms of alcoholism among the various populations of the world. It will be a long time before sufficient data become available to conduct a valid comparative study of alcoholism and other commonly used addictive poisons. The most indisputable fact is that, much as with magic poisons, the effect of addictive poisons cannot be investigated separately from the beliefs, myths, and folklore related to them, and it is often difficult to distinguish between the clinical effects of a poison and the part played by collective autosuggestion arising from the beliefs.

This fact applies even to the most common of intoxicating drugs, which is alcohol. When a man gets drunk, he not only experiences the physiological effects of alcohol but also plays the role of the intoxicated man, as learned from example, habit, the behaviour of his friends, and the entire cultural tradition. A curious example has been observed by M. Leenhardt (personal communication). The Kanaks of New Caledonia were ignorant of alcoholic beverages, which they learned about from Europeans only recently. Around 1890, in a remote area, a few Kanaks who had seen the behaviour of white people when they got drunk decided to act like them. They got a table, and some chairs and glasses, and started to drink water, imitating the attitudes of white people. Very soon they became so drunk that there was a scuffle, their hut was set on fire, and the police had to intervene. The same incident was reported by Félice (1947, 24). Some sober observers who joined in drinking parties in our countries without drinking anything themselves assure us that it is at times very difficult to avoid a state of intoxication through psychic contagion. This same psychic factor explains the possibility of collective delusions during intoxication; such delusions are probably more frequent at drinking parties held according to well-defined rites, such as those of the ancient Greeks. Athenaeus relates, in his *Banquet of the Learned* (II:37), the story of a group of young people in Agrigento who, after getting drunk together, believed they were in a ship shaken by a storm, and threw out all the furniture from the windows of the house. The next morning, they persisted in their collective delusion. It is not yet possible to evaluate precisely the role of cultural factors in the semiology of effects produced by this absorption of addictive poisons.

The third aspect relates to the *clinical effects produced by the said poisons* in various populations. Take the example of a poison absorbed by millions of human beings: Indian hemp. Are there specific hemp and hashish psychoses? That is, are there psychopathological conditions specific to people who become intoxicated with these poisons? Some authors claim not only that hashish psychoses exist but also that they are very common. Dhunjibhoy (1930) describes three forms of hashish psychosis: one is acute excitement with visual and auditory hallucinations, aggressiveness, and complete amnesia after the attack; another is prolonged mania with euphoria; and the third is terminal dementia. Chevers described a rare variety of hashish psychosis, characterized by a complete loss of speech for a long period of time. One of Dhunjibhoy's patients remained in this condition for eight years, after which he recovered the faculty of speech, at which point he explained that he had understood every word uttered in his presence during those eight years without being able to utter a word himself. Other authors claim that among the effects attributed to hemp, many are conditioned by the personality of the patient and the culture to which he belongs. In a critical study on the subject, H.B.M. Murphy (1963) concluded that the specific syndromes probably exist but are not common, and that consequently the clinical effects of Indian hemp remain insufficiently known.

Another problem we shall mention only briefly is that of the *choice of poison*. Why did Western populations adopt, as their main addictive poison, alcohol; Chinese people, opium; and Hindus and the inhabitants of Asia Minor, hemp and its derivatives? Some authors seem to draw an analogy between the effects of opium and the philosophy of Confucius, between the effects of alcohol and the activist philosophy of Europe and North America, and so on. It will be a long time before such hypotheses can be elaborated upon.

(4) *Diseases of unknown origin*. At this point, two clinical entities whose causes remain mysterious must be mentioned: *kuru* of New Guinea, and *bangungut* of the Philippines.

Kuru seems to exist solely in the Fore tribe in the Eastern Highlands of New Guinea, which were explored only in 1932 and were opened to white visitors only in 1949. The Fore people number between 10,000 and 15,000; they are the only group in which *kuru* is known to exist. The disease occurs so frequently among them that Zigas and Gajduseck (1957) were able to count about one hundred cases; they provide not only a clinical description of the disease but also the results of some autopsies. The illness starts like a locomotor ataxia, soon followed by trepidation of the trunk, limbs, and head and athetoid movements. The patient's emotional condition is seriously disturbed; he has spells of uncontrollable laughter, alternating with states of severe depression and aggressiveness. Then paralysis progresses and the patient dies from intercurrent complications. The few post-mortem examinations performed so far show a diffuse degeneration of the brain and of the extrapyramidal system as well as various other lesions of the nerve centres. No treatment is effective, and the patient always dies within six to nine months. Berndt (1958) pointed out that the illness develops in a highly unique atmosphere in which belief in sorcery exists alongside a kind of conditioning so that when an individual is affected by it, the illness follows a predetermined pattern governed by collective beliefs. Mitscherlich (1958) voiced the hypothesis that it is a psychogenic illness, which he compares to psychogenic death with acute progression as encountered in certain peoples. It appears very difficult to reconcile this hypothesis with the very serious and precise lesions found in the autopsy and the fact that to date kuru has only been observed in the Fore tribe or in individuals of other tribes who have a Fore among their ancestors, which makes one think of a genetic factor.

Another syndrome with as yet unexplained origins is known in the Philippines as *bangungut*. It is also rife among Filipinos working in Hawaii. According to the descriptions offered by Majoska (1948) and Stalcruz (1951), the syndrome is found only in men between twenty and forty years old, who appear to be in good health and most of whom are manual workers or unskilled labourers. Most often, the individual dies in the night; he had complained of nothing the previous evening, except sometimes of slight abdominal pain; in the night he could be heard moaning or groaning, and then he was found dead. Popular belief blames the death on a nightmare. The few autopsies performed to date have revealed nothing specific except, in some cases, an acute hemorrhagic pancreatitis; it is debated whether this should be viewed as a cause or an effect of *bangungut*.

MENTAL DISEASES THAT HAVE NO KNOWN ORGANIC CAUSE

Morbid Reactions

Depressive reactions. One of the most frequently discussed issues in ethnopsychiatry is the frequency and forms of mental depression among different peoples.

Some authors claim that mental depression is very rare in primitive peoples. Kraepelin (1904) noted the rarity of depression in Java. Carothers (1947) in Kenya, Laubscher (1937) among the Tembu in South Africa, and Stainbrook (1952) in Bahia found that depressions are far less frequent among populations of the black race than among Europeans and North Americans. Other authors think that depression in primitive peoples is no less frequent but either is not seen by European doctors, or is not recognized due to the atypical symptoms, or is short-lived (due to certain customs that have a cathartic effect or to effective intervention by native doctors).

In reality, it appears that depressive reaction can take several different forms and that the severity, length, and nature of the symptoms are determined by cultural factors.

(1) *Depression* in primitive peoples is distinguished, it appears, by the enormous influence of suggestion both in its genesis and in healing practices. Depression, here, often presents itself in violent and dramatic forms – intense grief or sorrow but open to rapid abre-action. At other times, however, depression is marked by a gloomy apathy, to the point that the subject allows himself to die unless there is an intervention. Native doctors are often a more effective interve-nors than white doctors. Another feature consists in the absence or slight intensity of *feelings of guilt*.

There is abundant literature on customs that have a cathartic effect on depression, mainly regarding the mourning customs of various peoples (theatrical grief, funeral cries and songs, hired mourners, funeral meals, mourning clothing, and so on). Sometimes people lose sight of the fact that these mourning behaviours can go too far, thereby shedding any therapeutic benefit. Mourning customs in Corsica, for example (Stephanopoli, 1950), with their concerts of cries and sobbing by the women in the family and the neigh-bourhood, their improvised funeral songs (a *ballata* or a *vocero* depending on whether the defunct died a natural death or a violent one), their rigorous and quasi-eternal mourning imposed upon the widow, and so on, in no way leave the impression that these customs have beneficial effects. In other peoples, we sometimes find reactions that are downright destructive (to the point of suicidal). As we will see later with regard to aggressive reactions, among some peoples homicidal reactions provoked by psychic pain have been noted.

Native doctors' actions can be illustrated by the practice of the Navajos, one of the best-preserved and best-known indigenous groups in North America. They are known for their weaving, their sand painting in various colours, their music, their mythology, which is as rich and complex as that of the ancient Greeks, and their religious ceremonies, during which their artistic talents are given free reign. Ethnologists assure us that mental illness is practically unknown among the Navajos, and they attribute this to the cathar-tic and preventative influence of the rites and ceremonies through which their shamans deliver sufferers promptly from their fears and obsessions (Coolidge and Roberts, 1930, 152). A Navajo falls easily into mental depression following a bad dream or when he believes he has met a ghost or offended a sacred animal. When this happens, the shaman heals the patient through a simple and brief magic rite; however, if the depression is more serious he will resort to one of the great ceremonies such as the "Nine-Day Chant" (Matthews, 1902), which involves an extremely complex ritual that includes coloured sand paintings recounting the history of the creation of the world and the history of the Navajo gods. Through this ritual the patient is reconciled with the powers he offended and is gradually reinstated in his family, clan, and people as well as the universe of his gods.

(2) Among peoples of the Middle East there existed a different form of depression. According to Staehelin (1955), we can find remarkably literal expressions of the most intense *melancholy* among the Sumerians, the Egyptians, and the Hebrews. However, it is unlikely that these were true melancholics who were able to express themselves in that way (our current melancholics, at least, would be incapable of giving such poetic expression to their sufferings). Staehelin thinks that among the ancient peoples of the Middle East,[4] serious physical diseases were accompanied by a deep conviction that the sufferers were being punished for sins against the gods (from which there arose the possibility of healing through reconciliation with the offended gods). Staehelin added that in the present day even the melancholic who is furthest removed from the idea of God is often open to the idea that his sufferings are part of a whole that is governed by the great loves of Nature (as are, for example, night, winter, old age, and death), that these are not an absurd things in a chaotic world but belong in one way or another to the order of the Universe.

(3) In Greco-Roman antiquity, in the Christian Middle Ages, and until quite late in modern times there existed a form of psychotherapy for depressive reactions that would seem incomprehensible to most of our contemporaries: *consolatio*.[5] It was a kind of philosophical exhortation addressed to a distressed friend, explaining to him, for example, that suffering and death are inevitable and are the lot of everyone, that there is no point in rebelling against the inevitable, and so on. Little by little, *consolatio* became a literary genre in verse and in prose and was sometimes even addressed to oneself (as in Boethius's *Philosophiae consolatio*); one of the last examples and perhaps the most beautiful is *Consolation à Monsieur Du Périer*[6] by Malherbe. This literary genre would not have flourished had *consolatio* not originally been a form of psychotherapy that was applied, apparently effectively, to a depressed individual by his dearest friends.

(4) Today we no longer conceive of a psychotherapy of melancholy through contemplation of the laws of nature or through philosophical exhortation. Staehelin believed that modern-day feelings of guilt

are vestiges (that are now diminishing) of the intense conviction of being punished for one's sins – feelings that distressed patients in Middle East, a culture saturated with religion. Most of our classic psychiatry textbooks continue to indicate that the presence of guilt feelings is an essential sign of mental depression; however, some research indicates that the frequency of these guilt feelings varies from one individual, place, and time period to the next.

Ruffin (1957) observed clergymen suffering from melancholy: those among them who, in a normal state, showed rigid and severe piety suffered, after becoming melancholy, from intense feelings of guilt. The reverse was true for clergymen who, in a normal state, were inclined toward indulgence and optimism. Ruffin added that melancholy was more often accompanied by feelings of guilt in southwestern Germany than in the middle of the country, where, by contrast, delusional ideas on themes other than guilt were more frequent.

Andreas von Orelli (1954) conducted a statistical study on the content of delusional ideas among melancholics hospitalized at the Clinique psychiatrique universitare in Basel from 1878 to 1952. He noted that during those seventy-five years, a steady decrease in delusional ideas on the theme of guilt was observed, especially in relation to religious themes (sinning against God or religious laws); this decrease was more marked in Catholic patients than in Protestant ones. Yet over the same period, there was an increase in ideas of inferiority and, to a slighter degree, hypochondriac ideas.

The Book of Job serves as an excellent example of a depressive reaction treated successfully in a people of the Middle East (Ellenberger, 1959).

A wealthy and happy man, Job was plunged from one day to the next into misfortune. Messengers came to inform him that he had lost all his assets and all his children. He immediately gave way to an emotional abreaction: he tore his clothing and covered his head with ashes. Then a second blow struck: he came down with ulcers, which added horrible physical suffering to the previous emotional suffering. Job sat on a heap of ashes, plunged into sorrow, but avoided cursing God, thus being very careful not to exceed the limits of a healthy abreaction. Job did not understand how he, a fair man, could be struck this way by God. Eliphaz, Bildad, and Zofar, his three friends, came to him then to engage in a kind of multiple therapy. First, they sat close to him and remained silent for seven days and seven nights, showing him that they shared his suffering and establishing emotional contact with him. Then the discussion began on the meaning of his misfortune: each of the three friends spoke in turn and presented arguments to Job, some of which resembled those later contained in the Greek and Roman "consolations." Job answered them each time, and as he was a strong dialectician, his friends soon ran out of arguments, at which point a fourth, Elihu, intervened without any more success. Then God spoke from atop a cloud, playing the role of "great consultant." He raised the debate by describing the marvels of nature and the mysteries of Providence. Job, convinced, yielded unconditionally, so to speak, and accepted his fate. At that moment he was healed, and had only to proceed with a sacrifice that we may consider as "act of completion" (to use Janet's expression). The entire disease had scarcely lasted two weeks.

Diffuse aggressive reactions. These are violent impulses that suddenly take hold of an individual after a preliminary period of depression. The violence can turn outward or against the individual himself. When the subject has a weapon within reach, he may use it to strike, wound, or kill people nearby, or turn it on himself. Once the crisis has passed, he no longer remembers what happened.

Among other examples of such reactions, we note those that have been incorrectly called *hysteria of the Pacific*. Goldie describes these as follows:

> The patient, after a preliminary period of depression, suddenly falls into a state of violent excitement. He grabs a knife or some weapon, dashes throughout the village, slashing everyone he meets and causing endless damage until he ends up dropping, exhausted. If he has not found a knife, he may rush toward the reef, plunge into the water and swim for miles until he is either rescued or drowned. This state of violent hysterical excitement is common to all the islands, as well as the opposite state of sudden deep depression. (Goldie, 1904, 81)

Such impulses are not found solely among primitive people. In the late seventeenth century, two English doctors, Stubles and Oliver, described a morbid condition, today essentially forgotten, which they referred to as calenture. For a long time it was considered a special disease of sailors. Boissier de Sauvages described it in his *Nosologie méthodique* (1770–71) as "a disease that suddenly strikes patients into a frenzied delirium. It ordinarily attacks people who travel in scorching climates under the equinoctial line. This frenzy is violent, especially at night, when the ship is enclosed on all sides and all the heat is concentrated in it. It erupts suddenly, and several patients throw themselves into the sea with no one noticing." Calenture was a prominent aspect of naval medicine in the eighteenth century, and it is often discussed in works about navigation and travel of that era. Sometimes it took the form of an epidemic. British authors sometimes called it "the horrors."

Boudin (1857, vol. 2) gives many examples of it. A ship tried to enter the Senegal River when about thirty men, all struck with calenture, including the surgeon on board, threw themselves into the ocean, where they perished. In 1823, on the brig *Le Lynx*, near Cádiz, eighteen sailors out of seventy-five succumbed to it. Boudin himself witnessed an epidemic in 1829 on the *Duquesne*, stationed in Rio de Janeiro. The sailors, as many as twenty at a time, were struck "with extraordinary instantaneity," often in their sleep, became incoherent and furious, feeling themselves devoured by a burning fire or pursued by ghosts armed with glowing brands. They tried to rush into the water, assaulting and biting people who tried to stop them; convalescence took a long time.

Various other aggressive reactions, more lethal, were considered to be frequent among the Turks. A British traveller, Henri Barkley (1876, 240), describes seeing Turks several times, on the streets of Constantinople, struck by frenzied delirium, running and striking passersby with knives. He observed one of these individuals as he grew tired; his run turned into a walk, then he collapsed in a corner with a hangdog expression. Barkley thought these fits were often feigned, but they resulted in casualties nevertheless. At that time, in Constantinople, serious criminality was frequent and almost always unpunished.

Sometimes, crises of aggressive impulsiveness were governed by well-defined motivations. Roth, in his work about Sarawak (1896, vol. 2, 100), recounted the story of a Mohammedan of the region who, having lost his two grandchildren, found comfort in going off to massacre a tribe of harmless savages. Clark Wissler (1912, 32) wrote that when a Blackfoot realized he was suffering from an incurable disease, he took up his weapons and tried to kill as many people as he could. This is why, when a Blackfoot was suffering from a serious disease, every effort was made to conceal his condition from him until he was close to death. Wissler believed that this Blackfoot

custom was a relic of the old tradition of going on the "warpath."
He found the same custom among the Teton with the difference that
here, the patient would kill only one other man. Denig, cited by
Ruth Benedict (1932), stated that among the Assiniboine the loss of
a child was experienced by the father in such a cruel way that anyone who offended him at that time would be certainly killed by him,
as he sought to find comfort by taking the "warpath."

In these last cases we see the beginnings of a ceremonialization of
crises of aggressive impulsiveness. This ceremonialization is far more
extensive in other forms of crises, which we will now examine.

Ceremonialized aggressive reactions. In diffuse aggressive crises, tradition, custom, and social factors play a role. In calenture, a disease
generally attributed to heatstroke, psychic imitation and contagion
are important factors. In some Indian groups, the homicidal impulses
provoked by mourning were more or less modelled on war customs.
We now come to cases where the aggressive impulse is channelled by
social factors and conforms to a model rigorously defined by tradition, which gives it the aspect of a specific morbid condition. Such
was the "fury of the berserks" of the old Scandinavians, and such is
still the "running *amok*" of the Malay.

The fury of the berserks (*Berserkerwut* in German) is no more
than a memory of history, but it is still of great theoretical interest. It is likely that the *harii* among the ancient Germans, described
by Tacitus were a sort of furious people who smeared their faces,
shrieked, and committed acts of violence that were identical to those
of the Scandinavian berserks. The chroniclers of the Middle Ages,
in turn, spoke of warriors stricken with *furor teutonicus*. But it is
mainly old Icelandic texts that inform us about the berserks. The
descriptions vary across the centuries, and it is likely that the word
berserk changed in meaning throughout that time. Among the many
works on this subject, we mention those of Hermann Güntert (l912),
Martin Ninck (1935, 1937), and J.D. Scriptor (1935).

The original berserks were especially courageous warriors and
dear to Odin, the god of war. They were struck, on certain occasions,
by fits of fury: they would begin to howl horribly, showing their teeth
and foaming at the mouth, while their eyes turned in their sockets
and shone with thunderous brightness. They threw themselves on
anything nearby, uprooted trees, demolished dwellings, and bit their
shields while stamping their feet. When the crisis took hold during

a battle, they became practically invincible and killed great numbers of enemies. During certain crises they sometimes walked on fire or swallowed hot coals without burning themselves. The berserks often lived in groups, which were especially dreaded.

In later writings, the berserks were described as solitary individuals who sowed terror among sedentary populations. A berserk would provoke a rich landowner, demanding that he immediately hand over all his property. If the landowner refused, the berserk provoked him into a fight in which his strength almost inevitably gave him the advantage. The height of heroism for an ordinary man was to defeat a berserk. Apparently, the berserks degenerated into common bandits and disappeared after that part of the world was Christianized. What distinguished the furor of the berserks from an ordinary fit of fury was the subjective side. It was said that the berserk believed himself to have been transformed into a wolf or some other ferocious animal that tore to pieces anything that got in his way.

Several opinions have been expressed on the nature of the fury of the berserks:

(1) Some have suggested that these fits of fury were artificially provoked by alcohol or by a mushroom in the *Amanita* family. It is not impossible that this was sometimes the case, but it is hard to imagine the berserks resorting to this behaviour during a battle or an unexpected naval battle like the ones the Sagas mention so often.

(2) According to another theory, the fury of the berserk was a special case of a more widespread phenomenon known as "holy furor." Through a kind of autosuggestion, an individual would ignite within himself all his energy, imagining himself suddenly filled with superhuman, divine, and destructive strength, often accompanied by a sense of invulnerability. According to Victor Bérard (1928), the same phenomenon was found in ancient Greece, represented by the anger of Achilles, the furies of Ajax, and many other mythological tales. The exploits of Samson killing a thousand Philistines with the jawbone of a donkey, and those of other heroes of the classic Middle East, belong to the same category.

(3) According to Dumézil (1939), the berserks were simply gangs of young people who in Germanic societies rebelled violently against the social conservatism of their elders. (We could almost say that it was an institutionalized form of juvenile delinquency.)

These theories are not incompatible. The fits of fury, with their subjective state determined by religious beliefs, were a form of social

behaviour dictated by the people surrounding those afflicted. The
berserks were not simply feared – they were also tolerated, even
admired, and if need be they were used against the enemy. This was
therefore a means of discharging aggression that for a long time
remained socially accepted and ceremonialized.

Running *amok* was a famous manifestation of "exotic psychiatry."
Abundant and ancient literature exists on this topic, going back to
the first written accounts of the Portuguese explorers of India and
the Malay Archipelago. Metzger (1887) and Stoll (1904), summariz-
ing earlier authors, presented the history of *amok* and indicated that
it probably originated in southern India. By the early sixteenth century, travellers there were noting the existence of *amuco*, or a furious
crisis cast as carrying out a vow to God. A man named Correa,
quoted by Metzger, tells how during the war between Calicut and
Cochin (1503), two hundred followers of the defeated Prince of
Cochin shaved their heads and eyebrows, kissed one another, and
became *amucos*, then disappeared among the troops and population
of Calicut to kill at random as many men, women, and children as
they could until they themselves were killed. In other circumstances,
a debtor who was going to be sold by his creditor preferred to die
a hero than live in slavery, and got himself killed by killing as many
men as possible. It was only later that similar accounts were provided from the Malay Archipelago.

The French traveller Tavernier (1717) recounts that he himself
with two companions was attacked, during a stay in Batavia, by a
man who was running *amok*:

> Behind the palisades there hid a Bantamois, newly come from
> Mecca who was upon the design of *Moqua*, that is, in their
> language, when the rascality of the Mahometans return from
> Mecca, they presently pick up an ax, a kind of Poniard, with a
> half-poisoned blade, with which they run through the streets, and
> kill all those which are not of the Mahometan law, till they be
> killed themselves. These fanatics think they are serving God and
> Mohammed by having enemies of his law die this way, and that
> in doing so, they will be saved. As soon as they are killed, all the
> Mahometan rabble buries them like Saints, and each contributes
> to make them a fine grave. Often, there are a few big beggars
> who dress up as dervishes and makes a hut near the grave, which
> they take care to keep clean and on which they scatter flowers.

As people give alms, they add an ornament, because the more beautiful the grave is, the more devotion and holiness there is, the more the alms increase.

Boissier de Sauvages, in his *Nosologie méthodique* (1770–71), blamed opium for this display, which he referred to as "Indian demonomania" or "rage of Hamuck." He provided the following description:

The Negro Indians abuse opium punishingly to give themselves intrepidity and daring, to commit homicides; when bored of life and the insults afflicted upon them, they devote themselves to death, taking revenge, dipping their hands in enemy blood: these people eat opium to arouse their imagination, cloud their reason, and to become animated to the point of appearing in public with a dagger in hand, like rabid tigers, in order to kill everyone they meet, friend or enemy, until they fall, choking. This course of action, quite ordinary among the inhabitants of Java and more eastern lands, is called *hamuck*. Anyone who hears this name uttered shudders in horror; for anyone who sees a homicide, cries aloud *Hamuck* to warn anyone who is unarmed to take flight, and to keep themselves safe, while those who are armed, and are courageous, must come forward to kill this beast.

In the nineteenth century, *amok* was spoken of as a phenomenon specific to Java and the Malay countries. We could probably extract a strange anthology of the abundant literature, much of it written in Dutch, that exists on *amok*. One of the best-known descriptions was given by the naturalist Alfred Russel Wallace in 1869. He distinguished an individual form and a collective form. The latter sometimes appeared in times of war, when soldiers decided to "run *amok*":

They devoted themselves to death and charged the enemy with uncontrollable fury. The individual form was particularly frequent on the island of Celebes. In Macassar there are said to be one or two running amoks a month on the average, and five, ten, or twenty persons are sometimes killed or wounded at one of them. It is an honourable way of committing suicide among the natives of Celebes, and of escaping from their difficulties.

Emil Metzger (1887) believed that the frequency of *amok* in the Malay Archipelago varied by racial group, reaching its height among the Bugi of Celebes, a people known for their dangerously aggressive temperament. Metzger related *amok* to Malays' predisposition to commit collective murder. A person who ran *amok* used a bladed weapon; firearms were reserved for murder. The cause almost always involved a woman, typically a dancer or a prostitute. Sometimes humiliation was involved, in which case the *amok* was preceded by a period of rumination that could last from a few days to a few weeks. According to Metzger, the subject only intended to kill one person, but as soon as he began running, he lost all control of his actions. During the crisis, he displayed extraordinary strength and persistence; however, he sometimes collapsed suddenly for no apparent reason. On regaining consciousness (if he had not been killed), he declared that he was *mata glap* (that is, his eyes had grown dark). Metzger added that when the *amok* occurred without apparent motivation, mental illness was likely to manifest itself soon after.

Gilmore Ellis (1893), the senior doctor at the Singapore mental hospital, wrote that in the early nineteenth century *amok* was so common throughout Malaysia that the people of a village would keep a long pole ending in a fork with which to immobilize the maniac, after which he was almost always killed. If he survived, the Rajah decided his fate, generally taking him for a slave. If the *amok* was an influential man, he could redeem himself for a sum of money. According to Ellis, the incidence of *amok* decreased a great deal in British Malaysia after the colonial authorities decided to treat these individuals as criminals. Among the usual causes of *amok*, Ellis lists a wife's infidelity, gambling losses, a more or less imagined insult suffered by the subject, mourning, and sometimes the sight of blood. Running *amok* was sometimes preceded by a period of mental rumination called *sakit-hati*, comparable to the sulking of a badly raised child, which could last as long as five days, though in some circumstances it spontaneously disappeared. Running *amok* was sometimes a consequence of malaria.

Rasch (1894, 1895) insisted that suggestion and autosuggestion played a role in *amok*, which would explain why it was virtually endemic in certain regions. During the fit, the individual had a troubled conscience; he saw everything in red or black, which did not prevent him from striking his blows with a great deal of agility. The existence of *amok* was explainable by the Malay character, which was inclined to depression and to heroic bravery.

Van Brero (1897), director of the Buitenzorg mental hospital in Java, wrote that out of thirty-nine insane criminals confined to his mental hospital, eight had run *amok*. He too explained *amok* by the Malay character and national customs. Malaysians, he wrote, were both hypersensitive to minor suffering and remarkably tolerant of physical pain. They had little self-control, attached little value to human life, and were always armed. For these reasons, the carnage, wounds, and mutilations produced during running *amok* were horrifying. Doctors called to the scene were so busy caring for the wounded that they didn't have time to deal with the *amok* runner or to examine his mental state after the crisis.

Van Loon (1926–27) insisted that *amok* was frequently caused by infections such as malaria and syphilis. Epilepsy scarcely played a role; none of the epileptics known to Van Loon had had an *amok* episode. The subjective state, during running *amok*, was a kind of acute confusion, an agony of terror during which the patient, hallucinating, imagined he was being attacked by a tiger, a snake, or a human enemy. Van Loon added that while the customary reaction of a Malaysian who felt frightened was to grab his weapon, often the runner simply ran away or threw himself into water. Acts of aggression often began only when he encountered obstacles. Sometimes the subject turned his rage against himself in the form of suicide, self-castration, or some other form of mutilation. Sometimes he stripped naked, broke everything, or set fire to the house. The two main causes of *amok* were Malaysians' general absence of self-control and their deep-rooted habit of always having a knife within reach.

According to Van Wulfften Palthe (1933, 1948), *amok* was a psychogenic illness that developed under the effect of conflicts that appeared unsolvable, particularly of a sexual nature or that resulted from difficulties experienced by an individual in a new setting. Following an incident, a "period of meditation" began, with narrowing of the field of consciousness, during which the individual often recited to himself texts that he knew and was overcome with emotion. These overflowed suddenly and unfolded according to a preformed pattern. *Amok* was found elsewhere in Java, among the Chinese and the Arabs, but never among Malaysians living in Holland and never among Europeans. Indeed, Europeans easily expressed and released their feelings, while Malaysians inhibited them completely until the moment they burst forth like an avalanche.

Van Wulfften Palthe provided one of the very rare precise observations that medical literature possesses of an *amok* runner. One day, Ali Moesa (pronounced Moussa), the servant of a Chinese family, grabbed a shotgun and used it to kill his master and his master's wife; he then attacked the other inhabitants of the house, seriously wounding three girls with the butt of the gun before shooting one of them in the back, who soon died. A police officer who tried to stop him was shot in the stomach. After an all-out pursuit, Ali Moesa found himself cornered behind the house, where he shot himself in the head, but it was only a superficial wound. After a few hours, he regained consciousness and stated he remembered nothing. He was then transferred to the psychiatric hospital.

During the examination, Ali Moesa gave the impression of being an intelligent and polite young man, superior to the social stratum into which he had been born. He presented an amnesia that extended from the day before the running *amok* until he awoke in the hospital. Except for that, his mental faculties seemed normal, and he had no difficulty telling his story. The son of a poor peasant from Bantam, he had been placed at a young age as a servant to Europeans, had acquired a taste for their way of life, and had entered into the service of a wealthy Chinese man in Batavia. There he lived well above his means, dressing elegantly in European style, attending football games and boxing matches, going to the movies, and seeking to attract the admiration of his young companions as well as that of his family, who remained in the countryside. He ended up going into debt and owed his master a large amount of money.

One evening, the master called for his bath earlier than usual. Ali Moesa was at a football game. He was called by another servant and showed up late. After sharply reprimanding him, his master fired him on the spot. Ali found himself without a job, without money, and deep in debt. His only recourse was to return to his family, to whom he felt far superior. At that time, according to his account, he felt overwhelmed by his thoughts, experiencing dizziness and troubled vision. He thought he was dishonoured and that it would be better to kill himself by cutting off his genitals. He wrote a brief message, then felt sleep overcome him and his eyes grow dark. At that point he fell, and remembered nothing more of what followed until he woke up in the hospital. The investigation showed, however, that he had gone outside to have a meal and then got a large knife, which he took into his room. He continued to ruminate, slept from one until five in the morning, and then the tragedy began: he entered the room of his masters, and there, inexplicably, exchanged his knife for a shotgun he saw hanging on the wall, killed his masters point blank, and then indiscriminately attacked the servants and other inhabitants of the house. The farewell letter, quite confused, written in Malay, alluded to the war between China and Japan and contained curses against his master. It was accompanied by a drawing in which he depicted himself, a knife in hand, his genitals exposed, and his name written on his chest.

Van Wulfften Palthe concludes by insisting on the role of Malaysian customs and saying that *amok* must be understood as a rite. "The population has sacred respect for *amok* runners. Certainly, they try to kill them during their crises, but not as criminals."

Van Bergen (1953, 1955) pointed out the deep affinities between *amok* and *latah*, two conditions typical among Malaysians, the first among the men, the second among the women. Though very different externally, both presuppose a similar mental attitude. Among the Malay, writes Van Bergen, the emotionally "static" attitude predominates as opposed to the "dynamic" attitude of Europeans. The Malaysian is less capable than the European of distinguishing between subject and object; that is why he only perceives of the outside world what is reflected in the moment of his state of mind, and why he projects his emotions outside himself. The complexes accumulate in their active state beyond the threshold of consciousness and can manifest themselves, depending on the case, as *amok* or as *latah*. The typical situation of a man who runs *amok* is that of an individual who, having left his birthplace, finds himself battling the difficulties of an unfamiliar environment, most notably a big city.

Much has been said about the existence of *amok* outside Malay-language countries. Remember that Europeans first observed it in southern India and that it was also described in the Philippines. Musgrave and Sison (1910) found that *amok* was very common among Muslims on islands, where it existed in two forms: one followed a preliminary period of rumination and seemed similar to Malay *amok*; the other took a religious form. *Juramentado*[7] is the name given to a Muslim fanatic who, after binding himself by an oath, kills everyone he meets until he himself is killed in turn.

In the Philippines, *amok* has a counterpart, fortunately less dangerous, among women. This condition, called *dalahira*, may follow a specific incident or may erupt without apparent motive. A woman begins to quarrel with a friend or stranger and quickly falls into a frenzy of shouting and gesticulating that can last for hours until complete exhaustion. This sort of habit is not even accompanied by anger.

Octave Collet (1925) wrote that in Sumatra, among the Batak and especially among the Karo, there exists a custom called *moesoch berngi* in which an individual who thinks he is a victim of an injustice publicly declares himself an enemy of the community, warning it of the ravages he is prepared to commit if he is not given justice: the presumed enemy receives a figurative threat, called a *poelas*, which indicates with a miniature gun, hut, hand, foot, or the like, the way in which he will carry out his vengeance. This custom has been compared to a form of *amok*, although it is far less primitive.

Amok has also been compared to the rather grim institution of *kanaima*, which is found in Indian tribes in Guyana and northern Brazil (Koch-Grünberg, 1923, 3:216–19). Kanaima is the spirit of vengeance; with the help of certain ceremonies, it becomes embodied in an individual who wishes to take revenge. A man disappears into the forest, showing himself to no one, submitting to certain prohibitions. He spies on the deeds and actions of his future victim for months or even years, and when his time has come, he hurts him in such a way that the victim dies after three days. Then he goes to the grave of the victim and inserts a stick and drinks some of his blood, after which the perpetrator goes back home, where he is purified by a sorcerer and returns to the world of the living. Radin (1946, 68–72) views *kanaima* as a socialized form of *amok*, as proved by the terror it inspires in both its victim and the aggressor, as well as in the community at large.

In conclusion, *amok* may be considered both a form of suicide and an extreme form of vengeance; it involves a process of self-hypnosis, and from a social point of view a ceremonialization that, by dint of the prestige associated with the custom, perpetuates it. At the same time, it is encompasses certain practices and worldviews (disregard for human life, easy recourse to violence, the routine carrying of a dangerous weapon).

Reflex or reflexoid crime. Some have claimed, following Lombroso, that primitive man hid within him an instinct that led him to kill whenever he had the opportunity. Hives (1942), who spent many years in Australia, living in close proximity to Aborigines, declared that his neighbours were gentle and peaceful and that it would never occur to them to make an animal suffer, but that a homicidal instinct could emerge at any moment if circumstances allowed it. He gave the following example:

> I had a black servant who was in my service for about eight years. He was a capable cattle keeper – inasmuch as an Aboriginal can be – for naturally we can never fully trust them. One day, I found myself with him behind a herd, and since I was thirsty, I dismounted my horse near a stream to drink its clear water. The boy also put his feet on the ground to keep the horses whiles I lay flat along the shore to reach my mouth to the water. Suddenly, obeying an instinctive movement, I turned and looked up, and what I saw frightened me tremendously: leaning above me was the boy, his face contorted with hatred, shaking from head to toe so much so that his muscles were convulsing. In a flash I jumped to my feet. Unsurprisingly, with the greatest politeness, I asked him what was happening. At first, he had trouble getting even a word out. After a moment, the crisis seemed to have passed and he simply said to me: "Sir can never do that, or else I will kill him. Why? I do not know, but I must." I am convinced that he would have killed me immediately if he had had in his hand some object with which to strike me. He probably would have been saddened afterwards, but at the moment hereditary instincts would have won out.

In such a case, we do not have sufficient data for a precise appreciation of the facts. We would have to know more about the young Australian, his white master, and their relationship during the eight previous years. In addition, the incident would have to be placed in its social, economic, and cultural framework. If it is true, as we are assured, that the white colonists in Australia seized Aboriginal people's territories by driving them back into the desert and demanding their labour, it would not surprise us that they nursed great resentment. That being so, we would have no need of Lombroso's fanciful theories to interpret the incident described by Hives.

This type of reflex crime probably happens more easily in impulsive and aggressive populations. Ling Roth (1896, 2:162) describes how in 1857, when the Chinese occupied Sarawak, the Whites were evacuated by steamship. During the voyage, the travellers were soon bothered by a horrible stench; soon after, they discovered, hidden in a basket, the rapidly decomposing head of a Chinese man. The basket belonged to a young Dayak, who proudly explained that before the evacuation, he was walking in the fort occupied by the Chinese when he noticed, in a room, a Chinese man looking at himself, bending over a mirror. Instinctively, the Dayak drew his sword and cut of his head in one stroke, hid it in a basket, and walked through the fort to reach the boat. We know that the Dayaks of Borneo were fearsome head-hunters. For this Dayak, the opportunity was too tempting for him to resist, despite the danger to which he exposed himself.

Note that reflex crimes are well-known among civilized people. Such crimes were described by the Austrian criminologist Hans Gross (see the article "Criminologie" by Ellenberger and Dongier in *L'Encyclopédie médico-chirurgicale*, 37760A507,[8] 8).

Rapid psychogenic death. One psychopathological reaction that has aroused great surprise and incredulity is rapid psychogenic death (which some have referred to, very incorrectly, as "thanatomania.") It may seem incredible, indeed, that a vigorous, healthy man can die in a few hours or in one or two days from purely psychic causes. This phenomenon, long described by travellers, missionaries, and ethnologists, has found little credence among doctors. A summary of some of these cases appears in the well-known work by Oesterreich, *Die Besessenheit*, and in another by Stoll (1904). But it was Marcel Mauss (1926) who first drew attention to the great importance of this phenomenon: he also indicated the difference between the Australian cases and the Polynesian cases and emphasized the role of collective suggestion. In 1942, Cannon proposed a physiological hypothesis. I have tried to demonstrate that the cases known to date can be divided into three main groups, the African, the Polynesian, and the Australian-Melanesian, which differ from one another in significant ways (Ellenberger, 1951). We now review them, with their respective characteristics.

(1) *The African Form.* Here is a typical example, taken from a book by a missionary in the former French Congo, Pastor Fernand Grébert (1928, 172–3):

In Samkita, a pupil by the name of Onguïe was suddenly seized by convulsions and was carried into the dormitory where he fainted. When we came back to see him, he was surrounded by boys; some were holding his rigid arms and legs, others were trying vainly to open his clenched fists at the risk of breaking his fingers. Frightened as they were, it did not occur to them to them to remove the foam that was choking him. The little body was arched, but it soon relaxed. We were given a few hasty explanations: "He ate bananas that were cooked in a pot that had been used previously for manioc. Manioc is 'elci' for him; his grandparents told him that if he ever ate any of — even a tiny little bit — he would die." The violation of the ancestral command causes them such fright, such visceral anguish, such an organic collapse, that the sources of life are rapidly exhausted. "Look," they said pointing to the diaphragm that was shaking as if a small animal were struggling beneath the skin, "he has an 'evur,' which is getting excited." There was no doubt about the seriousness of the case. Alas! No medication would pass through the obstructed throat. The poor child had lost consciousness and was beginning to rattle. A man of the tribe ran to the neighbouring village to get the medication against *evur*, an egg mixed with certain other substances. We, in the meantime, were struggling against asphyxia by performing rhythmic tractions of the chest, but were unable to get hold of the tongue. It was all to no avail. The overtaxed heart ceased to beat, and the boy died in our arms.

Most accounts of this type relate to the same region, that is, the former Belgian Congo, from Gabon to Uganda. Acute psychogenic death is far rarer in Nigeria and appears to be unknown among the Bantu peoples of South Africa and among the black tribes of the Sudan. The Americans refer to it as "Voodoo death," even though it appears to be completely unknown in Haiti. It is difficult to assess its real incidence. John Roscoe (1921, 121), writing about Uganda, spoke of it as something that was once frequent. The essential fact, for the cases in Africa, is that death follows violation of an important taboo. Depending on the tribe and the individual, it can involve any kind of plant or animal, or the taboo can be unrelated to food. Very often, European medicine seems powerless, whereas the indigenous witch-doctor is able to heal the patient surprisingly quickly. The members of the tribes in question are convinced that the violation of a taboo inevitably results in death, but that the witch-doctor has the power to save the one who is dying.

(2) *The Polynesian Form.* In Polynesia, psychogenic death seems considerably more frequent than in central Africa. The New Zealand ethnologist Goldie (1904, 72–82) described it as the "rapidly fatal melancholia of the South Sea Islanders." Andrew Lang (1887, 104–5, vol. 1) gathered some interesting examples. In 1926, Marcel Mauss pointed out its frequency and importance in Polynesia, as well as its differences from the Australian form. Here, psychogenic death is connected to an idea of guilt; the predominant symptom is not fear, but rather a strong feeling of guilt and humiliation. The fear of magic plays only a secondary role. Polynesians had a refined system of commands and moral and religious rites, the violation of which could result in death.

Elsdon Best (1905, 221–2) tells how among the Maori of New Zealand religious taboos were extraordinarily numerous and important during the funeral ceremonies of chiefs. The son of the deceased or the person leading the ceremony had to be extremely careful, for the slightest error could be followed by psychogenic death. The same applied to a man who, while reciting the history of his tribe, committed an error. Goldie adds that a Maori who inadvertently entered a sacred place was convinced he had committed an unpardonable sin. He would wrap himself up in his mat and refuse to eat, and soon die. Taylor (quoted by Goldie, 17) recounts that the great chief Tanoui lost his fire-related instruments; these were found by common men, who used them to light their pipes; then, when they learned to whom these instruments belonged, they died of shame.

It appears that occurrences of this type have not disappeared completely. E. and P. Beaglehole (1946, 221) reported a case they learned about in New Zealand, in a town in the south of New Zealand's North Island:

Old Karé spent the day in a hotel before going to Taupata to attend a *tangi* (funeral ceremony). He probably got there drunk and absolutely wanted to make a few speeches, in which he uttered foolish remarks about the tribal people and customs. He was severely criticized and ridiculed in public by some of the elders. Karé, ashamed and mortified, got angry at people. He refused to spend the night with his relatives in the *pa* and went to sleep with strangers, as if to humiliate his family. He slept without any covers and probably caught cold. The next morning, he was calm but very angry and ashamed. He refused to eat in Taupata, saying he had been insulted by the inhabitants of the place. He got on his bicycle, saying that he was returning to his village where he was more respected. Halfway there, he was stopped up by a Maori in a car who offered him a ride because he appeared weak. He refused the offer. When he arrived home, it was clear that he was very sick. His family wanted to call a doctor; Karé refused, saying he had been deeply insulted by the ridicule and shame cast upon him. The following morning, when they went to see him, they found him dead. We would say that he had been killed by mental fatigue provoked by an attack of shame and the mortification resulting from having been publicly ridiculed in front of a crowd at a *tangi* because of inappropriate conduct contrary to custom. We who had known old Karé could not help but see in his death something of the justice of an ancient Greek tragedy. Karé had always been a fanatical adherent of old customs and a valiant defender of Maori tradition. There is irony in the fact that his death occurred because he had broken old customs, he who had always fought valiantly to maintain them and in whose interest he himself had so often unleashed streams of ridicule on some poor wretch.

We see in this example how greatly the Polynesian type of psychogenic death differs from that of central Africa. Whatever the role of fatigue and cooling relations may have been in this case, the main cause of death was certainly psychic in nature. This account is not about a man overwhelmed by fear, but about a man who gives himself over to death because the humiliation he has experienced has made life unbearable for him. Mauss notes[9] that the Maori language possesses a precise word for "mortal sin"; however, it does not refer, as it does for us, to "a sin that kills the soul," but rather, quite literally, to a "sin that kills man." Yet as M. Leenhardt remarked (personal communication), the feeling of guilt in itself is not enough; the reprehensible act must be made public and thus involve humiliation before the community.

Among Polynesians, psychogenic death can result from other causes as well, such as the certainty that one is the victim of a spell. Goldie also tells of how in the Fiji Islands, a young man and a young woman who have a secret affair may die when this is discovered and they are separated.

Mauss insisted that in Polynesia, psychogenic death can become a collective phenomenon. Goldie (1904, 79) thought it played an important role during the great epidemics, and that that was how massive crowds perished during an epidemic that ravaged the Sandwich Islands (Hawaii) in 1807. People simply gave themselves up to death and died in droves. An epidemic of that kind can exterminate an entire people.

The most typical example is that of the Moriori: Mauss recalls their history as it was told by Shand (1892, 1894). The Moriori, a branch of the Maori nation, had a few centuries earlier occupied the Chatham Islands, east of New Zealand. One of their ancestors, Nunuku, had abolished war and cannibalism. They no longer had weapons and could not defend themselves. In 1835, groups of Maoris disembarked, conquered the island without resistance, and reduced the population to slavery. Many Moriori perished in two days from an epidemic of an unknown nature. The others died gradually, with no apparent cause. One Maori said: "it is not the number of those that we killed that exterminated them, but the fact that we reduced them to slavery. We found them one morning dead in their houses. It was the fact that we broke their own taboos that killed them." (Apparently, the Maoris forced them to violate their own taboos).

The Australian–Melanesian form. The clinical picture here is completely different from that of Polynesia. Mauss showed that this form of dramatic death was all the more remarkable as the Australians' physical strength, health, and ability to recuperate were extraordinary, whereas Polynesians, even the stronger and healthier among them, were more delicate and less resilient. Among the Australians, the symptoms of psychogenic death greatly resembled those of central Africa, but here there was almost always a well-defined cause: magic.

The ethnographic literature contains numerous cases of this kind, most of them originating in Australia, with some from New Guinea and Melanesia. First off, the description of psychogenic death as described by Herbert Basedow (1925, 174–82) in Australia indicates that death there was produced by practices of magic that varied from one tribe to another; such magic was known by only a small number of insiders. The methods used may be divided into two groups. At times, something from the victim was used, for instance, his excrement or his footprint – or even, as among the Arrundta, his shadow. An old Arrundta custom was to "cut the shadow" of a man who was to die. In the second group, the larger one, death was brought about with a special instrument often made from human bones – thus the expression *pointing the bone* or *boning*. In this way, people condemned to death might actually be executed:

> Facing the doomed man's habitation, they lift the bone, or stick, to shoulder height and point it at the victim. The long piece of hair-string, which is attached to the instrument is tightly tied around the charmer's arm, above the elbow. This is done to endow his system with the magic influence of the pointing-stick he is holding; and that magic, he believes, passes into the destructive words, which he is uttering: "May your skeleton become saturated with the foulness of my stick, so that your flesh will rot and its stench attract the grubs, which live in the ground, to come and devour it. May your bones turn to water and soak into the sand, so that your spirit may never know your whereabouts. May the wind shrivel your skin like a leaf before a fire, and your blood dry up like the mud in a clay-pan." The effect of such a charm is immediate and infallible.
>
> The man who discovers that he is being boned by any enemy is, indeed, a pitiful sight. He stands aghast, with his eyes staring at the treacherous pointer, and with his hands lifted as though to ward [off] the lethal medium, which he imagines is pouring into his body. His cheeks blanch and his eyes become glassy and the expression of his face becomes horribly distorted, like that of one stricken with palsy. He attempts to shriek but usually the sound chokes in his throat, and all that one might see is froth at his mouth. His body begins to tremble and the muscles tense involuntarily. He sways backwards and falls to the ground, and after a short time appears to be in a swoon; but soon after he writhes as if in mortal agony, and, covering his face with his hands begins to moan. After a while he becomes very composed and crawls to his wurley. From this time onward he sickens and threats, refusing to eat and keeping aloof from the daily affairs of the tribe. Unless help is forthcoming in the shape of a counter-charm administered by the hands of the "Nangarri," or medicine-man, his death is only a matter of a comparatively short time. If the coming of the medicine-man is opportune he might be saved.

Basedow completes this picture with a detailed description of the procedures used by the indigenous doctor. After directing various phrases and incantations toward the patient and his family, he would crawl up beside the patient, bite him, and suck for a long while a place on his chest, until he had "extracted" a foreign body such as a small stick, a piece of bone, or a pebble, which was triumphantly presented to the patient and those surrounding him as the *corpus delicti*:

> The effect is astounding. The miserable fellow, until that moment well on the road to death, raises his head to gaze in wonderment upon the object held by the Nangarri, which, in all serious-ness, he imagines has been extracted from the inside of his body. Satisfied with its reality, he even lifts himself into a sitting position and calls for some water to drink. The crisis has now been passed, and the patient's recovery is speedy and complete. Without the Nangarri's interception, the "boned" fellow would have worried himself to death for a certainty, but the sight of a concrete object, claimed by the recognized authority of the tribe to be the cause of the complaint, signifies recovery to him.

Basedow adds that such a cure far surpassed anything that faith healers can do in our countries. Furthermore, Mauss points out that European medicine can do nothing in a case of this kind.

In New Guinea, examples are reported by C.G. Seligman (1929), relying on the authority of Campbell, who affirms that a sorcerer may hit a man on the back, telling him he is going to die and the man indeed dies. However, by no means have such facts been observed often or everywhere. F.E. Williams (1928, 214) affirms that they are unknown in the Orokaiva region.

Facts observed in certain parts of Melanesia closely resemble those in Australia. Here is a typical case, according to Codrington (1891, 205–6):

> Another remarkable engine of mischief is called in the Banks' Islands *tamatetiqa*, ghost-shooter. Since this is used also in Florida it may be supposed to be common to all these islands. A bit of bamboo is stuffed with leaves, a dead man's bone, and other magical ingredients, the proper mana song being chanted over it. Fasting in the Banks' Islands, but not apparently in the Solomon Islands, adds power to this and other charms. The man who has made or bought one of these holds it in his hand, with the open end of the bamboo covered with his thumb, till he sees his enemy; then he lets out the magic influence and shoots his man …

A striking story was told me by Edwin Sakalraw of Ara of what he saw himself. A man in that islet was known to have prepared a *tamatetiqa,* and had declared his intention of shooting his enemy with it at an approaching feast; but he would not tell who it was that he meant to kill, lest some friend of his should buy back the power of the charm from the wizard who had prepared it. To add force to the ghostly discharge, he fasted so many days before the feast began that when the day arrived he was too weak to walk. When the people had assembled, he had himself carried out and set down at the edge of the open space where the dancing would go on. All the men there knew that there was one of them he meant to shoot; no one knew whether it was himself. There he sat as the dancers rapidly passed him circling round, a fearful object, black with dirt and wasted to a skeleton with fasting, his *tamamiqa* within his closed ringers stopped with his thumb, his trembling arm stretched out, and his bleared eyes watching for his enemy. Every man trembled inwardly as he danced by him, and the attention of the whole crowd was fixed on him. After a while, bewildered and dazed with his own weakness, the rapid movements of the dancers, and the noise, he mistook his man; he raised his arm and lifted his thumb. The man he aimed at fell at once upon the ground, and the dancers stopped. Then he saw that he had failed, and that the wrong man was hit, and his distress was great; but the man who had fallen and was ready to expire, when he was made to understand that no harm was meant him, took courage again to live, and presently revived. No doubt he would have died if the mistake had not been known.

Many explanations for these remarkable facts have been proposed. It is difficult to accept, as some have claimed, that these individuals were poisoned by the sorcerer or his accomplices. F.E. Williams (1928) thought that people who died in this way were already ill and, while believing they were going to die due to magic, in fact died of the unsuspected disease affecting them. This explanation is hardly in keeping with cases where it is expressly mentioned that the individual was robust and healthy.

As Mauss indicated, an explanation must be sought in the threefold domain of psychology, physiology, and sociology. These are cases in which "social nature directly interconnects with the biological nature of man." In other words, these are "total facts"[10] in which the biological, psychological, and sociological aspects are but three sides of a fundamental unit.

A biological explanation, founded mainly on the Australian cases, was proposed by W.B. Cannon (1942), who referred to his previous work (1929) on physiological shock: prolonged hyperactivity of the sympathico-adrenal system results in a reduction in the quantity of circulating blood, a collapse in blood pressure, and lesions in the heart and nerve centres, resulting in a vicious circle. These problems are aggravated by the lack of food and lead to death. Acute psychogenic death is thus a specific case of shock through excess emotion. Finally, note that acute psychogenic death is not completely unknown in our countries. We find it described under the name of "terror" in Emilio Mira's treatise on war psychiatry (1943, 3l–5), in which it constitutes the sixth and most extreme degree of terror.

Cannon's hypothesis does not explain the Polynesian cases where an individual simply lies down on the ground, wraps himself in his mat, and soon dies; even less does it account for cases where a Polynesian calmly declares, at the sight of some unlucky omen, that he will die at the end of such and such a day, which indeed arrives. Facts of this kind more closely resemble what happens in an old married couple when one of the two dies, and the other, who may have been in good health, follows the first to the grave one or two days later, or the story of an old poet who, having completed his last work, prepares to die with a clear conscience.

From a psychological point of view, Mauss emphasizes that such a man dies because he is convinced he is going to die. In primitive man, the sense of the sacred is infinitely more pronounced than in most civilized people. Breaking an important taboo, committing certain forbidden acts, or being the victim of a specific act of magic produces a psychic disruption of an intensity unknown to civilized people. Even the least religious civilized man is not exempt from cultural idiosyncrasies. Clyde Kluckhohn (1949, 19) tells of a woman in Arizona who enjoyed serving her guests excellent sandwiches with a taste similar to that of tuna or chicken. When they had eaten, she informed them that they had just eaten rattlesnake, at which point most began vomiting violently. We can now imagine that the reaction of the primitive man was infinitely more intense and that he was conditioned by the idea that certain circumstances would unfailingly lead to his death; this belief was shared by all members of his tribe, and when an event of this type occurred it only reinforced his belief.

The sociological explanation has been well-regarded by all authors from Mauss to Cannon. Primitive man was far more closely integrated into the social organism than civilized man; being excluded from it was for him a much more serious psychological trauma. But once again, a complete explanation of psychogenic death can only be bio-psycho-sociological.

Mauss has also shown the powerful role of psychogenic death as a collective expression, as in the example of the Moriori. We know how many peoples have been wiped off the map after the arrival of the white man. Often, the effects of epidemics or alcohol are blamed, but gradually we have come to understand that things are more complex. As Mannoni writes (1950, 219): "In some Pacific islands it was not economic exploitation which decimated, or even exterminated the population, but our moral attitude, the conscientiousness with which we condemned beliefs and customs which were in fact the life-blood of the native peoples." It would be difficult to exaggerate the significance of these facts.

Slow psychogenic death. Slow psychogenic death appears to be more frequent than acute psychogenic death; we observe it among many populations where acute psychogenic death appears to be unknown. In a first group of cases, the circumstances in which they occur are exactly the same as those of the acute form (violation of a taboo, act of magic), the only difference being that instead of dying in a few hours or at most in a few days, the patient dies in a few weeks or a few months. In a second group of cases, death occurs following well-defined psychological motivations, to the point that specific disease entities have been established. Two of these deserve individual mention: *lovesickness* and *nostalgia*.

Lovesickness. It may seem extraordinary that a disease that has been described in medical treatises for twenty-five centuries and that has given rise to an extremely abundant literature is today totally forgotten. However, this is what has happened with lovesickness (synonyms: *amor insanus, Liebeskrankheit, l'amour-maladie, mélancolie amoureuse,* and so on).

This subject does not appear to have been dealt with in its entirety by a historian of medicine. As described by the ancient authors, love sickness consists of a romantic attachment so deep and so exclusive that the impossibility of its realization leads to death, not by suicide,

but by slow and unconquerable wasting away; yet the mere promise
of its impending realization can lead to a kind of resurrection.

Innumerable authors, both doctors and non-doctors, have dealt
with this disease since antiquity. We know the story of Perdiccas
II, King of Macedonia, who was afflicted with a strange sorrow
that did not respond to any therapy, and how Hippocrates, called
upon to consult, was able to heal the monarch after guessing his
secret love for Phila, the former mistress of his late father, the king.
Equally famous is the story of Antiochus and Stratonice told by
Plutarch in his *Life of Demetrius*. Setting aside these more or less
legendary anecdotes, famous doctors such as Galen, Aëtius, and
Paul of Aegina[11] devoted chapters to this disease and indicated
ways of recognizing it through changes in the patient's pulse when
the person he secretly loved appeared or even at the mere mention of her name. Avicenna and the Arabs dealt with it extensively;
so did the doctors of the Renaissance. In the novel *Lucretia and
Euryalus* (1445) by Aeneas Sylvius,[12] the story is told of a married
woman who dies of sorrow after being abandoned by her seducer.
In the seventeenth century, Zacchias, the founder of psychiatric
legal medicine, distinguished lovesickness from rational love: the
lovesick can be recognized by their anxious, sad, downcast, and
meditative appearance, and by their eyes, which are sunken, ringed,
and lifeless. The sufferer has lost sleep as well as his appetite; he has
lost weight and is deeply unstable emotionally; he is taciturn, open-
ing his mouth only to speak of his love. His pulse changes when
the object of his love appears. From a medical-legal point of view,
Zacchias views such a patient as having no responsibility (Vallon
and Génil-Perrin, 1912). In the early nineteenth century, Esquirol
classified lovesickness as a variety of erotomania and thought it to
be quite frequent:

> There are few physicians who have not had occasion to observe
> and propose a remedy for it; which is sometimes too late, when
> the disease has a very acute course. A young lady from Lyons
> falls in love with one of her relatives, to whom she was promised
> in marriage. Circumstances oppose the fulfillment of promises
> made to the two lovers, and the father requires the removal of
> the young man. He has scarcely gone, when the young lady falls
> into a state of profound sadness, says nothing, confines herself
> to her bed, refuses all nourishment, and the secretions become

suppressed. She repulses all the advice, prayers, and consolations of her relatives and friends. After five days, vainly employed in endeavors to overcome her resolution, they decide on recalling her lover; but it is now too late. She sinks, and dies in his arms on the sixth day. (Esquirol, *Treatise on Insanity*, 339)

It would be interesting to investigate why lovesickness disappeared during the nineteenth century, indeed, so entirely that its existence seems to have been forgotten. It is described in a few nineteenth-century novels: *Wie Anne Bäbeli Jowäger haushaltet* by Jeremias Gotthelf (1843); *Little Women* by Louisa May Alcott (1869); *L'automne d'une femme* by Marcel Prévost (1893). Also, the geographical distribution of the disease seems not to have been examined closely; perhaps it is simply a legend, albeit one that today is still rife in Japan and Polynesia.

Nostalgia. Lovesickness has been known since the time of the ancient Greeks. The medical history of nostalgia began only in the seventeenth century in the form of a "Swiss disease." According to Fritz Ernst (1949), who devoted a thorough historical study to it, it was described for the first time by Johannes Hofer of the University of Basel Faculty of Medicine in 1688. This thesis was phenomenally successful, and authorities such as Haller, Auenbrugger, and Boissier de Sauvages all repeated and magnified its description. Nostalgia was rife, they said, among Swiss soldiers serving foreign princes. A soldier was gripped with an obsession for his faraway homeland; as a result, he lost sleep and appetite, wasted away, and inevitably died unless he was sent home expeditiously.

Toward the end of the eighteenth century, it was noticed that nostalgia reigned in other countries as well. The Revolutionary and Napoleonic Wars provided an opportunity to observe it, sometimes in epidemic form. As Bachet (1950) observed, in this period it was noticed that nostalgia struck mainly troops from certain provinces, especially Bretons, Corsicans, Basques, Savoyards, the Flemish, and soldiers from provinces where the people were deeply attached to their dialects and traditions.

During the nineteenth century, to the preceding descriptions were added those of young servants sent into service in cities. Esquirol had already reported the case of a young servant who, under the effect of nostalgia, on two occasions set fire to her master's house. Jaspers

(1909) in his thesis compiled around thirty cases of crimes committed in Germany under the effects of this disease: the sufferers were
girls aged eleven to sixteen, from poor rural families, most of them
illiterate, who, on being placed in service in the city, suffered from
unbearable nostalgia. One day, they set fire to the master's house or
killed the baby of the house[13] by drowning or poisoning. After committing the crime, they declared they did not know why they had
acted this way. The subsequent study does not show a progression
toward mental illness. Such cases, already exceptional in times past,
today seem to have disappeared completely.

The interest in nostalgia as a nosological entity has been intermittent for a century, disappearing in times of peace only to reawaken
with each war. The Second World War again provided the opportunity to study the disease, especially in the form of mental disorders
of captivity, of which Bachet (1950) provided an excellent general
review. Characteristically, they found among French prisoners the
same preponderance of ethnic factors (a predisposition among the
Bretons, the Flemish, and so on) that had been noted a century and a
half earlier. The interest of pediatricians was also drawn toward the
unknown frequency of nostalgia in children (Lippert, 1950). Martin
(1954) attempted to distinguish two forms of nostalgia: one was virtually biological in nature and comparable to the instinct of certain
animals to return to their previous habitat; the other was a particular form of obsession. Seguin (1956) thought that nostalgia played a
considerable role in the psychosomatic maladjustment syndrome of
mountain Indians who migrated to Lima, Peru.

We hope that ethnopsychiatry, by enriching our knowledge of the
diverse varieties of psychogenic death, will enable us to more accu-
rately evaluate certain psychic processes, the frequency and importance
of which have been forgotten or ignored by classic psychiatry.

Suicide. Space limitations prevent us from addressing here the question of suicide seen in light of ethnopsychiatry. We can only refer the
reader to specific works, notably to the book by Wisse (1933). See
also the article by Ellenberger (1953).

Morbid Developments and Neuroses

In this vast field, we will limit ourselves to a few types of well-defined neuroses: the cleaning neurosis of Swiss housewives, the kayak

angst (or dizziness) of the Eskimos, imitation neurosis, the *koro* of the Malaysians, and the *windigo* of the Indians of the Canadian northeast.

Cleaning neurosis. As Kroeber has shown (1948, 600), great differences exist from one people to another with regard to cleanliness of the body, clothing, and dwellings. In civilized countries, there have been variations over the course of history. The Romans revelled in their public baths, but this changed in the Middle Ages. The Crusades brought about a resurgence in cleanliness from the thirteenth century to the fifteenth, but this was followed by another decline, and it was only in the eighteenth century that habits of cleanliness became solidly established in Europe, where they took root differently from one country to the next. Today, do we not still speak of "Dutch cleanliness"? Yet it is difficult to establish what separates normal cleanliness from a collective obsession. Depending on the point of view, the Hindu Brahmans and the Japanese have been praised for their physical cleanliness or described as obsessive maniacs. The difficulty of tracing this boundary is demonstrated by the fact that a cleaning neurosis of extraordinary intensity was able to go practically unnoticed in Switzerland and German-speaking countries up until recent years despite its extreme frequency. I think I was the first to give a systematic description of it under the name *Putzwut* (pronounced *pouts-voûte*), or "cleaning mania" (Ellenberger, 1950). Stekel, however, alluded to it under the name *Hausfrauenneurose* in his book *Nervöse Leute*.

Putzwut, or cleaning mania, refers to the need to clean in an exaggerated and unreasonable way. It is almost exclusive to the female sex. Immediately striking is the excessive amount of time a woman with *Putzzwut* devotes to cleaning. From morning to night the housewife exhausts herself with her broom and her rags, no matter what the size of her dwelling. On Saturday afternoons, when everyone is free, she sends her husband out walking with the children so that she can devote herself entirely to cleaning. This activity reaches its annual peak generally in the spring (in Austria it is called die *Grundräumerei*, in northern Germany *das grosse Reinemachen*, and in German-speaking Switzerland *die Useputzete*); at that point life grinds to a halt and the house is cleaned from basement to attic with fanatical zeal. In some parts of Switzerland, men take part in it, cleaning the exterior of the house and brushing the tiles on the roof one by one. No less striking is the exaggerated care with which everything must be cleaned: cleanliness alone is not enough: everything must shine (*blitzblank*).

A characteristic feature of *Putzwut* is the utter unawareness of these women, who, while complaining abot the exhausting work, see it as a necessary evil and view themselves as sacrificing themselves for their families. Nothing is more typical than their indignation when it is suggested to them that the sacrifice is pointless. "We cannot very well always live in filth," is the usual response, accompanied by an expression of wounded dignity. These women have the deepest contempt for those women who are free of this neurosis, scornfully describing them as lazy, unclean, and incapable. No less characteristic is their stubborn resistance to any suggestion of ways to make their task easier, whether it is new cleaning products, time- and effort-saving machines, or furniture and utensils that are easier to maintain; the response is immediate, accompanied by an anxious expression: "too expensive," "not practical," "terribly complicated," "takes up too much room," "isn't safe," "in the end, doesn't save that much work"; all such objections are expressed sincerely and with full conviction.

Often these women present *other personality traits*. When they are not "putzing," they indulge in other obsessional-type occupations, such as interminable knitting and the meticulous repairing of tattered clothing; also, they have great difficulty leaving their four walls. One of my patients, for example, had only gone out once since her marriage ten years earlier, to attend a concert by the village brass band. Furthermore, their houses are often filled with clutter: old-fashioned things and damaged or broken and useless objects "that could maybe be useful one day." Finally, we note that this cleaning neurosis is not necessarily connected to personal cleanliness.

In France and England, this neurosis is not unknown, though it is infrequent, except in parts of northern France and in Alsace. In Germany and Scandinavia, it is very frequent, as it is in Holland, Luxembourg, and the Flemish part of Belgium. But the country of choice for *Putzwut* is German-speaking Switzerland. Some French tend to think the French-speaking Swiss are exaggeratedly clean, but they are commonly considered slovenly in German-speaking Switzerland. Indeed, the French-speaking Swiss, besides the verb "nettoyer" (to clean, used for normal cleaning) also have the verb "poutser" to indicate excessive and absurd cleaning. In some villages in German-speaking Switzerland, children are even obliged, at regular intervals, to bring to school a brush and soap to clean their desks under the watchful eye of the master.

Among the causes of this neurosis, we may place the blame on:

1 *Feelings of inferiority*, which are always present among these women.

2 *Feelings of guilt*, generally resulting from an extremely moral upbringing that drives them to purify themselves, even though this purification is directed toward the exterior ("instead of cleaning one's soul, one cleans pots and pans"). This cleaning is carried out as a self-punitive act.

3 *Resentment*, that is, according to the conception of Nietzsche and Max Scheler, an intoxication of the soul as a result of constant repression of feelings of hatred and vengeance. Note that neurotic cleaning is carried out in a way that weighs heavily on the lives of the husband and the children, upon whom are inflicted strict taboos regarding the cleanliness of floors, furniture, clothing, curtains, and so on. What is more, these women are almost constantly in a foul mood, ostensibly brought about by the overwork they are forced to carry out to maintain the house in a state of cleanliness.

4 *Lack of sociability*, which among these women is constant. The house is basically off-limits to visitors (especially unexpected ones), to the husband's colleagues, to the children's friends, and so on.

Note that in families where this neurosis resides, the husband occasionally complains about the excessive cleaning but pretty much accepts it; he finds it a good pretext to spend his evenings elsewhere, taking it for granted that his wife will be confining herself to the house. The couple's relations are often complementary: the woman feels a need for submission and subservience, and the man for superiority and self-centredness. Other socio-psychological factors are often at work. If she has a maid, the mistress of the house overburdens her with all the cleaning work. I knew a hospital[14] where a particularly tyrannical head nurse exhausted nurses with excessive cleaning, to the great detriment of the patients.

In regions such as German-speaking Switzerland, where the "cleaning mania" takes hold we can easily identify the *cultural factors* that are at work. First, we note a strange fusion of the concept of duty with the concept of work. It emerges from interviews with these women that they identify their conception of duty with work that is hard and interminable, even unproductive. If they should have to stop work, due to illness, they suffer acutely from guilt. They are always ready to accuse people who do not have the same concept of work of being irresponsible. As for their conception of work, it is extremely simplistic: in their mind, the more unpleasant and tiring a job is, the more praiseworthy it is. No less striking is their way of identifying morality with cleanliness. For all of these reasons, these women in no way suspect that their need to clean is a neurosis, or that it may present any sort of danger to their children. In German-speaking Switzerland, nothing is more difficult to treat than a cleaning neurosis, for the psychotherapist has against him not only the resistance of the patient but also that of the family and above all the entire weight of tradition and cultural values.

Kayak angst or dizziness (kayaksvimmel). When the Danes colonized Greenland, they noticed that a very specific psychopathology existed among the Eskimos there. The administrators, missionaries, and doctors wrote their observations in works in Danish that today are difficult to access. The mental anomaly that attracted the most attention was "kayak angst or dizziness" (*kayaksvimmel* in Danish), which has sometimes been described as a neurosis exclusive to the Eskimos. We base our description on the observations of Alfred Bertelsen, first published in 1905; he subsequently reworked and updated them (Bertelsen, 1940).

To be properly understood, *kayaksvimmel* must not be isolated from the other neuroses that afflict the Eskimos, or from the character of this people. Bertelsen attributes to the Eskimos features such as impulsivity, great suggestibility, emotional lability, and fickleness, which together explain why they often make important decisions on the spur of the moment. The Eskimo lives from day to day, concerned with neither the past nor the future. He is inclined to plunge into violent emotional crises. At such times, he may run away, tear his clothing, commit acts of violence, or fall into a kind of half-sleep, from which he awakens with no memory of what he did during his crisis. At other times, crises occur that may resemble the hysteria of Charcot. Another pathological reaction consists of "going to the mountain": after a bout of anger or sorrow, an Eskimo leaves his community for higher ground, supposedly to meet a supernatural being, though in reality it is a sort of walk toward death. The essential characteristic of the Eskimo, according to Bertelsen, is a profound anxiety, which is understandable, given the hardships they encounter in their precarious lives. Add to that the impact of the silence of the world in which they live, and their austere natural surroundings, all of this accompanied by the darkness of the Arctic's winter nights.

It is against this background that the appearance of kayak angst must be understood. If this neurosis has attracted more attention than others, it is simply perhaps because *kayaksvimmel* affects the Eskimo's ability to make his livelihood. Here is an observation summarized by Bertelsen:[15]

> An Eskimo, age twenty-nine, an excellent whale hunter and a good paddler, found himself on one July day around noon fishing cod. He was not far from the coast, the weather was relatively warm, the sky clear, and the sun shone directly in his eyes. He began thinking about his late father and his brother who had died the previous year. He himself had not learned the art of righting the kayak should it capsize, and that is why, in his words, he prepared for death on a daily basis. He feared it, however, not knowing what punishment awaited him in the beyond. He had caught several fish when he noticed something biting him. He raised the line, from which a sea cucumber was dangling (*Cucumaria frondosa*). The creature seemed horrifying to him. He threw it back in the water and his whole body began to shiver violently. He felt as if something hot were flowing down his back and legs. He began to sweat, had a splitting headache, saw spots whirling around in his visual field. The tip of the kayak seemed to him to be doubled and farther away than usual. The entire kayak seemed to grow longer and lean to one side, and for that reason he leaned to the other side. Remaining as still as possible, he began paddling with small strokes in the direction of land, still under the impression that something unknown was following him and hovering around him. He called another kayak paddler, and when he was nearby, his anxiety disappeared. However, something continued to dance before his eyes even after he disembarked, and he felt an urgent need to move his bowels. Shortly thereafter, he once again felt capable of paddling and continuing to fish.

About a year later, he had another such crisis. This time, he was farther away from the coast; the sea was rough; he was afraid of being unable to reach land before the wind increased. Suddenly, he lost the strength to paddle and experienced the same condition as before. Several such crises occurred at increasingly shorter intervals. He threw back what he fished and splashed his head with cold water but it did not help at all. Now, eight years later, he readily experiences a similar sensation when, on high ground, he approaches the edge of a cliff. On flat ground, he sometimes feels as if he is sailing. He is startled at the slightest sound, frequently has palpitations, feels suffocated and ruminates about his concerns, has trembling in his hands and his pulse is unstable.

In 1902 and 1903 Bertelsen had the opportunity to examine sixty Eskimos suffering from kayak angst in western Greenland. One quarter of them said they had their first crisis immediately after having been frightened, either by a real danger or by an imaginary danger. Sometimes, the first attack followed by a few days the death of a relative or fishing buddy by accidental drowning. Often the attack began with a fear that the kayak was about to capsize or that a foreign object was about to overturn it, or that there was a hole in the kayak. An Eskimo told him that he seemed to feel water filling the kayak; he paddled as hard as he could, but the kayak seemed to grow heavier and slid deeply into the water. When he finally reached the shore, he was surprised to find the kayak perfectly intact. More often still, the paddler felt as if the kayak was higher and narrower than usual (which naturally increased the danger of it capsizing and sinking). Some people had the impression that "something" in the sea has caught onto their kayak, or on the contrary that the paddle had suddenly become extraordinarily light and unusable. For a few of them, the attack began with feeling cold in their legs; for others, with violent trembling. The patient felt paralyzed, unable to manoeuvre his paddle or even to turn his head. The attack stopped as soon as he felt a human presence or the kayak reached land.

Such attacks are liable to recur. A man who experiences kayak dizziness lives in the fear of a recurrence, which inevitably occurs, first in similar circumstances, then in less and less dangerous ones. Also, he starts to experience dizziness on firm ground, just by looking at the sea or simply thinking about it, until one day he finds

himself unable to return to sea. A statistical study by Bertelsen of
130 Eskimos suffering from kayak dizziness demonstrates that the
frequency of *kayaksvimmel* increases with age.

Bertelsen carefully analyzed the factors blamed in for causing this
neurosis. He rejected epilepsy or nicotine addiction. In his view, the
appearance of the neurosis was conditioned by the Eskimo's character,
his impulsivity, suggestibility, emotional lability, and his predisposition
to hysteria and mental contagion. Moreover, the frequency of *kayaks-*
vimmel increased with the seriousness of the real danger, attaining its
maximum on the west coast of Greenland, where the danger of ice-
bergs is greatest and where the Eskimos are not such good paddlers.
Bertelsen concludes that kayak dizziness is basically a psychogenic
neurosis, comparable to various other phobias that are contained in
the chapters on neuroses of our classic treatises.

We may compare *kayaksvimmel* to the siderodromophobia
described by Rigler (1879), which developed among locomotive
engineers and other railway employees following a railway accident.
Besides back pain with no detectable organic substratum, these individuals presented neurotic troubles and an insurmountable aversion
to their job. We know that comparable troubles are known among
aviators.

Neuroses of imitation. These neuroses are characterized by the fact
that the patient feels compelled to repeat what is said in front of
him and to imitate the gestures and actions carried out in front of
him. Also, there is often an impulse to utter obscene words *(copro-*
lalia). This neurosis is widespread in several parts of the world, but
three major focal points exist: the first extends over Indonesia and
Malaysia, where it is known as *latah.* The second is among indigenous peoples of eastern Siberia, where it is called *myriakit.* The third
is restricted to the Ainu, a small tribe[16] in northern Japan, where it
is called *imu.*

Latah, despite its frequency, appears to have been noticed rather
late by Europeans. According to Yap (1952), it was described by
Logan in the *Journal of the Indian Archipelago* in 1849. O'Brien
spoke of it in 1883 as a little-known disease; after that description,
more of them came out.

Metzger (1882) described it in Java under the name *sakit latah*,
which referred people of the Malay race who, when called aloud
or when someone made a sudden movement in front of them, were

startled, could not look away, and begin imitating unintentionally and against their will everything that was said or done in front of them, often even continuing to carry out a movement that they had seen begin. A young servant, for example, who was *sakit latah*, entered the dining room carrying a stack of plates that her mistress had told her not to drop. The servant began to repeat these words with greater and greater emphasis, and when the mistress of the house unintentionally extended her hands before her, the servant did the same and dropped the plates. Metzger added that his own cook, during attacks of *latah*, was capable of repeating foreign words and understood sounds unknown in Malaysian, which she was incapable of doing when she was her normal self.

O'Brien (1883) wrote that the disease is very frequent in Malaysia, but only among Malaysians – it is rare among other peoples. Several forms of it exist. In its, more basic and more frequent form, impressionable subjects are startled by the slightest unexpected noise and invariably utter an obscene expression and seek to strike the nearest object or person. In a second form, individuals panic intensely the instant that certain words are uttered, such as "alligator," "tiger," or "serpent." This anxious reaction has been provoked by the word rather than by the animal itself. An indigenous servant will not hesitate to draw from the shore an alligator that has just been killed and open its mouth, but at the utterance of the word "alligator," she will fall into an insane terror. A third group comprises individuals who, with or without the symptoms displayed by the other groups, compulsively begin to carry out actions performed or begun in front of them, even very unpleasant or very dangerous ones. A Malaysian woman of respectable character and advanced age found herself, when facing a man who was taking off his coat, compelled to undress completely in front of him, all the while protesting against this outrage, swearing at him and asking witnesses to kill him. Still worse, a ship's cook who was playing with his young child was joined by a man who began throwing a log in the air and catching it; the cook then began to imitate him with his child. Then the man deliberately failed to catch the log, at which point the cook dropped the child, who was killed falling on the floor. In a fourth group are extreme cases where the individual, having lost all traces of will, completely gives himself over to the wishes of anyone who wants to dominate him. This form of *latah* increases in frequency with age, and many older women suffer from it.

The naturalist Henry Forbes (1885) described *latah* as he observed it in Java. One day as he was biting into a banana, a *latah* servant who was carrying a bar of soap bit into the soap. Another time, while taking care of his plants, he found a caterpillar, which he threw at her in a joke, unaware that the natives were terrified of them. The servant trembled in fear, tore the clothing from her body, rushed naked outside, and ran until she dropped of exhaustion. A Malaysian servant of Forbes, who did not hesitate to take hold of snakes with both hands, became *latah* the minute he touched a caterpillar. A Malaysian woman, encountering a lizard, fell to the ground and began crawling like it through the water and mud until the animal disappeared into a tree, at which point she returned to normal. The same woman, encountering a venomous snake in a field, began moving her fingers, imitating the tongue of the reptile, remaining face to face with the snake until the animal bit her; she died less than an hour later. The most appalling aspect of *latah*, Forbes added, was that patients were constantly tormented by those around them.

Van Brero (1895), a doctor at the Buitenzorg[17] mental hospital in Java, made eight observations, unfortunately rather brief, of women suffering from *latah*. He emphasized the role of heredity, predisposition, and nervous hyperexcitability.

Gilmore Ellis (1897) distinguished between two forms of *latah/* One of these he called the *mimetic form*, in which the patient imitates what he sees happen before him; the other, the *paroxysmal form*, in which the individual is startled at the sound of a noise, utters obscene words, and sometimes carries out indecent acts. Ellis likened *latah* to an advanced state of hypnosis. These patients, he wrote, ended up obeying all orders given to them while remaining perfectly aware of their own subservience and the ignominy of their persecutors. During a *latah* attack, the pulse accelerates and reflexes are normal. *Latah* is almost invariably hereditary, attacking a large proportion of mainly female members of the same family. It almost never appears before the age of twelve, and once it does the unfortunate victim is mercilessly tormented by other children. There is no link between *latah* and religion. The frequency of *latah* had not decreased since the British occupation and the founding of schools.

Hugh Clifford (1893, 186–201) offered almost incredible examples of the martyred lives led by individuals suffering from *latah* and of the horrible ways in which the people around them persecuted them.

One of his servants, for example, was compelled by a child to take in his hand a metal pot that was red-hot; he burned himself horribly. From the day the other servants noticed he was *latah*, he became their scapegoat, and in two months was a wreck; but around that same time, several of his companions found themselves afflicted in turn by the same disease. Clifford's view was that all Malaysians were predisposed to *latah* and capable of becoming typical cases if they were sufficiently persecuted and harassed. The first step was to startle them, which could be dangerous, for they sometimes responded by stabbing the offender. Eventually, the patient lost the capacity to act on his own volition and sought actions that would serve him as guides.

William Fletcher (1908), a surgeon in Malaysia, studied the medico-legal aspects of *latah*. During legal proceedings, the judge might find it impossible to question witnesses suffering from *latah*, for they would do nothing except repeat his questions and imitate his gestures. The judge had to have the witness sit next to him, calm him down, and speak gently to him until he was finally is able to answer him. Crimes committed under the influence of *latah* definitely exist. With the serious form of *latah*, it is possible to suggest to an individual that he commit a criminal act, which he then carries out. With the less serious form, the one involving startling someone or influencing that person by a sudden movement, the individual may respond with an act of violence. One day, for example, two Malaysians were walking in the jungle, each armed with a sharp knife. One stumbled and fell; the other, affected by *latah*, fell in turn. The first, become *latah* as well, stabbed his companion with his knife and cut off his hand. The court condemned him to six months in prison, reckoning that accepting *latah* as a cause of irresponsibility would have created a dangerous precedent. In a second case, a Malaysian, suddenly in the grip of *latah*, coming upon a stranger unexpectedly, cut off the man's head with his knife. Neither Fletcher nor the other authors already cited mention another aspect of the problem, that of individuals who are *victims* of a crime due to their *latah*.

Octave Collet (1905, 205) wrote that latah is very frequent in Sumatra. The crisis, he wrote, often ended with an attack of nerves. He continued: "Malaysians have many fables describing feats of *latah* that terrified tigers in their perfect imitation of the roaring and movements of the beast of prey."

Van Loon maintained that *latah* is first and foremost a disease of women from the poorer classes, and mainly of those that have been in close contact with Europeans as cooks or maids. According to the patients, *latah* often begins after a sexual dream that is terrifying in its details, for example the sight of erect male organs wriggling like worms attacking the dreamer. She is compelled to cook and eat them, at which time she wakes up startled and has violent bouts of nausea. The character of the Malaysians plays an important role in this; even in their normal state, they imitate one another, and they imitate Europeans even more.

Bruce Lockhart (1936) described how in his youth, spent in Malaysia, he and a few friends would play tricks on a poor woman suffering from *latah* who sold fruit to travellers in a train station. They amused themselves by throwing things on the ground; the old woman would react by throwing her fruit on the train platform. The pranksters paid her for them, but even so "it was a cruel amusement, the thought of which today fills me with shame."

Van Wulfften Palthe (1948), regarding the stereotypical dreams, sexual in nature, with which *latah* often begins, established a connection with *koro*, which, as we will see, is a sexual neurosis specific to men, and which, from this point of view, presents a characteristic directly opposed to that of *latah*.

Van Bergen (1955) stresses the fact that most cases of *latah* occur among women transplanted into a strange environment where they are unable to carry out the work expected of them.

H.B.M. Murphy mentions the predisposing role of games played by Malaysian children: they lead a boy, by singing, by playing tricks, or by covering his head, to imagine he is such and such an animal whose behaviour he will imitate; they lead a girl to feel possessed by a spirit. Such practices are an impetus to suggestion, and it is likely that they are conducive to the appearance of *latah*.

Neuroses similar to *latah* have been indicated in various parts of Southeast Asia. Adolf Bastian (1867, 296) travelled to Siam, where he noted the presence of *yaun*, a neurosis identical to *latah*. In the Philippines it has been described under the name of *mali-mali* (Stoll, 1904, 108; Musgrave and Sison, 1910). Jules Levi (1913) reported its frequency among the natives of Fezzan in Tripolitania, and Répond (1940) encountered it during a trip to the southern Sahara.

Myriakit. The second major centre of imitation neurosis is found in Siberia, where it occurs among several small primitive tribes that occupied that land before the arrival of the Russians.

In a travel narrative about the north of Siberia written by
Wrangell, Matiouchkine, and Kozmine (1843, 1:117) we find
mention of *miryak*, "a bizarre ailment to which all inhabitants of
northern Siberia are more or less prone: patients had all kinds of
supposed convulsions under the influence of an old and famous
witch from those parts." Another traveller, Richard Bush (1871,
202), gave a more precise description of it: entering a native house
where a group of Yakut and Tungusic were gathered, Bush's companion shouted and made a sudden movement in his direction.
Immediately, a very old woman who was there also shouted and
threw herself on Bush, grinding her teeth and hitting him with her
old fists. Bush's companion doubled up with laughter and seemed
surprised that Bush did not enjoy the joke. The poor old woman
then began to experience convulsions that continued for nearly
three hours. Bush learned that the disease was incurable (they had
tried in vain to treat the patient by flogging), that it was frequent
in the Far North, and that it could be dangerous to excite these
patients, for sometimes they would use any weapon that happened
to be in reach.

Three American navy officers, Buckingham, Foulk, and McLean
(1882), travelling by boat on the Ussuri River, saw the captain clap
his hands when they approached the chief steward, and the steward
clap his hands in the same way while furiously watching the captain. Incidents of this continued to recur, and they finally understood
that the wretch was suffering from a neurosis that made him the
scapegoat of the crew and the passengers. Some of them imitated
the grunting of a pig, said ridiculous things, threw their hats in the
air, and so on, and the poor devil repeated exactly the same things,
often several times in a row; he would beg the people to leave him
alone, or he would become furious but be unable to stop himself
from carrying out the orders of his torturers. Often, he would shut
himself up in his windowless galley, locking the door, but even there
he could be heard, repeating the grunting and shouts coming from
the people outside that were intended for him. One day, the captain, while provoking him, accidentally fell on the deck; our man
immediately fell exactly in the same way and just as hard. Our three
Americans learned that this ailment was called *myriakit* and was not
uncommon in Siberia, especially among women.

By then, Russian doctors had observed and described the disease in
detail. Catrou (1890) provides the translation of an article published

by Yankowsky in 1885 in the Russian newspaper *Vratch*. During a stay in 1876 in eastern Siberia as a medical officer, Yankowsky was called to the side of fourteen soldiers who had "gone crazy," all repeating in unison every question they were asked. They were highly agitated and in each, the pulse was racing. The next morning, all had returned to their normal state, remembering what they had done the day before as if in a dream. The investigation revealed that these fourteen soldiers had seen a Korean merchant who had *meryacha*. Two years later, in Vladivostok, Yankowsky observed a case of multiple *méryachénié* in a family in which the children, aged three to seven, repeated the words addressed to them or uttered in their presence, or the words uttered by one of them, and imitated the gestures in the same way. In isolated form, *méryachénié* was frequent in Siberia, and the sufferer would serve as a toy for those around him. In 1875, he saw a man who, at the command "throw your hat," threw it into the water; he was then ordered to throw himself in, and he would 'have done so and drowned had he not been held back in time. Yankowsky deemed this neurosis to be a hereditary disease specific to certain regions of eastern Siberia, mainly among poor natives and children.

The famous Russian psychiatrist Tokarski wrote a report (1890) on *méryachénié*, known to us by summaries of it in German. He observed that this neurosis existed mainly among the Yakut and the Buryats of eastern Siberia and among certain Russians who settled in the same regions. He reported the observations of the medical officer Kaschin (1868) in the Baikal area: during an exercise, a detachment repeated the orders of the officer instead of executing them, and when the officer got angry, swearing at them and threatening them, they repeated his swearing and threats. Tokarsky demonstrated *méryachénié*'s strong resemblance to *latah*, while distinguishing it from the convulsive tics of Tourette syndrome.

Myriakit was revisited by ethnologists as they conducted in-depth studies of eastern Siberian people for the "Jesup North Pacific Expedition." These observations were scattered throughout ten enormous volumes edited by Franz Boas between 1904 and 1910. These ethnologists introduced the concept of *arctic hysteria*, viewing it as a neurosis common to all Siberian tribes and appearing in various forms, one of which was *myriakit*. Its manifestations varied from one tribe to the next; all, however, were based on commonalities observed in the psychobiology of these Siberian tribes.

Waldemar Bogoras (1909, 38–50) analyzed the biopsychological characteristics of the Chukchi, which were also found in most other tribes: their extraordinarily sensitive sense of smell, the peculiarities of their taste and visual sensitivity, their reckless sensuality, their endurance of physical pain and of cold and hunger, their extreme irritability, and their suggestibility. Bogoras observed that Arctic hysteria manifested itself among the Chukchi through a serious disease, *ité'yun*, consisting of convulsions followed by crises of catalepsy that could last several hours and were then repeated at intervals of a few days, ending in death, sometimes after several years of suffering. Another ailment, *iu'metun*, was a kind of violent nocturnal nightmare during which the patient often died of suffocation. (Incidentally, this description is reminiscent of *bangungut* the Philippines.) Bogoras attributed both these diseases to evil spirits. The wretches who suffered from them were looked upon with abhorrence and avoided. The imitation neurosis itself was rare among the Chukchi.

Jochelson (1908, 416) described Arctic hysteria among the Koryak, among whom the two predominant forms were *meryak* and *menerik*. The first consisted of a kind of hysterical crisis that could end in epileptic convulsions or a cataleptic state. *Menerik* was the Koryak variety of imitation neurosis. In mild cases, the patient would jump at the slightest noise and involuntarily utter an obscene exclamation. In more serious cases, patients had no will of their own, carried out orders given to them, and repeated the words of others (even in a foreign language) as well as actions begun in front of them. These patients, most of whom were women, often old, were treated as playthings and made to perform indecent or dangerous acts. To these neuroses was added a drug dependency: the individual would become inebriated by drinking a concoction made of fly agaric.

Jochelson (1910, 30–8) described Arctic hysteria among the Yukaghir and the Tungusic, where it existed in various forms. One, called *carmoriel*, consisted of a kind of crisis of spirit possession and could last several days. The patient would sing, accompanying himself with rhythmic head and body movements, in this way expressing (so people believed) the desires of the spirit that had possessed him. The crisis might end with convulsions. *Omürax* (similar to the *meryak* of the Koryak) consisted in extreme impressionability that led the woman to be startled by the slightest noise, uttering obscene words and repeating words or noises that she heard and the gestures she saw. Jochelson provides examples of atrocious hoaxes inflicted on such patients; but sometimes patients took revenge on this abuse by suddenly attacking their perpetrator with a knife or any other weapon. A third variety, which, unlike the previous one, was more common among men, consisted of singing in one's sleep. The patient would begin singing in a sad, monotonous voice for hours and, once awake, would not realize he had been singing. A fourth form of Arctic hysteria consisted of a kind of apathy and general indifference. The patient would remain seated for entire days in silence, head bowed. Finally, Jochelson adds that these tribes were subject to psychic epidemics. In 1900, a large number of Yukaghir youth, especially girls, experienced crises during which they uttered inarticulate cries, tore their clothing, tried to drown themselves, looked for knives and axes, and, when people tried to control them, climbed to the tops of large trees, where they remained for entire days.

To these various manifestations of Arctic hysteria we should add *ikota* of the Samoyedic (Cerletti, 1904), a neurosis of married women that generally began on their wedding day: the bride would give a high-pitched cry, be seized with convulsions, tear her clothing, cry, sob, or laugh frenetically, swear or utter obscenities, and sometimes attack those present; at other times she would go into ecstasies, predicting the future on behalf of the devil that had possessed her. When the crisis had passed, the patient would remember nothing. Crises of this sort would repeat themselves well into old age. Obviously, neuroses of this sort presuppose a collective belief in demons and witches, and that the woman was anxious on her wedding day, especially if she had seen other women experience similar.

The last indication we have found of *myriakit* is found in a work by Shirokogoroff (1929, 327). It would be important to know whether this neurosis still exists in Siberia and what forms it now assumes. We sincerely hope that Russian ethnopsychiatrists will soon provide us with information on this topic.

Imu. A third instance of imitation neurosis, very limited in scope, is found in the north of the island of Hokkaido in Japan, among the Ainu. This is a primitive population that, it seems, occupied a large part of the country before the arrival of the Japanese, and that was gradually driven into the north, where they now number around 10,000. This ethnic group, which has nothing in common with the Japanese, has long attracted the attention of ethnologists. We do not know when the existence among this people of a specific neurosis, *imu*, was first reported. A brief description appears to have been given in German by Y. Sakaki in 1903. We also note a study by Winiarz and Wielawski (1936). The most thorough investigation appears to have been conducted by Professor Yushi Uchimura (1956), who examined 110 patients. It is his description that we will follow.

Imu is found exclusively in women and never starts before age thirty. Frequency increases with age. In daily life, at first the patients are not differentiated by anything in particular; but when suddenly excited, they fall into an intense crisis of agitation and anxiety of variable duration. The same applies to the sight or mention of a snake and occasionally another animal (frog, caterpillar, and so on). During the crisis, manifestations of imitation and automatic obedience upon command may be provoked. It is not unusual for women to injure themselves during the crisis or for pranksters to have them drink alcohol or perform erotic dances of which they are deeply ashamed when the crisis has passed. Uchimura adds that he has never encountered a case that resulted in healing.

Imu is very frequent among the Ainu. According to Uchimura, one quarter to one fifth of women over thirty are affected. However, the disease never occurs among the Japanese. A few women who are affected may take advantage of their disease by becoming female shamans.

Among the causes of the disease, we must take into account the role of religious beliefs and superstition, tradition, and the state of subservience to their husbands in which the women live. Winiarz and Wielawski place some importance on the fact that women have the privilege of being able to commit acts of aggression upon their husbands with impunity.

We note some differences between *latah*, *myriakit*, and *imu*. The first two occur sometimes also among men, while *imu* is exclusive to women. *Myriakit* is found in children, and also in collective form. As for *imu*, Uchimura adds that imitation sometimes occurs negatively: the patient executes the opposite movement or command to the one someone wants to have him do.

Conclusion. Much has been written about imitation neuroses, but they have yet to be studied as required. At this point it is impossible to assess the roles played by constitutional biological predisposition and by social and cultural factors. But whether we are dealing with Malaysia, Siberia, or Hokkaido, the same basic elements are found, not only in the clinical picture of the neurosis but also in the social structure. Neuroses of imitation are diseases of the poor, diseases of women in cultures that subject them to male domination, and diseases of the aged in communities where respect for the aged is lacking; finally, they develop under the influence of the harassment and persecution to which the patients are subjected, making their lives ones of constant agony. We may say that these diseases represent an extreme effect of collective aggression against certain categories of individuals, and in that sense there come to mind the witch trials that were endemic in Europe in the fifteenth century: then, too, the great majority of victims were women, especially poor and aged women, who were forced to confess and who ended their pitiful lives at the stake. There we find two different forms of a process similar to social victimogenesis.

Koro. According to Van Brero (1897), it was a Dutch medical officer, Blonk, who first described this neurosis in 1895, in the *Geneeskundig Tydschrift voor Nederlandsch-Indie.* This description was taken up again by Vorstman, and in particular by Van Wulfften Palthe (1935, 1948). New observations were published by Hsien Rin (1963) and by Yap (1964).

Koro consists of crises of paroxysmal anxiety accompanied by two ideas: (1) that the patient's penis is retracting and disappearing inside the body; and (2) that this will result in the death of the subject. For several hours, in order to avoid the fatal outcome, the subject holds his penis with all his might, sometimes with the assistance of people around him. Van Wulfften Palthe provides the description and the drawing of a special apparatus to which patients sometimes have recourse (1948, 266).

The frequency of this neurosis is difficult to assess, as the patient is ashamed to talk about it (Van Brero). The earliest observations dealt with natives in the south of the island of Celebes. Vorstman found it in western Borneo, and Van Wulfften Palthe in Batavia among the Malaysians and also among the Chinese, who called it *shook yong*. There was also a female form of the neurosis among women, who were afraid that their breasts would disappear into their thorax. Hsien Rin (1963) wrote that *koro* existed in southern China under the name of *suo yang* and reported two cases he observed in Formosa among Chinese émigrés: both belonged to traditional families and were eldest sons but lacked identification with the father;

both had masturbated, frequented prostitutes, drank, gambled, and suffered economic difficulties. Yap (1964) in Hong Kong collected nineteen observations of *koro* over fifteen years: thsee patients were all between thirty and forty and were anxious; they all believed that masturbation was the cause of *suk yeong*.

Several theories have been put forward on the subject of *koro*. Van Brero considered it to be a kind of cenesthetic illusion and compared it to those of neurotics who, for instance, have the impression that their head is increasing in size or that their body is decreasing in size. Van Wulfften Palthe saw it as a manifestation of the castration complex. In his book (1948, 258–65), he drew a parallel between it and *latah*, in which the woman is violently repelled by the male sexual organ, which, we may add, is on the contrary, overestimated in *koro*.

Some people have considered *koro* to be a form of sexual psychopathy. In the sixteenth century, demonologists accused witches of making male sexual organs disappear and reappear at will, and the *Malleus Maleficarum* provides two strange descriptions of what apparently was a kind of negative localized hallucination (Sprenger, *Hexenhammer*, trans. Schmidt, 2:78). Hammond (1883) cited the case of a hypochondriac who was obsessed with the idea that his organ was decreasing in volume and who believed it no longer existed. Bychowski (1943) described a patient who suffered from a feeling of localized depersonalization, first in his genitals and then extending to other organs; he committed suicide (we may wonder whether he was schizophrenic). In reality, none of these cases reflected *koro* precisely, and before light can be shed on how it came into being, an in-depth investigation will have to be conducted into the beliefs and superstitions regarding the sex lives of the peoples in which this neurosis exists.

Windigo. A great deal has been said recently about *windigo* (or *witiko*, *witigo*, and so on), and it has been presented as a form of mental disease specific to certain Indian tribes of northeastern Canada.

Windigo refers to both a fabulous being and a disease. The first is an anthropomorphous giant 8 to 10 metres high, with a heart of ice, who lives in the forest and is starved for human flesh. It is described sometimes as a man, sometimes as a woman, but always as a solitary being, naked, who strides through the forest and is terrifying to see. Endowed with prodigious strength, it can easily uproot a tree and has a blood-curdling shriek. It impossible to overcome it, except perhaps through witchcraft. The belief in this monster's existence is deeply rooted among the Indians. It is reported that in 1950 a group of 1,300 of Saulteaux Indians, panicking at the rumour that *windigo* was approaching, fled in terror (Teicher, 1960, 4).

The existence of *windigo* was noted as early as the seventeenth century by Jesuit priests, but the first precise ethnological studies were written by Saindon and Cooper in 1933. Morton Teicher's excellent monograph (1960) includes a general summary and an anthology of everything that has been written on the folklore of *windigo*, with statistics on all known clinical cases, the texts of all descriptions related to such cases, a map, and a complete bibliography.

To understand the genesis of *windigo*, we must place it in its geographical context (Teicher). The desolate regions of northeastern Canada, dotted with lakes and conifer forests, are subject to harsh winters, the length of which precludes any farming. The Indian tribes (Cree, Ojibwa, Montagnais-Naskapi, Tête-de-Boule, and so on) that lead precarious lives in these regions can only feed themselves on what they have hunted, and game is not abundant. Thus they are exposed to two permanent dangers: hunger and cold. In winter, these Indians live in groups of one to three families at most. In summer, larger groups gather in villages, the social organization of which is vaguely defined. But tradition is very strong, as is the belief in ghosts, and the children themselves often play *windigo*.

The severe famines to which these Indians are exposed allow us to understand why cannibalism, which they abhor, nevertheless sometimes occurs. But with the disease of *windigo*, the fundamental phenomenon is not so much cannibalism as the sufferer's conviction that he has been possessed by the cannibalistic monster's spirit. According to Teicher, the Indians distinguish several ways in which the illness can occur:

1 Sometimes it follows a real act of cannibalism committed in the course of a famine: the man who ate the human flesh developed a taste for it and became *windigo*.
2 Sometimes a metamorphosis occurs, which basically creates a heart of ice.
3 Sometimes the guardian spirit is involved: every Indian in these tribes, at a given moment in his life, is said to acquire a guardian spirit whose arrival is revealed to him in a dream; it can happen that this spirit is *windigo*.
4 Finally, a person may become *windigo* through witchcraft.

The individual affected with *windigo* disease experiences, besides a hunger for human flesh, a state of anorexia and chronic nausea. He often falls into a deep depression, loses sleep, isolates himself from other men, and remains silently seated, surrendering to his imaginings of virtual cannibalism. Sometimes he announces to those around him that he has become *windigo* and asks that they kill him, and the terror aroused by this illness is so great that his request is quite likely to be granted. At other times the patient acts upon his threat; the victim will usually be a member of his family. Sometimes the patient merely eats corpses, which, in a harsh climate, keep rather well. Finally, he may heal, through the intervention of either the native doctor or a missionary. Teicher's statistics include seventy cases, forty-four of which actually ate human flesh and twenty-six of which abstained. Out of these seventy, thirty-three were killed by those around them, nine were banished, ten were healed, one committed suicide, and two others were eaten in turn; the fate of the fifteen others is not known.

The data we possess are not sufficiently precise for us to diagnose every case based on the principles of Western psychiatry. Probably we would end up with a whole range of intermediate diagnoses between obsessional neurosis, serious depression, and paranoid schizophrenia. In any case, there is no doubt that the content of the disease and its outward expression are moulded by cultural factors. Among these, the intensity of belief in the *windigo* monster plays a predominant role. From a young age, these Indians are conditioned to the idea that they may become *windigo*. Cooper (1933) mentions that parents forbid children from eating ice, telling them that if they do so, they will be transformed into *windigo*.

Saindon (1933) stresses the role of psycho-biological factors such as nutritional imbalance, tuberculosis, consanguineous marriages, and lack of discipline. Indians, he adds, are impressionable, hyper-sensitive, and subject to their imagination; they have more memory than reasoning, are gullible, and are subject to numerous nervous conditions. Hysteria is frequent among the women and manifests itself as symptoms such as sleepwalking, lethargy, and catalepsy. Cases of hallucination are frequent, and so is a specific kind of obsession commonly termed Indian fear. It would appear, according to this picture, that *windigo* is merely a psychopathological manifestation among others that to date has not been sufficiently studied.

Is *windigo* really a mental illness specific to a few Indian tribes in Canada? Those who claim so seem to have forgotten the resemblances between this condition and the vast group of "delusions of body transformation," particularly transformation into a ferocious animal. Leaving aside the tendency toward cannibalism determined by the specific living conditions of the Canadian northeast, we cannot help but be struck by the resemblances between *windigo* and lycanthropy, a clinical entity largely forgotten today. We know that the werewolf was an individual who believed himself to have been transformed into a wolf, either temporarily or permanently. This delusional idea was based on the near-universal belief in the existence of werewolves (men transformed into wolves through the power of witchcraft or of the devil). The analogy between lycanthropy and *windigo* is reinforced by the fact that some werewolves seem indeed to have committed acts of murder, even of cannibalism, under the influence of their delusion. Esquirol still spoke of this in his *Treatise on Insanity* (1845, 251). Another clinical variety consisted of pseudo-hydrophobia of patients who, without having been bitten by a rabid dog, thought they had caught rabies; not only they but their doctors imagined they found certain characteristics specific to the nature of the wolf, such as eyes that glowed in the dark (Boissier de Sauvages, 1770–71, 2:704).

Finally, we may wonder whether the delusion of body transformation into a ferocious animal is not the complete actualization of a myth[18] that remains in the latent state in all human beings, appearing occasionally in various forms. A strange self-observation by G.E. Morselli attests to this. Morselli (1950, 1:105) reports that while experimenting on himself with mescaline, he experienced this type of feeling:

> As the attacks recurred, I experienced a new, fundamental feeling; it played a dominant role until the toxic action subsided: a tawny-coloured monster was on the verge of suddenly appearing in me ... Some wild thing was about to explode inside me, and, strangely, this retrospective intuition was combined with the image of a tawny colour.

Other clinical entities. Lack of space prevents us from addressing here the study of some neurotic or psychotic psychogenic conditions such as possession syndromes (for which the reader may refer to the fundamental work by Oesterreich) and those of the "loss of soul" (in particular *susto*, so well described in Peru by Sal y Rosas, 1958).

MORBID PROCESSES

What, throughout the many populations of the earth, becomes of the two morbid entities so well described in our classic treatises and so well represented in our psychiatric hospitals: manic depressive psychosis and schizophrenia? We are compelled to recognize that despite a great many studies, the subject remains one of the most obscure in all ethnopsychiatry.

The psychiatrist first comes up against difficulties in terms of diagnosis that are almost insurmountable. To which frameworks in our nosology do the depressions of the primitives correspond? The majority of descriptions make one think of reactive depressions, rarely neurotic or symptomatic. As for endogenous depression (melancholia), thus manic-depressive, some suspect that they take on the mask of psychosomatic disorders, which makes studying them quite uncertain. For schizophrenia, the difficulty is worse, for the term has become one of the vaguest in all the pathology. Depending on whether it is included or not under the name "acute schizophrenia," temporary acute states of confusion, or brief delusional and schizophreniform disorders, we are inclined to think of schizophrenia as very frequent or as very rare in Africa. The paradox is that clinical pictures that are very similar to various clinical forms typical of clinical schizophrenia may be reproduced by trypanosomiasis (Tooth) or hashish addiction (Dhunjibhoy, Lewin), or may appear as a reaction to emotional trauma and heal rapidly by suggestion (Lewin), while in the same regions, schizophrenia can take atypical or pseudo-hysterical forms. Any comparative study of schizophrenia requires the use of rigorous diagnostic criteria and reliable statistics, conditions rarely fulfilled. Recently, the transcultural study group at McGill University in Montreal conducted an international study with the help of questionnaires containing very precise rules and criteria. Despite still being incomplete and imperfect, this investigation has shown that the distribution of schizophrenia and above all of the symptomatic manifestations of schizophrenia vary throughout the world in correlation with certain social and cultural factors (Murphy, Wittkower, Fried. and Ellenberger, 1963). (For details, consult the contribution of H.B.M. Murphy.[19]) Already, we can state that the image of schizophrenic illness, as described in our classic textbooks, must be seriously revised in light of the facts that ethnopsychiatry has acquired.[20]

Psychopathological Personalities

There are at least five types of psychopathological personalities worthy of an in-depth ethnopsychiatric study: the transsexual, the "holy fool," the charismatic healer, the prophet, and the criminal fanatic. Due to restrictions of space, we will limit ourselves to a brief of examination of the first two.

The transsexual. Ethnopsychiatry knows of numerous cases of individuals experiencing gender identity disorders who identify with the opposite gender to their own. This is the case with the *berdache*[21] in North America, the *sekatra* of Madagascar, and many others, the existence and nature of which present problems of the greatest interest. In the great majority of cases, these are men who adopt the women's way of life. The reverse also exists but is rarer.

First, we should clarify some concepts. In sexual pathology, we must distinguish between deviations related to the *object* and those related to the *subject*. Among the former is homosexuality, which consists of attraction to an object of the same sex with aversion for the object of the opposite sex. Among the deviations related to the subject is transsexuality, which is an identification with the opposite sex. There are several forms of transsexuality of variable intensity:

1 The most benign is *transvestism* or cross-dressing: a simple desire to dress in the clothing of the opposite sex.
2 A more pronounced degree of it is when the individual experiences the desire to permanently adopt the clothing, lifestyle, or a job of the opposite sex.
3 The individual suffers from an intense desire to physically transform himself into the opposite sex, to such an extent that some men have themselves castrated.
4 Finally, there is a psychosis characterized by the delusional conviction of having been transformed into the opposite sex (what Krafft-Ebing calls *metamorphosis sexualis paranoiac*).

Transsexuality and homosexuality are sometimes associated, but they are fundamentally different. A century ago, Ulrichs defined male homosexuality as a "female soul in a man's body," an unfortunate definition if ever there was one because it is the precise definition of transsexuality. Ulrichs introduced a regrettable confusion that after a century has not been completely cleared up. Magnus Hirschfeld deserves credit for being the first to radically differentiate these two deviations in his book *Die Transvestiten* (1910). Since then, numerous studies have helped shed light on the genesis and phenomenology of transsexuality. We will mention those of Hans Binder (1933), Bürger-Prinz et al. (1953), Hans Thomae (1957), and Bowman and Engle (1957).

The ethnopsychiatric study of transsexuality began with the Hippocratic treatise on Scythian disease. We find similar facts in the writings of the doctors of classical antiquity and the Arabs. With the discovery of America, the Spanish noted that in the Caribbean, in Louisiana, and in Florida, there existed among the natives a category of men who live dressed as women with the approval and even the respect of the community (Lovén, 1935). These individuals were taken for hermaphrodites or homosexuals and killed mercilessly by the Spanish. The French traveller Le Moyne, who explored Florida in 1564, wrote that among the Indians, these individuals were despised by the community but were used, in time of war, as porters, stretcher-bearers, and nurses. As explorations extended throughout the world, a host of comparable observations were made in the most diverse countries, although the facts themselves tended to disappear following the extermination or deculturation of indigenous peoples.

The founding of a science of sexual psychopathology in Europe by Krafft-Ebing brought renewed interest to this problem. In 1901, Karsch published a copious but uncritical review of these facts, in which he constantly confused cross-dressing with homosexuality. His work is of interest as a collection of documents. Other summaries are the work of ethnologists, in particular Ernest Crawley (1931). J. Winthuis (1928) tried to integrate these facts into a theory that postulated a primitive belief in a supreme bisexual being. These rash theories, backed up by unconvincing arguments, were rejected. A work by Hermann Baumann titled *Das doppelte Geschlecht* (1955) contains a meticulous review of the facts of institutionalized transsexuality throughout the world, accompanied by maps; in it, the author studies the relationship between these facts and rites as well as the myths of various peoples.

Ethnopsychiatry can contribute to the study of transsexuality, because of the abundance and variety of observations it has accumulated; also because it provides observations on the institutionalization of transsexuality, something unknown in our regions;[22]

and, finally, because it can provide new elements for the construction of a theory of normal and pathological sexuality.

We will now very briefly review the main ethnic groups in which facts of transsexuality that are particularly of interest are found.

In *North America*, men who adopted the lifestyle of women have been observed in a great number of Indian tribes. Generally, they are called *berdache*, although their name naturally varies from the language of one tribe to another. The few doctors who had the opportunity to examine some of them, such as Holder (1889) and Hammond (1883), believed that these were sexual perverts. Ethnologists then demonstrated that things were not that simple. In fact, transsexuality is or was an institutionalized phenomenon, that is, the individuals were tolerated and given a specific place in the community. According to Lowie (1948, 244), among the Crow Indians, they were assigned to cut the sacred tree for the Sun Dance.

According to Powers (1877, 132), among the Yuki of California, they memorized the history and legends of their tribe and taught them to youth. According to Kroeber (1925, 497), among the Yokuts of California, they had the privilege or obligation of preparing the dead for burial and conducting the song for the funeral ceremonies. James Teit (1927–28, 384) reports that among the Salish, they became shamans and treated the sick. According to M. Opler (1941, 416), they were ridiculed although tolerated among the Apache. However, among the Navajo, according to W.W. Hill (1935), they were viewed favourably and took care of the children, directed the work of the women, and oversaw the kitchen during great ceremonies. We could extend this list a great deal without altering the general picture, which is, that the *berdache*, whether honoured or despised, everywhere were accepted and assigned certain social functions. It is quite likely that their role changed over the course of centuries within a given tribe.

In Siberia, among the Chukchi, the psychological process of sex change was closely associated with the vocation of shaman. Bogoras (1909, 449) described the stages of this. A young man, at the time of his "election" by a spirit guide, received from him the dreaded order to change gender. First he had to fix his hair the way that women do. In the second stage, the spirit ordered him to don female clothing. In the third stage, the young shaman was forced to abandon all activities and habits of his gender and adopt those of women. He learned to sew, and took care of the children; his appearance, voice, and pronunciation changed and became feminine. He came to give the impression of being a woman, and sometimes "married" a man with whom he led the life of a married couple. Sometimes the process was reversed, with equivalent transformations.

It appears that in Siberia this form of psychic transformation from a man to a woman was closely associated with religious ideas. The individual's shamanic powers grew in proportion to his psychic sexual metamorphosis. Similar facts were described in Sarawak by Ling Roth (1896, 266). Among the coastal Dayak, there existed a superior category of shaman, the *manang bali*, who was said to have changed sex. As among the Chukchi, this transformation happened in stages and on the spirits' orders. A shaman of this category was highly honoured, and grew rich thanks to the medical treatments he dispensed to the sick. He served as a justice of the peace and often became the village chief.

Another form of institutionalized transsexuality existed in Madagascar. The explorer Flacourt, who visited the island in the seventeenth century, mentioned the *sekatra* as a category of "effeminate men." French medical officers who stayed on the island in the late nineteenth century spoke of *sekatra* and *sarimbavy*. Lasnet (1889), among the Sakalava in the northwest, described the *sekatra* as physically normal men who, from an early age, due to their fragile and frail appearance, were treated as little girls; they gradually began to perceive themselves as women and adopted women's dress and lifestyle. "Their condition of gender surprises no one, people find it very natural and no one dares make any remarks, for the *sekatra* may take revenge by casting a spell and bringing disease to people discussing his case." Rencurel (1900) examined in Imerina several *sarimbavy* (a word that, he says, means "image of woman"). He wrote that these people conformed anatomically to the normal male but had completely assumed the attitude, appearance, voice, and movements of a woman, so much so that it was difficult not to mix them up at first. This psychic transformation had taken place in childhood, either of the subject's free will or after he was compelled to undergo it by his parents (as in a family where the father, having seven sons and no daughters, decided that one of the boys should do the work of a daughter). The *sarimbavy* were found mainly among the poor. Rencurel emphasized their ultra-feminine nature as well as their modesty, which often contrasted with the ways of other Malagasy women. Laurent (1911), like the previous authors, claimed that the *sarimbavy* were in no way homosexuals. He recounted that this deviation was often the result of the mother's decision; having had several sons, she would desire a daughter, and when her hopes were dashed, she would dress one of her sons as a girl, give him a girl's name, treat him like one, and accustom him to living as if he were one. Maternal suggestion and autosuggestion make him forget his true gender.

In *Polynesia*, this anomaly was well-known. According to John Turnbull (1807), there existed a class of individuals in Tahiti called the Mahu "whose open profession is of such abomination that the laudable delicacy of our language will not admit it to be mentioned." According to Mühlmann (1932), transsexuals played an important role in the secret society of the Arioi. However, modern authors describe the Mahu as simple transvestites who are not homosexuals (Loursin, 1960; Mazellier, 1964).

The reverse form of transsexualism – a woman dresses as a man and lives like one – is far less frequent. Kroeber (1925, 749) writes that among the Yuma and the Mojave, sometimes a girl adopted the life of a man, but it was quite a rare occurrence. Devereux also cites an example among the Mojave. However, the collective phenomenon of Amazonism is better known. Without speaking of the Amazons of antiquity, about whom Herodotus and the Greek historians gave us so many details that are more or less legendary, Dahomey's Amazons were seen by objective observers (Herskovits, 1938). Every three years, representatives of the king travelled to all the villages and all girls had to be shown to them. The sturdiest were chosen and raised in kinds of barracks adjacent to the royal palace. They were dressed as soldiers, fed as such, did exercises, and learned the art of war, including how to handle weapons. In their songs, they declared, "We are men, not women." They were forced to remain virgins, on pain of death. In war, they were the most valiant soldiers, the cruellest and the most feared by the enemy. Their numbers reached four to eight thousand, according to estimates. They were divided into several regiments. The Agoge, according to Le Hérissé (1911, 67), were the most fearsome; their refrain was "Let the men stay at home and grow corn and palm trees! We will return the entrails with our hoes and our machetes." After the French occupation, the Amazon regiments were dissolved. Le Hérissé says that he met several who became mothers. "They seem to have maintained their former state with a kind of belligerency that was waged particularly against their husbands."

This brief summary of comparative transsexuality among various peoples allows us to distinguish *several categories*:

(1) Transsexuality attributable to *early education*. As we have seen, at least some of the *sarimbavy* were little boys whose parents decided to raise them as girls, and Dahomey's Amazons were little girls upon whom the king imposed a male warrior upbringing.

(2) Transsexuality through deliberate choice and social renunciation. *Berdache* existed among peoples affected by very strong "gonochorism," where the life of men was so harsh and dangerous that some preferred to adopt the lifestyle of women. This change, accepted and institutionalized, was sometimes consecrated with a special ceremony. Powers (1877, 133) recounts how among certain Indians in California the subject appeared before a public assembly, where he was presented with a bow and a women's work tool; if he chose the latter, the status of woman was officially assigned to him.

(3) In some cases, *inverted homosexuals* seem to have been involved, as perhaps for the ancient Tahitian Mahu.

(4) In a final group, the transformation was associated with a *psychotic* or *quasi-psychotic* process. The Siberian shaman felt his mysterious powers increase insofar as his psychic transformation from man to woman was completed. We recall the case of President Schreber,[23] who said that "God had transformed him into a woman in order to save the world." Had Schreber lived among the Chukchi, he would have become a very respected shaman; having had the misfortune to be born in Germany, he was institutionalized. That shows us how the same sexual deviation can have different origins, which ethnopsychiatry allows us to distinguish in a kind of magnifying mirror.

"Holy fools." Classic Western psychology knows two clear-cut cases: the "true fool," and the "simulator." To these, some add an intermediate case: the exaggerator or oversimulator. Ethno-psychiatry reveals the existence of other situations, completely foreign to our way of thinking, in which the problem of the "role" of the mental patient appears in all its complexity.

We encounter in various places, and with varying attributes, an individual foreign to our Western mentality, the "holy fool." This is someone who deliberately acts the fool for a long period or for the rest of his days, generally driven by religious motives.

Probably the best-known type of holy fool is the one the Byzantines called *salos* (plural *saloï*), and after them the Russians called *yurodivy*.

The Byzantine type of "holy fool" was analyzed in detail by Ernst Benz (1938). The *salos* himself was heir to an ancient Middle Eastern tradition not well-known. Benz laid out the social and cultural conditions that made possible the existence of such an individual: first, the unshakable belief, shared by the entire society, that demons exist and that they have a vast sphere of operations in the world. Add to this the notion that insanity is one among many manifestations of the demon, and the result is that the fool is rejected because he is inhabited by demons but recognized as not responsible. Finally, a specific social status is assigned to the fool. He disgusts people and is despised, ridiculed, and subject to a great deal of ill treatment. He is rejected by society but is tolerated within a well-defined territory that includes the street, the public square, the market, the church front, the portico; he shares that domain with people possessed by the devil, tramps, and dogs. But at the same time, the fool is mistreated only to a certain degree, for people fear him and good souls take pity on him. He is given food and alms, and above all he enjoys a degree of freedom and the privilege to say to everyone whatever he likes.

That is how the "fool" lived in Byzantium. We may wonder now what could bring certain men to play such a role. According to Benz, the first motive is asceticism, the desire for heroic self-discipline; the life of the holy fool is indeed more unpleasant that that of the anchorites and the desert monks. Second, the holy fool is able to bring unobtrusive but effective help to certain people who are difficult for the church to reach (people possessed by the devil, thieves, tramps, prostitutes, and so on). Third, the holy fool has the ability to yell out what common mortals only think and do not say. In public, he gives merchants, the wealthy, hypocritical Christians, and the powerful a piece of his mind. Finally, sometimes the holy fool, by way of revelation, is able to publicly predict misfortunes.

So the holy fool plays an excessively tiresome and difficult role, one that requires vigilance at every moment and for which he must immediately adapt his conduct to everyone he meets. Thus he leads a double life. By day, he plays his role of fool; at night, he withdraws to pray. His incognito is known only by one or two people who are very faithful to him and who are bound by absolute secrecy.

Benz described in detail the role the holy fool is forced to conform to, a role that makes its way into everything he says and does. He does not walk like everyone else; instead he hops, limps, dances, and turns in circles, often uttering inarticulate cries. He speaks like a drunken man and eats disgustingly, often unappetizing things. He dresses in rags and is sometimes almost naked. He lives in a sordid hut lacking furniture and books but often spends the night outdoors. He sometimes speaks in long monologues, or utters biting witticisms and insulting remarks. He addresses others as if they were the fools and speaks of himself in the third person. His words seem incoherent but in fact have a double meaning, and the person he addresses sooner or later realizes their hidden meaning. He often speaks in parables or expresses his message through symbolic acts. Among the holy fools of Byzantium, some were considered to be saints, such as Simeon (sixth century) and Saint Andrew (ninth century). Tradition accorded them all kinds of virtues and supernatural gifts.

When Russia, evangelized by Byzantine missionaries, adopted the Orthodox religion, this figure came to Russia under the name of *yurodivy* and played an important role in Russian piety. Several among them were canonized. Among the studies written about them, we note that of Madame Behr-Sigel (1938). Descriptions of them all resemble that of the Byzantine *salos*; in Russia, however, they played a more pronounced role socially and politically. They defended people against the nobility, the poor against the rich, and even went so far as to criticize Czar Ivan the Terrible for his crimes. In the seventeenth century, they began decreasing in numbers, though they still existed, we are told, well into the nineteenth century.

The holy fool was a very foreign figure in Western Christiandom, but he was not completely unknown, and people claimed that Saint Philip of Neri and Saint John of God had a similar quality. It is likely that the "madness" for which the latter was institutionalized in the hospital of Granada was an actual attack of psychosis.

The Byzantine "holy fool" is but one specific instance of a much more general phenomenon – that is, insanity acted out for motives and in forms that are culturally determined. There exist innumerable varieties of it that are difficult to classify. "Role psychology" could be useful here, were it not for the regrettable semantic confusion it perpetuates around the concept of "role"[24] by indiscriminately adapting the term to very different facts. This word is in fact applied:

1   to the role played by someone who knows he is acting in front of an audience that knows he is acting (like an actor in the theatre);

2   to the role played by someone who knows he is acting in front of an audience that doesn't know that he is acting (like the role played by a spy);

3   to the role played semi-unconsciously by someone in front of an audience that lets itself be taken in (like the compulsive liar, the hysteric, or in Moreno's histrionic neurosis);

4   to the role played unconsciously (as in possession or mediumism);

5   to the normal functional role (as when people say that an individual is acting his role of father, husband, office employee, and so on);

6   to the functional role imposed upon a mental patient by those surrounding him or by culture.

Ethnopsychiatry provides many illustrations of these diverse varieties of roles.

Many peoples hold celebrations in which certain individuals dress up and play the buffoon in front of a gathering, entertaining them and sometimes insulting or ridiculing them; they are often paid in return. Lowie (1913, 207–11) gave detailed descriptions of them for certain Sioux tribes. In other cases, an individual finds himself compelled to act for some time the role of a fool in daily life. Clark Wissler (1912, 82–5) described among the Teton Dakota, the "*heyoka* cult." An individual dreams, for example, that lightning has struck his parents' tent. To ward off the curse that may result from this, the interpreters of the dream decide that the subject will become *heyoka*; from then on, he must wear a grotesque disguise and act out all kinds of eccentricities in the company of other *heyoka*. Becoming a *heyoka* is a dreaded misfortune, but the person who manages to perform the role well may earn general respect.

At other times, an individual plays the role of a fool as a penance or out of sorrow. Thus Don Quixote (in Part I, Chapter 25) decides to imitate Amadis, who, due to a heartbreak, has been acting the fool for some time. Likewise, Don Quixote retreats into the mountains, tears his clothing, and does somersaults, which essentially (seeing that Cervantes describes Don Quixote as a fool from the beginning of the book) figuratively represents madness. When Plutarch recounts that Solon feigned madness in order to draw attention with impunity to the political situation in Athens, and in other similar cases, we may wonder if simulated madness is not a means for a citizen to say things out loud that are normally forbidden.

Madness acted out by an individual to trick those around him has often been reported. In the Bible, David simulated faith with Achish, King of Gath, to save his life. Saxo Grammaticus recounts how Hamlet simulated madness in order to save his life and prepare his vengeance, and how he managed to foil all strategies for unmasking him. We read in the story of Tristan how that hero disguised himself as a fool in order to approach Isolde, and so on. It is also among the ranks of those who simulated madness (i.e., did not simply act) that the Byzantine and Russian "holy fools" should be classified.

More complex is the case of certain shamans of Siberia, Alaska, and elsewhere with whom it seems quite difficult to distinguish intentionally simulated madness from real psychosis.

The problem with the channelling of psychosis into a functional role deserves a longer study. It seems that even the most authentic mental patient has a tendency to act out his mental illness according to a role assigned to him by tradition and by those around him. Alongside other imposed roles (such as that of diabolical possession), there is another that we may call "classic madness," which consists of: (1) committing acts and uttering words that are absurd; (2) doing or saying the opposite of what is expected; (3) sometimes uttering amusing words or painful truths. This is the role that, throughout history, we see played by David, by Solon, by the Byzantine *salos,* by Hamlet, by Tristan, by Don Quixote, and so on, and that still appears in our countries in the form of Ganser syndrome.[25] In India, as we have seen, the schizophrenic may socialize his illness by adopting the preformed role of *fakir* or *sadhu,* with all the eccentricities that entails. In modern psychiatry in civilized countries, the chronic patient in a mental home has long been reduced to playing a role in which catatonic stupor, stereotypes, mannerisms, and pseudo-dementia are dominant.

A more in-depth study of such facts could likely help psychiatry sort out the part that "roles" play in mental diseases and in neuroses.

COLLECTIVE PSYCHOSES

Definition. The term *collective psychosis* has been applied to disparate facts. We exclude from this study psychoses involving two, three, or four people, or that extend to a family or a small number of individuals. We reserve the term for psychopathological manifestations that present the following characteristics:

1 They strike a number of individuals that surpasses ten and can reach hundreds, thousands, and sometimes millions.
2 The psychopathological manifestations that strike these individuals are not identical to the neuroses and psychoses of conventional psychiatry, despite some superficial resemblances; they are distinguished through certain specific traits from the moment they strike a crowd or a community.
3 The specific features of collective psychoses are related to a specific category of complex interpsychological phenomena summarized under the term *mental contagion.*

Classification. We can classify collective psychoses under two broad rubrics: (1) *rapid and passing* forms, and (2) *extended* forms, either continuous or intermittent, which may sometimes extend over several generations. It is often difficult to define the scope of these two forms. Sometimes collective psychopathological manifestations that appear to be new and spontaneous are merely revivals of prolonged collective psychoses become latent.

History. The study of collective psychoses has gone through several phases and cannot be separated from the development of concepts concerning group psychology.

Certainly, Greco-Latin antiquity was familiar with collective psychoses, the memory of which was often distorted, even at times mythologized (Heiberg, 1927); it is to one of these psychoses that the cult of Dionysus probably owes its origin. Reiwald (1946, 566) demonstrated that the Romans had ideas about group psychology very similar to those of Gustave Le Bon – for example, the idea that a "crowd" was worse than the sum of individuals constituting it: "Senatores omnes boni viri, senatus romanus mala bestia." According to Hagemann (1951, 101–15), this may be explained simply by the fact that the wealthier Romans, who owned slaves, shared the anti-democratic sentiments of Le Bon: the very term "soul of crowds" expresses a negative value judgment, similar to Horace's *odi profanum vulgus et arceo.*

The oldest collective psychoses about which we have details are those of the Middle Ages, whose chroniclers left us brief accounts.

Hecker (1845, 1865) extracted all useful data from these diffi-
cult-to-access works and summarized them.

A truly precise knowledge of historical collective psychoses begins
with the "witchcraft psychosis" (*Hexenwahn*) of the sixteenth, seventeenth, and eighteenth centuries, for which we have numerous
judicial documents. Many historians have described that particular phenomenon (Roskoff, 1865; Soldan, Heppe, and Ries, 1880;
Hansen, 1900; Delcambre, 1948–49, and so on).

In the nineteenth century, people began publishing compilations
that reviewed the history of the great collective psychoses, either
from a psychiatric point of view (Ideler, 1848; Calmeil, 1845), or
simply from an anecdotal point of view (Mackay, 1852).

A crucial step was taken by Taine, who, in his works on the Ancien
Régime (1876) and the French Revolution (1876–85), did not merely
describe the riots preceding and accompanying the Revolution, but
meticulously analyzed the proximate and distant causes.

In the 1890s, sociologists attempted to unearth the general laws of
collective psychopathy. The great pioneer in these studies was Gabriel
Tarde with his book *The Laws of Imitation* (1903). According to
Reiwald (1946, 131–42), Tarde described under the name of *imitation*
everything that later was called *identification*. For Tarde, the father
is the first Lord, priest, and model for his son, and the "imitation" of
the father by the son is the vital phenomenon at the origin of society;
this "imitation" is based not on strength or guile but on "prestige."
"Prestige" is a phenomenon comparable to hypnotism; it stems from
the father, from the leader, and later from entire communities (that is
how Tarde explains the fascination people from the countryside have
with large cities). Later, Tarde elaborates on his thoughts: "prestige"
does not depend on intellectual superiority, it is not even explained by
will, but is based on "an unanalyzable physical action," which "may,
by an invisible link, be connected to sexuality" (1893, 81). According
to Reiwald, Tarde was the first to show the role of the unconscious, its
coercive force, and of repression in social psychology. Tarde describes
the crowd as intolerant, hypersensitive, and ridiculously proud; as
lacking a sense of responsibility, and as intoxicated with the feeling of
its own power. He distinguishes crowds united by hatred from others
united by love.

Inspired by Taine and by Tarde, Scipio Sighele published a book
called *The Criminal Crowd and Other Writings on Mass Society*
(1892, English translation 2018). Reiwald (1946, 124) writes that

Sighele, while in Sicily, had witnessed a riot during which police officers were killed and partly devoured by infuriated women. The analysis of some crimes committed by the crowd led Sighele to formulate two conclusions: (1) the crime of a crowd cannot be judged if we do not know exactly the historical and social context in which it occurred; and (2) collective crimes do not depend solely on collective suggestion, moral intoxication, or other causes indicated by Taine; above all, they depend on the specific composition of the particular crowd.

The third annual Criminal Anthropology Congress, held in Brussels 1892,[26] heightened the already considerable interest in group psychology, which some seem to have confused with the study of riots and the crimes of crowds. This conception of group psychology was then established by Gustave Le Bon with his *Psychology of Crowds* (*Psychologie des foules*; 1895), a wildly successful book. Le Bon was strongly inspired by Taine, Tarde, and especially Sighele, though he does not quote them. His principal merit is that he presents in an appealing way the concepts developed by his predecessors, though unfortunately he greatly oversimplifies them. Where Tarde speaks of a highly complex "prestige" of nature, Le Bon simply compares the action of the leader on "the soul of crowds" to that of the hypnotizer upon the hypnotized. Following Taine, Tarde, and Sighele, Le Bon describes the collective psyche as a state of regression: the civilized becomes a barbarian. This collective psyche, intellectually, is below that of the individual; emotionally, it is sometimes better but most often worse. The crowd is suggestable, unstable, impulsive, gullible: it thinks in images and not in logical concepts, it exaggerates and distorts, is subject to collective hallucinations; its sense of power makes it dangerous. Le Bon does not go deeper into the psychology of the leader; he succinctly describes the means by which he acts upon the crowd – through sweeping statements, relentless repetition, and mental contagion. The essential stupidity and malice of crowds is the great leitmotiv running through Le Bon's book.

Le Bon's ideas were accepted by many authors as ironclad scientific truths. He established a system of group psychology that may be summed up as follows:

1 Any man placed in a crowd momentarily loses his individuality and acquires another, that of the crowd.
2 A "soul of crowds" exists, from which emerge psychological phenomena irreducible to those of individual psychology.

3 This collective soul is inferior to the individual soul, more rudi-
   mentary, and less sound.
4 The "soul of crowds" cannot be understood without recourse
   to the data of pathological psychology: hypnosis, regression.
5 The psychology of human groups is described based on that
   of crowds. Le Bon applies it, for example, to the psychology of
   juries and parliamentary assemblies.
6 We can thus explain the great vicissitudes of history and the
   destinies of humanity.
7 This is a highly topical problem: "We are in the age of crowds,"
   proclaimed Le Bon. The psychologist will be the doctor.

In fact, "crowd psychology" cannot be understood except as a
historical phenomenon. Dupréel (1934) writes instead about a
vague "anti-democratic pessimism," stirred up by the riots of the
Commune de Paris and maintained by strikes, often bloody, of that
period when "socialism still appeared as street politics, of which
riots were the usual instrument." He emphasizes that it was Tarde
who began a new school of thought with his book *L'opinion et la
foule* (1901): "Our time," said Tarde, "is no longer the time of the
crowd, which has become diffuse, but the time of public opinion,
thanks to the progress in means of communication such as newspapers and telegraphs."

Whereas previous authors attributed the action of mental contagion to a particular psychic mechanism ("prestige," "hypnosis"),
Hellpach (1906) distinguished three forms of psychological interac-
tion: *Einredung* (persuasion), *Einfühlung* (empathy), and *Eingebung*
(suggestion). The contagion between hypochondriacal neurotics
occurs mainly from the first, among manic depressives from the
second, and among hysterics from the third. In psychic epidemics,
these three mechanisms may be found isolated or associated in variable proportions. Unlike Le Bon, Hellpach believed that in collective
psychoses the role of participants' individual characters was more
significant than that of the "collective soul."

Unlike the French and Italian authors, McDougall (1920) adopted
a positive attitude toward the crowd. He recognized the existence
of a primitive fool, such as described by Le Bon, but he saw in it
the point of departure for an evolution leading to the constitution
of increasingly organized groups. This evolution occured under the
effect of a continuity of existence leading to the creation of a group

consciousness, which might be reinforced by relations (conflictual or not) with other groups, by the existence of shared traditions, uses, and habits, and by the differentiation of individuals or specialized groups within the community.

A new chapter in the history of group psychology began with its reshaping within the great systems of dynamic psychiatry (Janet, Freud, Jung, Adler).[27]

For Janet, imitation is the basic psychological phenomenon linking the individual to the group. Imitation is an action driven by the sight of another action. It is twofold behaviour, one part of which is the action of imitating, the other the action of being imitated. Imitation is an economical action, that is, it does not cost much in terms of psychic energy; inducing imitation requires a great outlay of energy, but the imitator is rewarded by the stimulation he receives in return from those who imitate him. That is all the more so in more complex dual conduct, one term of which is the command, and the other, obedience. It is on this basis that rites and myths and then religion are developed, whose function is to extol the strength and elevation of the participants' mental level. Seeking such an effect leads to behaviour such as collective mystical ecstasy and religious fanaticism (Horton, 1924). Unfortunately, Janet did not present these theories in more detail. They account for some collective psychoses, such as the religious frenzy of certain Anglo-Saxon revivals.[28]

Freud presented his ideas on group psychology in his essay *Group Psychology and the Analysis of the Ego* (1923), a complement to *Totem and Taboo* (1912–13) and to his articles on war. Freud cites Le Bon and was inspired by him, but as Reiwald indicated, his ideas mainly resemble those of Tarde. In Freud we find, recast in psychoanalytic language, the principles first developed by Tarde, Sighele, and Le Bon. First, the idea that the individual's psyche becomes transformed in the crowd and takes on its specific characteristics. Then the idea that mental contagion is exerted by the effect of a dual identification, that of the individual with the leader and with the other members of the group (Freud calls "identification" what Tarde called "imitation"). Like Tarde, Freud has this phenomenon of identification derive from a primary model, that of the son's relationship with the father. Third, Freud rejects the notion of the libidinal structure of the crowd, calling "libido" what Tarde and Le Bon called "magnetism" or "hypnotism." Freud adds that aggressive instincts play a role alongside the libido, which corresponds to the distinction Tarde makes between crowds united by love and crowds united by hatred. Finally, Freud too considers the collective psyche of the crowd to be the result of a regression from the civilized to the barbarian (in psychoanalytic language this would be the "primitive hoard" of *Totem and Taboo*). Reiwald criticizes Freud for overestimating the role of the leader and for not taking the crowd's feedback to the leader into account. Freud's theory gives an account mainly of the panic and rapid social disorganization that follow the sudden disappearance of a leader, a situation that occurred in Austria when the Hapsburg Empire collapsed in 1918.

C.G. Jung, representing extreme individualism, paints just as unflattering portrait of crowds as does Le Bon; he calls them "blind beasts" (*blinde Tiere*) and speaks of the role of collective suggestion and "imitation." In the crowd, the individual is subjected a process of "psychic inflation" due to his identification with the crowd and the feeling of increased power resulting from it. These considerations would have introduced no new elements to the subject had Jung not added to them his original views on the revival of archetypes. These are powerful collective images, normally latent, that can grab hold of an individual and make him psychotic, or a crowd, producing a collective psychosis.[29] In a famous article, "Wotan" (1935), Jung explained the advent of Hitlerism by the resurgence of an old archetype, dormant for centuries in the German soul, the archetype of Wotan, god of storms and war, but also of prophetic inspiration and secret sciences. Jung distinguishes between two sorts of leaders: the anonymous leader without any sense of responsibility (*Massenführer*), who lets himself be guided by the crowd that he pretends to guide, and the "true leader" (*wahrer Führer*), who rises above the crowd and leads it. Jung, like Janet, understood that the leader depends upon the crowd and that prestige is far more than a mere individual quality. Prestige raises not only the leader but also the group; however, when it reaches its saturation point, it loses its positive value and a regression occurs. Jung takes up the Sighele's idea that a collective psychosis cannot be understood outside its historical and social context; it extends to all the circumstances made up of the cultural and even vital situation of humanity. In a short book on the myth of flying saucers, Jung (1958) declares that these apparitions, whether or not they are physically real, constitute psychic realties for the people who believe in their existence; he analyzes their structure as symbols and finds in them archetypical characters (symbols of mediation between two immeasurable worlds); this is a myth generated by the fear of atomic destruction and other scourges that endanger the physical existence of humanity.

Adler's theories are in sharp contrast to those of Tarde, Sighele, Le Bon, and Freud. These authors, especially Le Bon, consider the crowd to be intellectually and morally inferior to the individual, as well as dangerous. Adler instead adopts a conception of the community similar to the one held by the German Romantics and even more so by the Russian Narodniks. That is, he sees in the community the source of all public good: language, national culture, logic, the feeling of justice stemming directly from the community. The "sense of community" (*Gemeinschaftsgefühl*) is the basic instinct connecting the individual to the community. But social equilibrium is disrupted by the instinct of superiority, which drives the individual, under the effect of feelings of inferiority, to rise up against the community and want to expand at the expense of other men. It is difficult to account for collective psychoses with this theory. Adler (1934) was compelled to admit that the masses continually allow themselves to be led astray by leaders who trick them with the intention of satisfying their selfish desires for personal domination. Reiwald thinks that Adler's greatest contribution to collective psychology was his description of a certain type of leader, one who exercises "leadership through resentment" (*Führer aus Ressentiment*).

The rise of Hitler and the Second World War revived interest in the study of collective psychoses. We may differentiate two tendencies: one draws on the theories of Tarde, Sighele, and Le Bon and develops or contradicts them. The other seeks new ways for us to renew our understanding of collective psychoses.

Le Bon's scathing opinion of crowds was pushed to its extreme by Ortega y Gasset (1930), spokesman for an individualism almost as radical as that of Stirner.[30] But the great majority of authors ruthlessly criticized Le Bon, whose theories were declared not just false but even dangerous. Stieler (1929) wrote that the crowd was not an organism but a "process," always temporary, one that must be understood based on its location in time and space. He meticulously analyzed the interpsychological relationships between the crowd and the leader. Baschwitz (1951) went over the history of a number of riots Le Bon used to illustrate his theories, showing that Le Bon not only misinterpreted the facts but also often distorted the facts themselves. He wrote that riots and collective crimes are caused merely by a small number of aggressive individuals or criminals, who take advantage of a "paralyzing idea" (*lähmende Idee*) and ensure the neutrality or reluctant participation of the majority by imposing on them a "silent panic" (*stumme Panik*). Add to this the inertia of public authorities (who are sometimes terrorized by their belief in the invincibility of the frenzied mob), and the actions of hidden groups who use the riot for their own secret ends. Hagemann (1951) declared that spontaneous crowds, unorganized, of the type described by Le Bon, were exceptions among the great number of groups he listed as having distinctive characteristics.

Other authors have sought to open new avenues to collective psychology. Cantril (1940) successfully applied sociological research methods to the study of a collective panic. Demographic analysis methods, applied by Bouthoul to a limited field, that of the etiology of war, constitute another avenue of approach. Ethnology introduces us to phenomena such as "cultural mutation" and "mythical liberation movements" that shed new light on collective psychopathology. The same applies to zoology, which has revealed to us the existence of collective psychoses among certain species of animals, linked to biological cycles, which are themselves perhaps linked to cosmic cycles.[31]

Several authors have sought to summarize our knowledge of collective psychopathology. Reiwald (1946) offered a presentation of the various tendencies, seeking to do justice to each. Meerloo (1950) studied in particular the symptoms, causes, and effects of the collective psychoses of war.

Collective psychoses in rapid and passing forms.[32] In this group we must mainly consider collective hallucinations, panics, attacks of mass hysteria, riots (bloody or not), crimes of crowds, and epidemics of collective self-destruction.

Collective hallucinations. The classic example of a collective hallucination is that of the crew of the frigate *La Belle Poule*, which broke out in 1846, and which we will first cite in the version provided by Le Bon:

The frigate *La Belle Poule* was cruising to find the corvette *Le Berceau*, in the middle of the day, under a sunny sky. Everyone, officers and sailors, noticed a raft filled with men signalling for help. A rescue craft was sent out, which noted "masses of men, restless, lifting up their hands, and ... the muffled, indistinct sound of a great many voices." In reality, it was merely a few tree branches covered in leaves, pulled from the nearby coast.

At first glance, the anecdote seems to confirm Le Bon's opinion on the stupidity or intellectual incompetence of a "crowd," if we give that name to a ship's crew. But Le Bon neglected to take into account the principle put forward by Sighele: no phenomenon of collective psychopathology can be evaluated separate from its antecedents and its historical and social context. By isolating it from its context, Le Bon rendered this event unintelligible. To understand it, we must reference the account given by the sailor Félix Julien (1861). From that, we learn the following details:

(1) The crew of *La Belle Poule* had been stricken hard by malaria and was physically exhausted.

(2) *La Belle Poule* had for a long time been moving in convoy with *Le Berceau* before the two were separated by a terrible hurricane. It was feared that *Le Berceau* had foundered, engulfing three hundred victims.

(3) On the day of the hallucination, *La Belle Poule* had been looking for *Le Berceau* for a month; during that time, the crew of *La Belle Poule* had been very anxious, besides sailing with a makeshift mast. At the time of the hallucination, the presumed death of so many comrades and friends was at the heart of all conversations.

(4) That evening, the sun was bright and warm air shimmered on the horizon. It was on that side of the ship that the sea current was carrying along a mass of large trees (not just "a few branches"), which probably had been uprooted from the coastal forest by the hurricane.

The sailor on watch, seeing in the intense light objects whose nature he could not make out, cried: "Disabled ship ahead!" That was the point of departure for the collective hallucination. The sailors and officers, indeed the admiral himself, thought they saw a ship in distress as well as boats filled with men, whose gestures they soon saw and whose cries of distress they soon heard. We see in this case that the collective hallucination was explainable by a series of causal factors: physical exhaustion, mental depression, overriding concern that over a month had developed into an obsession, and finally sensory factors that contributed to creating an illusion (floating trees hard to make out under intense light). But the alignment of all these causal factors does not imply that the collective hallucination was inevitable. It is very possible that, had the sailor on watch not sounded the alarm with so much conviction, the crew would not have been victim of the illusion. Nor does Le Bon mention the important detail that the collective hallucination was not instantaneous; it was at first that of just one man, then a few, before it became generalized.

Another classic example of collective hallucination is that of the "Angels of Mons."

In August 1914, the British were pulling back from Mons when the retreating soldiers saw in the sky long lines of mysterious cavalrymen, armed with bows and arrows, who for long hours accompanied them. Some recognized St George, England's patron saint, at the head of a celestial army, but most saw angels or "mysterious beings." That is, at least, the common version of this event.

This episode led to heated debate. The writer Arthur Machen (1915) claimed involuntary responsibility for the collective hallucination. Machen relates how, when he learned the news of the disastrous retreat from Mons, he wrote a short story in which he showed British soldiers comforted by a strange light, in which could be made out a long line of "shining beings." This tale, published by a newspaper, was taken by many readers as authentic testimony and reproduced widely with variations. The "shapes" became saints or angels, then the *Occultist Review* began collecting accounts from eyewitnesses (Shirley, 1915). Harold Begbie (1915) investigated and came to conclude that the hallucinations had begun a few days before the publication of Machen's short story. But after extensive research, he could find only one witness, a wounded officer, who told him that during the retreat, he had noticed in the sky "a strange light" in the middle of which three "shapes" could be made out, one of which, in the centre, featured "something resembling open wings." These apparitions – less spectacular than in the usual account – lasted about three quarters of an hour.

Among the causal factors for these hallucinations, we find the following:

1 The *physical exhaustion* of troops defeated and harassed by the enemy.
2 The *mental exhaustion* of soldiers who had thought the war would be brief and glorious and who were experiencing the shock of an unexpected defeat.
3 *Optical phenomena*. A particularly luminous sky toward evening, which seems to have contributed to the illusion.

But these various elements do not explain everything. Begbie notes that the British soldier was hardly prone to mystical hallucinations and that these did not arise among the French, who at the time were undergoing an equally difficult ordeal. We are thus led to suppose that among the British there was an initial source of the hallucination, perhaps the hallucination of just one man – perhaps someone who had read Machen's story – which spread by mental contagion. In contrast to the hallucination of *La Belle Poule*, there seems to have been here a series of collective hallucinatory episodes, occurring in several places and over several days.

Another type of collective hallucination is that in which visions, initially perceived by one or two people, are repeated before growing numbers of spectators, who individually give differing versions that end up merging into a common legend.

An example is a supposed appearance of the Virgin Mary in Dordogne in 1889, which Marillier (1891–92)[33] went to study on site. A girl, aged eleven, Marie Magontier, said that the virgin had appeared in a deserted place surrounded by celestial light. A second girl, Marguerite Carreau, then said she had had the same vision. Then it was the turn of a third, Marie Gourvat. The appearances increased and recurred in front of crowds, which grew eventually to 1,500 people. Marillier was received by the "seer," Marie Magontier, "with an expression of mocking hostility." He learned that she was the daughter of an epileptic father and a psychotic mother: the parish priest described her as "full of ambitious ideas" and "thinking she knew better than the priests," for she was a friend of the Holy Virgin. According to Marillier, the second visionary was kind and shy, and the third was pretentious and insolent.

To clearly understand these hallucinations, we must place them in their local context of superstition and folklore, and in the broader context of the controversies of this time between Catholics and free thinkers, between conservatives and "republicans." If the epidemic did not develop further, it is probably due to the lack of encouragement it encountered in ecclesiastical circles.

In most accounts of collective hallucinations, we find that each of the participants, when questioned separately, saw the hallucination in a different way. At times it is not seen by one or some of the participants, who, worried they will not see like the others, end up experiencing the contagion. Sidgwick (cited by Schjelderup, 1964, 172) describes how the famous Italian revolutionary Mazzini one day

witnessed the collective hallucination of a crowd who saw a cross
in the sky; only one man appeared unbelieving. "What do you see?"
asked Mazzini. "The cross, here," replied the man. "But no, there is
no cross," Mazzini told him. Upon which the man seemed to awaken
from a dream and said: "No, it's true, there is no cross there."

Panics. A *panic* is an attack of collective fright or terror in which the
phenomena of mental contagion play a key role. We usually distinguish panics that occur due to a real danger (such as war panic) from
those that are triggered by an imaginary danger. There is also a more
basic and practically physiological form of panic, independent of the
clear representation of danger.

A typical example of "pure panic" is the disaster that cast a shadow
over the coronation day of Czar Nicholas II, on 18 May 1896.
Conforming to an old tradition, the government wanted the people to
share in the festivities, so it organized the distribution of small pack-
ages of food on a vast plot of land, Khodynka, near Moscow. The
authorities expected 400,000 people to attend, but double that number showed up, many of whom were poor *muzhiks* come from afar by
rail. As the night was fine and warm, the crowd gathered the evening
prior on the field where the distribution was to take place to spend the
night outdoors. The tragedy unfolded in three stages.

1 After the long hours of waiting through the night, the crowd
   was tired but happy.
2 Starting before dawn, a feeling of uneasiness emerged as the
   crowd continued to grow. Those who approached were as if
   snatched up by the throng, and it became impossible to leave.
   The newcomers pushed and shoved the others; there was a lack
   of space. People were anxious for the distribution to begin.
3 Suddenly someone shouted: "There are 400,000 portions
   and we are already twice that many. Forward!" A ripple went
   through the crowd, and, seized with a blind fright, it surged
   forward, trampling men, women, and children. The number
   of fatalities was estimated officially as 1,300, but as 4,000 to
   5,000 by enemies of the regime; the numbers of injured were
   considerable.

Causes of this catastrophe include the insufficient number of
policemen, the physical exhaustion of many of the participants, and

other unknown factors. Following the panic, there was a wave of unrest and demonstrations against the police, resulting in crackdowns. Political tensions increased. Superstitious minds saw in this catastrophe a harbinger of more serious tragedies to come. Just as in group psychology, an event takes on its full meaning only after it has been placed in its broader historical and social context.

The great majority of panics are connected to a clear representation of real or imaginary danger. But in panics that follow a real danger, the imagination often plays an important role.

The oldest recorded panics where real danger was involved were probably those that struck armed forces in the field. Yet we know there is no direct relationship between the panic itself and the actual seriousness of the danger (it is classic here to point to the inexplicable panic that struck the Persian army at Marathon and led to the victory of the Greeks). This is why many authors have sought to clarify the causes of these panics.

Brousseau (1920) cites many factors:

1 *Physical conditions*: exhaustion, poor diet, intoxication.
2 *Psychological conditions*: long waits, isolation, darkness, the disadvantages faced by some units.
3 The *seriousness of the danger* and its duration. He cites Ardant du Picq's assertion: "Man can tolerate a given amount of terror; beyond that, he is overwhelmed."

To these conditions, Meerloo adds the *surprise factor*, which appears in panics provoked by unknown weapons: gas attacks in 1915, tanks in 1917, *stukas* in 1940, and the atomic bomb in 1945. However, decisive importance must be given to *accidental factors* (false news, orders heard wrong) and to the example of isolated individuals or small groups who give in to the fear.

Brosin (1943) attempted to summarize the teachings of the Second World War. Excessively emotive people and unstable emotional people are predisposed to panic; the quality that best protects soldiers from panic is endurance. Panic can be prevented by the following: confidence in leaders, good training, maintaining of physical contact with friends, the constant dissemination of accurate information, avoidance of motor and spatial limitations and of "the unknown," engaging in constant activity, fighting against false news, and being trained to mask one's emotions. The soldier must be accustomed to the idea of killing and being killed, and maintain his individuality under "stress." Most panic-stricken soldiers react quickly and well to an atmosphere of security and reassurance. Sometimes it is their physical condition that requires care. In all cases, the treatment is individualized; if possible, they are to be treated by people who come from a cultural milieu similar to their own.

With a few minor variations, these conclusions apply to all sorts of panics, such as those that occur during a fire, a shipwreck, or a bombing. Sometimes the quick intervention of a person speaking with authority, giving clear and precise orders, is all that is needed to quell a panic at the start. Much more effective prevention is ensured by any trained and disciplined organization (firemen, ship's command, civil defence service, and so on), providing they act rapidly and firmly.

The impact of emotion and the imagination on panics is demonstrated by the fact that panics may occur in the complete absence of danger. One of the best-known examples is that of the "Martian invasion," of which Cantril (1947) conducted a model study.

On 30 October 1938 at 8 p.m., American radio stations broadcast an adaptation by Orson Welles of the famous novel by H.G. Wells, *The War of the Worlds*. For the radio production, the novel was presented as a series of broadcast messages, as if a real event were taking place. Astronomers reported that they had seen gas explosions on the planet Mars. Then they announced that an enormous cylindrical object had crashed in New Jersey. The cover of this cylinder, they added, had slowly come undone, and a kind of monstrous snake had emerged that killed the human beings present with a "heat-ray weapon." The broadcast was interrupted four times to remind the public that it was a fictional story.

Well before the broadcast ended, a panic of national proportions developed across the United States. It was estimated that 9,000,000 adults were listening to the broadcast, one third of whom believed it was true; 1,200,000 listeners were "worked up," and thousands were terror-stricken and began crying, praying, and taking to the roads to escape. Some believed they saw flames. However, there were no victims.

Cantril and his team carried out a study on the factors that had produced the panic. Among those who listened to the broadcast, they distinguished four types of reactions: (1) some people at no moment believed it was anything but fiction; (2) some had doubts but made inquiries and were quickly reassured; (3) some tried to make inquiries but were unsuccessful; and (4) some did not even think to verify the story's authenticity because they were so upset.

Cantril's team found that individuals who in normal circumstances had critical thinking skills had nevertheless believed the invasion was genuine. Therefore, in exceptional conditions, critical thinking is not enough. The factors conducive to panic were emotional instability, susceptibility, immaturity, phobias, lack of self-confidence, and fatalism. Differences in age and gender do not appear to have played a role.

According to Cantril, a factor that was powerfully conducive to the outbreak of panic was the political situation and fear of an impending war with Germany. Another factor seems to us to have been neglected, however: the broadcast took place the evening before Halloween, when American children dress up and often enjoy playing pranks and frightening the neighbours.

Mass hysteria. The term *mass hysteria* applies to all psychopathic manifestations where irrational movements and actions spread through mental contagion. We distinguish two broad categories: identical disturbances (the same among all participants), or multifaceted (aspects differ from one participant to another).

Some manifestations of mass hysteria are "socialized," that is, channelled and recognized by the community provided they occur on certain dates, in certain places, and within strict limits. We note the Saturnalia of the Romans, the Feast of Fools in the Middle Ages, and Carnival in the present day. But sometimes these manifestations break out of their institutional framework and degenerate into a collective uncontrollable frenzy accompanied by orgies or violence. This sometimes occurs during Carnival in some regions of northwestern Argentina (Dudan, 1953), and no doubt in other places.

Regarding mass hysteria, it is customary to mention the psychic epidemics that invaded convents in the Middle Ages, such as the story, cited by Hecker (1832), of the convent where nuns meowed like cats for several hours a day, and the one where they bit one another. Such anecdotes are unusable for collective psychopathology. Any epidemic of mass hysteria will be of enormous complexity, and its etiology can only be elucidated by an investigation that is at once psychiatric, psychological, sociological, and often ethnological. As an example, we look at the epidemic of mass hysteria that struck the girls of an American school in 1939. Here is the customary account, as summed up by others who have cited it:

In the spring of 1939, at a high school, a girl named Helen was overcome with involuntary twitching and twisting of her right leg. In the space of a month, many other girls in the same school temporarily experienced the same twitching, so much so that authorities were forced to close the school temporarily. The epidemic soon disappeared, and, alone, Helen and one of her friends still occasionally experienced twitching of the leg.

Presented in this way, the account is perfectly unintelligible. Fortunately, the authors published the results of a detailed investigation they conducted (Schuler and Parenton, 1943).

We must begin by situating the event in time and space as well as its social and cultural context. The psychic epidemic took place in the small city of Bellevue, 80 kilometres from New Orleans, Louisiana, in a parish inhabited by the descendants of French colonists who still spoke (at least at that time) a Creole dialect. These people were deeply attached to their religious and cultural traditions; Carnival, for example, was a time of great rejoicing, but Lent was strictly observed. The high school, which 275 girls attended, was excellent. Naturally, it followed the program and methods of similar American schools, in which great importance was attached to "social" activities and to one's own "popularity." All of the students lived at home; no one boarded.

Now let us look at the circumstances of the time. This was the spring of 1939, when there was much discussion of a possible war (remember the "Martian" panic had taken place a few months previous). Another circumstance: a new dance, the jitterbug, was all the rage in the big cities and had just appeared in Bellevue. Carnival was a few weeks away, and according to local custom, the school's students were supposed to elect a king, a queen, and a Mardi Gras court; there would be a dance at the school, for which a compulsory dance class for students had been organized so that the oldest ones (including Helen) could learn a new dance called the bunny hop. The school carnival was meant to take place on 16 February, but on 28 January another annual school ball, the Alumni Homecoming Dance, was held.

The psychic epidemic began with a seventeen-year-old girl, Helen. The authors tell us that she was pretty, intelligent, considered a good student, and "popular" among her classmates (we know that in American schools, the word "popular" has a specific meaning: it contains the idea of success in a permanent competition to be well thought of by others). Moreover, Helen belonged to a traditionalist family. Highly devout, she belonged to the Children of Mary. Like her parents and her older brothers, she was not at all interested in dance, and at the ball she was content to be a spectator. Nevertheless, that year, dance had been declared obligatory, so she had to take part in the class; but she began missing it, coming up with excuses. Two other recent events affected Helen. She was in love with a young man, Maurice, who had just dropped her, attracted by a German girl, Gretchen, who was a very good dancer. Finally, during the election of the Mardi Gras court, Helen was not elected for any of the duties of lady in waiting (which seemed to indicate a decline in her popularity).

The psychic epidemic unfolded in three stages.

In the first stage, it involved only Helen. On the evening of Saturday, 28 January, at the Alumni Homecoming Dance, she began to experience twitching in her right leg. The twitching recurred at intervals, arising each time Helen was forced to make an effort to do something, or each time someone spoke to her. It occurred less often at home than at school. Naturally, it prevented her from dancing. The school carnival was then held (16 February), and the public dances of the Mardi Gras took place in Ferryville, not far from Bellevue.

The second stage began the day after Mardi Gras. A sixteen-year-old student, returning from the celebrations in Ferryville, was overcome by twitching similar to what Helen had experienced. A third girl, also sixteen, was affected in class the following day. These two new patients belonged to families poorer than Helen's and were not popular like her. From that point on, the epidemic spread rapidly.

The third stage was triggered by the intervention of a family in Ferryville: the mother had openly just withdrawn her children from the school, and following her example other families did the same amid cries and anxiety. Other students had to be sent to the infirmary. Rumours spread outside about "strange events" occurring at Belleville High School. Given this situation, school authorities closed the school for a week.

The school then reopened, but for scarcely half the students. The head of the school board made a reassuring speech to the students, as did the doctor, and the other students gradually returned. The epidemic came to an end the following week.

Schuler and Parenton indicate that other etiological factors were associated with the ones mentioned above. The people of Bellevue had been preoccupied with an epidemic of measles, as well as with the unpleasant taste of the local drinking water, and there was a widespread fear of epidemics. At school, conflicts had arisen over a new gym uniform the students were being forced to wear. Finally, the new and fashionable dance, the jitterbug, certainly had some similarities to the hysterical twitching of the young patients.

We can now briefly reconstruct the process of this psychic epidemic. In the *first stage*, it only involved Helen and her personal problems: she was experiencing inner conflict about the dance, torn between her aversion (probably due to the family tradition) and her duty to take part in it, along with, most likely, the desire to not let herself be outshone by her younger rival and thereby lose her popularity. The twitching of her leg constituted a typical symptom, a kind of compromise between impulse and inhibition; it allowed Helen to find an escape from her conflict, an excuse not to dance, and this symptom attracted new attention to her at a time when she feared the waning of her "popularity." In the *second stage*, it was two girls, less privileged than Helen in terms of social status and popularity, who resorted to this means – hysterical twitching – to draw attention to themselves; the example of Helen was all the more willingly imitated as Helen was very popular at school. From that moment on, the psychic contagion came into play at school. In the *third stage*, the psychic epidemic reached environments outside the school: the families of students as well as public opinion. Outside opinion had been prepared by various causes: concern about recent epidemics, dissatisfaction in certain families (apparently) regarding the new gym uniform, and, finally, general concern about the international political situation.

It seems to us that Schuler and Parenton have not sufficiently highlighted the ethnopsychiatric side of the psychic epidemic. We think there was a *cultural conflict* at play, between, on one hand, the old French milieu, Catholic and traditional, and on the other, American education and ideology with the emphasis it places on the "social" aspect of the dance as an instrument of competition and popularity.

This example shows us the degree to which the simplest, shortest, and most localized collective hysterical epidemic can turn out to be complex once we begin to sort out the etiological factors. This is even more true for similar epidemics that extend over space and time and for those that arise in populations that are culturally very different from our own. Here ethnopsychiatry provides a great quantity of documents, but without in-depth investigation, most of them are only of anecdotal interest.

Nor is it always easy to distinguish the collective hysteria of a riot. Also, it is also not rare for a riot to begin with a stage of mass hysteria.

Riots. Riots are collective psychoses characterized by the fury of the participants and the destructive nature of the acts they commit. Sometimes only the destruction of material goods is involved, sometimes also aggression against people. We also distinguish between "pure" riots, which have no specific purpose, and riots directed toward a special purpose or against certain people. "Pure" riots are often spontaneous; riots with special purposes are generally organized by at least some of their participants (even if only a very small number, who influence the rest through mental contagion).

The scientific study of riots began with Taine and his writings on the French Revolution. Taine was the first to realize that the disorders of the Revolution could not be understood without considering the general causes that made them possible:

1 First there was the *food shortage*, which had been almost permanent for ten years and which drove enormous crowds to despair.
2 Then a kind of *hope* appeared. Under Louis XIV and Louis XV, people had suffered more, but the rioting they had engaged in had been repressed quickly and harshly. Now there was talk of reforms, and of parish, provincial, and other assemblies, and this made the people grow impatient to finally see them.
3 *The revolutionary ideology* had filtered down, level by level, from the aristocracy to the educated members of the Third Estate and even to the people, through countless revolutionary pamphlets.
4 There was a *core of agitators*, centred in the Palais-Royal, usually a centre of idleness haunted by loafers and adventurers. Being off-limits to the police thanks to the privileges held by the Duke of Orléans, to whom it belonged, it was an ideal place to stir up agitation and riots.
5 *Recruits for the riot* were at hand, who came from three

different ranks: the starving; the patriots, who were convinced they were acting for the common good; and suspicious elements. In fact, there had been in France for a long time under the Ancien Régime huge numbers of smugglers and other petty criminals, as well as vagrants, escaped or ex-prisoners, and beggars. These constituted a fluctuating and highly mobile mass, ready to place themselves at the service of the agitators.

6 All of the above would not have been enough without adding the *inadequacy of the central government*: the weakness of the king, the softness of the military leaders, and the ultra-polite manners of the upper classes made it impossible to adopt the appropriate response to violent unrest.

Taine wrote that when the government fell, a victim of its own weakness, everything happened as if to a living organism whose brain had been paralyzed. With the disintegration of society, each man fell back into his original weakness. The former social deterrent of the law and the inner deterrents of discipline and education disappeared. Gangs were formed, led by the worst and subject to the compounding effects of protests, drunkenness, and the spectacle of destruction. The agitators of the Palais-Royal and elsewhere provided the slogans, which their leaders translated into actions (apparently it was Taine who introduced the word *meneur* to French, as an equivalent for "leader").

We see how much more nuanced Taine's ideas were than Le Bon's. Le Bon borrowed from Taine his historical examples and part of his psychological description of crowds, but he attributed to the crowd a kind of psychic autonomy and essential malice, suppressing the historical and sociological aspects that made intelligible the riots described by Taine. Baschwitz (1951), basing his thought on the study of recent riots, showed that they often confirmed Taine's ideas and that this knowledge of their mechanism made effective prevention and suppression possible.

But Taine's descriptions concern only a particular type of riot. Certainly other types exist, the analyses of which reveal a different mechanism. This is so for certain riots, close to mass hysteria, that appear to be spontaneous and unorganized.

Take for example the riot that occurred in Stockholm on the evening of 31 December 1956. The Kungsgatan, a principal thoroughfare in the Swedish capital, was invaded by around five thousand furious teenagers and young people, who for several hours were masters of the street, roughing up passersby, throwing projectiles at police, smashing store windows, overturning cars, setting up barricades with materials at hand, setting a fire, and even desecrating graves in a cemetery. Only after a bitter struggle did the police bring the situation under control. Eyewitnesses were struck by the "silent frenzy" of the teenagers, who, judging from their nasty and impenetrable expressions, did not appear to be enjoying themselves. The investigators stated that the violence had not been directed against anyone in particular – it had erupted spontaneously and had no recognized leaders.

This riot generated numerous discussions, and no agreement as to its cause has ever been reached. Stieler's ideas (1929) about the spatial-temporal structure of riots provide the beginnings of an approach. From him we learn that episodes of the same type, albeit on a lesser scale, were far from rare in Sweden – indeed, they recurred every Saturday in some places. Moreover, for several years, New Year's Eve had been taking place in a carnival-like atmosphere, which strengthened from year to year, reaching its peak in 1956. Also, the crowd was less unorganized than had first been reported: it was comprised of groups of teenagers who often knew one another, at least by sight, and who had participated in previous disturbances of this sort. The 1956 demonstration, though a little more violent than usual, was part of a permanent state of affairs that required closer analysis.

The investigation revealed that these furious youths were often the sons and daughters of skilled workers and that many of them had jobs; none faced material hardships or had any personal concerns about the future. The destructiveness seems to have been directed not against people or institutions, but against the ideology of the former generations. The massive vandalism seems to have been directed against propriety itself. A desacralizing impulse was apparent in the choice of New Year's Eve (which had once been a religious holiday) and in the desecration of the cemetery. Following their own preconceptions, the authors suggested that the riot's causes included the damaging effects of widespread social welfare, the "era of affluence," the destruction of the family, religion, and morality, a demographic revolution that had distorted the age cohort of recent decades, and rapid cultural change that led to a generation gap. Going further, De Martino (1962) spoke of a manifestation of Freud's death instinct, comparable to the periodic outbursts during New Year's festivals in Babylon and in other cultures. At the very least, we can conclude that the Kungsgatan riot was one accidental manifestation among others of a collective psychosis far more vast than Sweden, one that extended to many other countries, and one that has barely been studied scientifically.

Crimes of crowds. Crimes of crowds are a specific variety of riot. With these, the people's fury rapidly seeks to assuage itself with the murder of one or several individuals. Some of the riots examined by Taine belong to this group. The first notable monograph devoted to such crowds was Sighele's *The Criminal Crowd and Other Writings on Mass Society* (2018). In-depth studies have been conducted in the United States by Raper (1933) and by other authors.

Two main points were demonstrated by Sighele. The first, which we have already referred to, relates to social context:

> We cannot pass judgment on a criminal by examining his
> conduct only in terms of the crime connected; we must try
> to discover his state of mind, his character, and the economic
> conditions – likewise, we cannot judge a crowd's crimes if we do
> not know the aspirations, leanings, and in a word the physical
> conditions and the morale of the people of whom this crowd is
> but one part. (85)

The second essential point is that a crowd's crimes are a function of the criminal elements it contains. During the French Revolution, crowds committed murders and atrocities, but that was because the crowds, as Taine has shown, were partly comprised of brigands and habitual criminals. But Sighele also refers to the riot of May 1760 in Paris, during which the chief of police was surrounded in his backyard; an officer, facing the assailants, opened the doors and by his attitude alone made the people retreat. Sighele reckons that in similar circumstances during the Revolution, the crowd would have killed that officer. In this instance, however, the riot had been provoked by the rumour that Louis XV was kidnapping children of the people and having their throats slashed so that he could take baths in human blood and thereby regain his health, which had been worn out by debauchery. Far from being a criminal crowd, it was comprised of fathers and mothers who were terrified for their children. To take more recent examples, Sighele relates how, during a strike in Decazeville in 1886, an engineer named Watrin was killed by the crowd; among the assailants were several former ex-convicts. However, during a riot of workers in Rome in 1889, a crowd of one thousand demonstrators let themselves be persuaded; thirty-two arrests were made, but none of those arrested were found to have a criminal record. Sighele adds that among the criminal elements of the crowd there were also latent criminals, soldiers, and butchers (who often played a bloody role in revolutionary riots).

Sighele did not delve deeper into how criminal elements manage to have a crowd carry out a crime. He wrote that it is often difficult to tell who is the leader and who are the led. Instead, an explosion of brutality occurs among the criminal elements, and the participants follow, be it voluntarily or reluctantly. Jean-François Marmontel formulated the pithy phrase, referring to Tacitus: "If among the people few men then dared crime, many wished and all suffered it."

Baschewitz (1951), as we saw earlier, reviewed the analysis of collective crime, adding the notions of "the paralyzing idea," "silent panic," and the subsequent devaluation of the victim by the inactive participants or passive spectators, who were seeking to rid themselves of the guilt they felt arising from their passivity.

Collective crime takes very diverse forms, depending on the country, the time period, and the ethnic and social environment. A collective crime that has been studied in great depth is the lynchings of Blacks in the United States; we will briefly sum up the characteristics of these crimes, based Raper's book about them (1933).

Raper begins by calling lynching a gang murder in the sense that it is premeditated, organized, and performed by a criminal organization, generally in secret. Yet lynching is also a spontaneous crime, carried out in the presence of a wide public, in open defiance of the law, and is conducted with certain rites. The word lynching is derived, apparently, from the name of the farmer Charles Lynch, who, in the absence of a local police force, founded in Virginia a small organization of dispensers of justice to fight outlaws and partisans of the British.

For a long time, lynching was only practised *on* Whites and *by* Whites, who claimed they were assuming the duties normally granted to the law, acting in its place when local courts showed too much leniency. As for the crimes committed by black slaves, they were punished by their white masters with the approval of the official system of justice.

After the Civil War, the victims of lynching were increasingly likely to be Blacks in the southern United States. The practice seemed to be disappearing elsewhere. It is estimated that in 1890, two hundred lynchings were conducted every year. After that year, they gradually decreased. Lynching is now very rare.

People have wondered why lynching has been non-existent in some countries, such as South Africa, where there is no less racial conflict than there is in the United States. Lynching can only be understood in relation to the historical and social circumstances that give rise to it. After the Civil War, the southern American states were ruined; unsolvable problems arose both for whites and for freed Blacks. Segregationists would tell us that excesses were committed by the Blacks and that the whites organized themselves to fight against what they saw as a mortal danger. It is from this perspective that segregation, the banning of Blacks from voting, secret societies such as the Ku Klux Klan, and the lynchings of Blacks should be understood.

From the start, the characteristics of lynching were sharply defined. The capital crime was the rape of a white by a Black. An alarm would be sounded, and a dramatic pursuit would ensue, sometimes with police dogs, sometimes with a semblance of resistance from the police. The arrested Black was often subject to a travesty of a trial. The execution was carried out with some ceremony, publicly, in the presence of a huge crowd (estimated at 15,000 in one case); the victim was often burned alive or killed after being tortured for a long time. Some spectators took photos, filmed the death, or picked up "souvenirs" (the victim's skull, for example). Often, the lynching was accompanied by destruction, including the torching of nearby black properties. One striking fact was the absence of guilt among the perpetrators and spectators: an act of "public justice" had been carried out, just as in times past an act of official justice.

There was also an indirect form of lynching: after a Black was arrested, a crowd would invade the courtroom and compel the judge to condemn the suspect to death. The judge would typically justify doing so by saying that the Black would be put to death anyway and that the official condemnation would spare him a crueller death.

Many sociologists have studied lynching. Raper conducted a meticulous analysis of all the lynchings carried out in the United States in 1930; there were twenty-one of them. Twenty of the victims were black, and one was white. Raper estimates that one third of the victims were certainly innocent of the crimes of which they were accused. The perpetrators of the lynchings were mainly under thirty years of age and included a great number of adults. Among the spectators, many women and children were noted. In one case, among the fourteen lynchers arrested, five were found to have a police record; none of them paid taxes or were landowners. The statistics analyzed by Raper show that lynching was a rural phenomenon or one of small towns, and linked to economic insecurity; graphs indicate that the number of lynchings increased when the price of cotton fell.

Among the instigators and perpetrators of lynchings, we generally find a number of criminals and psychopaths. However, the size of the crowd that typically participates in a lynching suggests that the event involves more than the silent panic described by Baschwitz; here it is "honest people" who are driving the phenomenon. Moreover, there is an almost complete lack of policing and local justice. Insurance companies never insure against murders and material damages that are the result of lynchings. Newspapers, when they do not directly approve lynching, take an "objective" stance, merely reporting the facts without comment. Clearly the phenomenon of lynching implies the tacit complicity of the authorities, as well as the general belief in a "right to lynch." Put another way, it is seen as a "democratic" institution intended to compensate for the inadequacies of official justice. The mindset of the spectators at a lynching may therefore be compared to that of spectators at an execution in the days when these were carried out publicly and with cruelty.

Cromwell [Cox] (1948) described a "lynching cycle" that included the following phases:

1 The White community is concerned, seeing the lifestyle and the independence of Blacks increasing; they are escaping their domination and becoming "insolent."
2 Racial antagonism increases, manifesting itself in discussions and criticisms.
3 Rumours circulate concerning certain so-called outrages experienced by Whites.
4 An incident occurs; the crowd goes into action and lynches a Black, while also mistreating other Blacks and burning their property.
5 The other Blacks hide, terrified.
6 After two or three days, emotions calm down; some people

demand justice, and an investigation is conducted, but
generally justice dismisses the case.

7 Life resumes, and the Blacks are humbler and more
circumspect.

8 The Blacks forget, smile at the whites, and hold no grudges
(at least in appearance); "social euphoria" is restored.

Today, lynchings of Blacks have almost disappeared. It is not
easy to establish the cause of this disappearance. For reference purposes we mention an opinion according to which "substitutes for
lynching" have developed: silent murders that are not revealed, an
increase in police violence toward Blacks, more frequent legal death
sentences, and so on.

Clearly, crimes of crowds are complex phenomena that come
under the realm of psychiatry, psychology, sociology, ethnology,
and law. From a legal point of view, they pose difficult problems.
Sighele strongly rejected the notion that the criminal crowd bears no
responsibility and declared that the instigators and the leaders must
be punished. The reason being that every collective crime establishes
a prototype, which, when added to a sense of impunity, has significant chances of serving as a template for subsequent crimes.

Collective self-destruction. Individuals who make up a collectivity
can destroy themselves in two ways: by commiting suicide together
(either in isolation or by helping one another), or by killing one
another without intending to kill themselves.

The best-known type of collective suicide is double suicide, which
is not part of our topic. In normal conditions, it is rare that a large
number of individuals commit suicide together, but history does
provides many examples, such of those of besieged cities whose
defenders, reduced to despair, killed themselves after killing their
wives and their children. Historians of religion report that in sev-
enteenth-century Russia, members of the Raskolniki sect, or Old
Believers, persecuted by the Official Church, committed suicide by
the thousands; they shut themselves up in their churches and set
fire to them, or sometimes buried themselves alive in vast graves
(Welter, 1950; Pascal, 1938). And we know that after the discovery
of America, native populations of the Antilles, reduced to slavery by
the Spanish, committed suicide en masse, as related by Las Casas
and Oviedo (Stoll, 1904, 146–9).

Self-destructions in the form of reciprocal murders perhaps belong more to the collective psychoses. These involve a blind, spontaneous outburst of aggressivity among a small group whose members kill one another. Here is an example, cited by the American writer Robert Payne (1945) in his Chinese journal:

> In a small town in Outer Mongolia, seven Japanese officers and businessmen lived together in the main hotel with their mistresses and their concubines. One day an extraordinarily beautiful Russian dancer arrived who consented to dance for them, fascinated them all, but scornfully rejected their advances. After three or four weeks, one of the Japanese officers managed to get a date with her. That evening, the other Japanese, gathered together at the hotel, decked out their mistresses in the same way as the Russian, and had them dance, watching out for their friend to return, became drunk, and then suddenly drew their swords, killed their mistresses, after which they killed one another. When their friend came back at seven in the morning with the Russian dancer to announce their upcoming marriage, he saw the scene of carnage, killed the Russian and committed hara-kiri.

The narrator concludes that these Japanese "killed without reason, without knowing why and without being able to stop themselves." Was this really an inexplicable eruption of the Freudian death instinct? Freudian theory alluded more to the "libidinal structure of a mass," that is, the aggressivity of these men had been neutralized when their libidos were focused on the Russian dancer; when she chose one of the men, a precarious balance was upset and their aggressive instincts were freed and vented. We must naturally take into account the disinhibiting role of alcohol, as the narrator specifies that these men were all drunk. We may also suppose that their aggressivity was inflamed by the fact that they were far from home and perhaps in danger due to the Sino-Japanese War, which was raging at the time. The principal factor was perhaps the military education of these men and a tradition that had taught them to scorn human life.

Self-destruction through reciprocal murders does not always occur as rapidly as in the preceding example; such an event may continue for months or years. The story of the Japanese on Anatahan Island obtained a kind of imfamy in this respect.

In 1951 the US navy discovered to its astonishment that a group of about twenty Japanese soldiers and sailors had been living for seven years on the small island of Anatahan in the South Pacific. They were the only survivors of the crews of three small vessels that had run aground after American aircraft had bombed and sank their vessels. The island of Anatahan had been evacuated and appeared deserted. The shipwrecked Japanese had adapted, not without difficulty, to life in the wild, but they managed to form a stable community. Their equilibrium was destroyed the day they discovered in the forest a cabin inhabited by a Japanese couple. Starting that day, everything changed. The Japanese woman, named Keiko, was at first cautious and reserved; then she took a series of lovers, and the murders and mysterious accidents began. After the discovery of a shipwreck on which pistols were found, gunshots were fired and the male population gradually began to destroy itself. A film was made about this that was very successful in Japan, and one of the survivors wrote an account, of which an adaptation exists in English (Michiro Maruyama, 1954). Unfortunately, the account is somewhat fictionalized and is illustrated mainly with photos from the film.

Conclusions. The limited scope of this article does not allow us to address the vast problem of prolonged collective psychoses, which are more a matter for sociology and political science than for psychiatry.

In all cases of acute collective psychosis – panic, collective hysteria, riots, and so on – it is not enough to invoke the misdeeds of a mysterious "soul of crowds"; the facts must be analyzed each time, taking into account mainly the following points:

We must be wary of confusing the precipitating event of a collective psychosis with its root causes; the spontaneous nature of riots, for example, is much more apparent than real.

Collective psychoses do not appear just anywhere and at any time; they are part of a temporo-spatial complex and a very precise social context and are in more or less visible relation to historical circumstances. That is why a collective psychosis, however new and spontaneous it may seem, may often merely be repeating a prototype provided by a former collective psychosis, and may also serve as a precedent and model for a subsequent collective psychosis.

It is important to remember that collective psychoses do not affect anonymous and homogeneous masses, whether they are driven by a leader or not. There will be a differentiation of roles among several categories of participants. A crowd is less a stable state than it is a process.

These facts are of paramount importance when it comes to organizing the prevention of collective psychoses and to warding off the immediate dangers they may present.

Notes

ETHNOPSYCHIATRY

Text finalized by Emmanuel Delille. This edition was made possible thanks to the support of the Maison des sciences de l'homme Paris-Nord (MSH-PN) and the Japan Society for the Promotion of Sciences (JSPS). Thanks to Samuel Lézé (École normale supérieur de Lyon) and Kosuke Tsuiki (Institute for Research in Humanities, Kyoto University). I dedicate this work to my friends and colleagues in Kansai (Japan). For the sake of clarity, all notes written for this new edition are indicated by (*Ed.*) (Editor's note).

1 As with other colonial or racist terms, "Eskimo" is no longer acceptable. Today these people are called Inuit. (*Ed.*)
2 *Transcultural Research in Mental Health Problems*: first series, nine issues from 1956 to 1962; became *Transcultural Psychiatric Research Review*, issues 14 and 15, 1963; a new series: *Transcultural Psychiatric Research Review*, volumes 1 to 33, 1963–96; became *Transcultural Psychiatry*, starting with volume 34, 1997–. (*Ed.*)
3 See H. Murphy, "Méthodologie de recherche." This booklet preceded the one by Henri Ellenberger, and the two texts were written simultaneously. (*Ed.*)
4 Modern term: Kickapoo people from the Great Lakes region, a branch of which settled in Kansas in the nineteenth century. (*Ed.*)
5 A voodoo priest. (*Ed.*)
6 According to the definition in the *Robert*, the word is of Melanesian origin: "impersonal supernatural force or power and guiding principle in certain religions." Claude Lévi-Strauss analyzed *mana* in his famous

preface to Marcel Mauss's book: "a zero symbolic value," which can be any value at all or possess all values at once, and has no other purpose than to establish the social institution it reveals. See Lévi-Strauss, "Introduction à l'oeuvre de Marcel Mauss." (*Ed.*).

THEORETICAL AND GENERAL ETHNOPSYCHIATRY

1 This systematic presentation was previously published in condensed form when Henri Ellenberger was part of the research team at McGill University. See H. Ellenberger, "Aspects culturels de la maladie mentale." (*Ed.*)

2 The Kwakiutl have been studied by Franz Boas (*The Kwakiutl of Vancouver*, 1909), who described their system of gifts and counter-gifts (*potlatch*). (*Ed.*)

3 Island located to the east of Papua New Guinea. (*Ed.*)

4 Modern term: congenital hypothyroidism. (*Ed.*)

5 Modern term: Down syndrome. (*Ed.*)

6 Modern term: children with developmental disabilities. (*Ed.*)

7 French West Africa (1895–58) was a grouped-together eight French colonies: Mauritania, Senegal, Mali, Guinea, Niger, Upper Volta, Dahomey, and Ivory Coast. (*Ed.*)

8 This term – totally unacceptable today – was still commonly used in North America in the 1960s. *(Ed.)*

9 This idea of an organic nucleus of mental illnesses and of a socio-cultural expression of symptoms is certainly not new, but it was taken up in an original way by Ian Hacking, in particular during his teaching at the Collège de France (chair of philosophy and history of scientific concepts), in terms of various syndromes that have taken the form of "transient mental illnesses" throughout history. Hacking was greatly inspired by the works of Henri Ellenberger and of Mark Micale, a specialist on Henri Ellenberger and a historian of psychiatry. But as opposed to the ethnopsychiatrists, Ian Hacking uses the analytical framework drawn from North American philosophy and inspired by the works of Michel Foucault to explain this type of composite phenomenon from the concepts of "interactive classification" and "the loop effect." See Delille and Kirsch, "Le cours de Ian Hacking." (*Ed.*)

10 The attitude of the family during the chronic illness of children of different socio-cultural origins was the first subject of study assigned to Henri Ellenberger by Eric Wittkower when he entered the transcultural psychiatry group at McGill University in 1959. (*Ed.*)

11 Gansu and Qinghai (current spelling) are Chinese provinces historically linked to Tibet, of mixed population. (*Ed.*)

12 Bantu people living in Tanzania. Tanganyika was a British protectorate before gaining independence and forming Tanzania. (*Ed.*)

13 Region in Uttar Pradesh, in the north of India on the border of Nepal. (*Ed.*)

14 The concept of schizophrenia was created by Swiss psychiatrist Eugen Bleuler (1857–1939). Simple schizophrenia (*schizophrenia simplex*, 1911) is a crude form of mental illness, that is, it presents few symptoms, except for some peculiarities that that are difficult to diagnose alongside a straightforward psychotic process (*Ed.*).

15 Ivan Alexandrovitch Goncharov (1812–1891), a novelist and high-ranking Imperial Russian civil servant. The novel was published in 1858. Oblomovism refers to an idle man immersed in a kind of apathy, lethargy, laziness, or procrastination; in the novel it is embodied by an aristocrat of Imperial Russia, haunted by a carefree childhood, which he relives in a dream. In particular, the sequence in the novel titled "Oblomov's Dream" has been interpreted as an expression of the hallucinatory delirium of disorganized schizophrenia. An immediate hit, the story also was interpreted as criticism of the Russian nobility, paternalism, and the inertia of the *ancien régime*. For an English translation, see Goncharov, *Oblomov* (Penguin Books, 2005). (*Ed.*)

16 We are referring to Mathilde and Mathias Vaerting; the English translation of their work (*Neubegründung der Psychologie von Mann und Weib. Die weibliche Eigenart im Männerstadt und die männliche Eigenart im Frauenstadt*, 1921) has recently been republished as *The Dominant Sex: A Study in the Sociology of Sex Differentiation* (Honolulu: University Press of the Pacific, 2002). (*Ed.*)

17 Today: bipolar disorders (*Ed.*).

18 In German, *Hutterer*, by Jakob Hutter (c. 1500–1536). This Anabaptist movement, born in the Tyrol, is notable for its rejection of violence. The community was persecuted by the Hapsburgs and dispersed after it settled in Moravia (1533). (*Ed.*)

19 Literally, "temptation," and in this context in the sense of being attacked, overcome by temptation. (*Ed.*)

20 The Eta belong to the *burakumin*, the caste of hereditary outcasts in Japan, comparable to the Untouchables in India. Considered to be "impure" during the medieval period, their descendants still experience a

high degree of social exclusion, even though they have enjoyed the same rights since the imperial restoration of the Meiji Era at the end of the nineteenth century. (*Ed.*)

21 The Yenish people still make up the largest travelling community in Switzerland. The spelling with only one "n" has become established. (*Ed.*)

22 Pastor Oskar Pfister (1873–1956) was one of the first generation of psychoanalysts and a personal friend of Freud. Henri Ellenberger underwent analysis (1949–52) with him while working in Switzerland, just before moving to the United States. (*Ed.*)

23 Henri Ellenberger was a friend and student of Professor Henri Baruk (1897–1999), a member of the Israel Medical Association, which helped reorganize Israeli psychiatric institutions shortly after the creation of the Jewish state – a topic they address in their correspondence. The correspondence between Henri Baruk and Henri Ellenberger is held at the Centre de documentation Henri Ellenberger (Paris). (*Ed.*)

24 An allusion to one of the most famous patients of the famous psychologist Pierre Janet (1859–1947): writer Raymond Roussel (1877–1933), presented as the Martial case in *De l'angoisse à l'extase* (1926). Wealthy and eccentric, he was diagnosed as neuropathic, and frequented private sanatoriums in the Seine and in Switzerland, but was never institutionalized in an asylum. Michel Leiris and Michel Foucault also devoted essays to Raymond Roussel. (*Ed.*)

25 Literally, the term pathoplastic means that which has power to give the form of the pathology, without being at the origin (pathogenic). The word does not appear in dictionaries, and does not exist in English, but we find it used in other articles about ethnopsychiatry, by other authors. (*Ed.*)

26 Brisset, "Anthropologie culturelle et psychiatrie."

27 Repressive psychiatric practices in the Soviet Union were not officially condemned until the 1997 World Congress of Psychiatry (motion at the Honolulu Congress). See Palem, *Henri Ey.* (*Ed.*)

28 H. Ellenberger, "Les mouvements de libération mythique." (*Ed.*)

29 On this point, once again, Henri Ellenberger was able to draw his documentation from the articles and papers of Henri Baruk, who presented clinical cases to the Société medico-psychologique (Medical and Psychological Society); medical and psychological literature on this topic also exists in English. (*Ed.*)

30 This is also a personal memory, as Henri Ellenberger settled in the United States at age forty-seven. (*Ed.*)

DESCRIPTIVE AND CLINICAL PART

1 The 1965 article mentions, between parentheses, "lack of space prevents us from addressing here," as Henri Ellenberger did not have enough space to address this topic. But the editors of the *Encyclopédie médico-chirurgicale* (EMC) insisted that he publish an additional article, which was delivered shortly thereafter and published in 1967; we include it here unmodified, in the order originally planned. (*Ed.*)

2 A doctor; not to be confused with bestselling author Carlos Castaneda (1925–1998), the American anthropologist originally from Peru. (*Ed.*)

3 Carl G. Jung's theory of archetypes. (*Ed.*)

4 Henri Ellenberger uses the term "Classic Orient." (*Ed.*)

5 On the history of this genre, see for example the works of Jackie Pigeaud. (*Ed.*)

6 A work by François Malherbe, composed as a tribute to his friend François Du Périer: *Stances. Consolation à M. Du Périer* (1599). (*Ed.*)

7 The word is derived from the Spanish *juramentar*, "to take an oath, to swear to God as a witness." As opposed to *amok*, these are ritual religious murders, planned in advance, against non-Muslims, conceived as a personal form of *jihad*. (*Ed.*)

8 Alphanumeric code (like those of the previously cited booklets by Charles Brissèt and Brian Murphy) used to classify articles in each specialized medical treatise of the EMC, when an update appears in the pre-established table of contents. Without this code, and especially without a summary of the year of the update, it is not possible to find an article that was published, even if one knows its title and the names of the authors, as the EMC contains about a hundred volumes and thousands of articles that are regularly updated. (*Ed.*)

9 Henri Ellenberger is referring to an article by Mauss published in 1926 in the *Journal de psychologie normale et pathologique*, cited in the bibliography. He takes up many elements from it, including the reference to Goldie, and the question of psychogenic death, but also the discussion of the concept of Arctic hysteria. (*Ed.*)

10 A concept of Marcel Mauss, this designates social facts "where all kinds of institutions are expressed at once: religious, legal, and moral" (for example, *potlatch*, in his famous "Essai sur le don" (1923–24). (*Ed.*)

11 Paulus Ægineta (AD 620–680 or 690), a Greek (Byzantine) doctor and surgeon of the seventh century. (*Ed.*)

12 The author of this "erotic" novel, Aeneas Silvius Piccolomini, was none other than Pope Pius II (1405–1464), who wrote it in Vienna in 1444,

fourteen years before his investiture. The story was inspired by the real love affairs of someone close to the Holy Roman Emperor. (*Ed.*)

13 It was this type of case that Michel Foucault and the research participants in his seminar dealt with based on the case of Pierre Rivière. Several cases are quoted for France, without connections being established with known cases in Germany. See Michel Foucault, *I, Pierre Rivière* (*Ed.*)

14 This singular intrusion of the *I* in an encyclopedia-type text is an opportunity to note Henri Ellenberger's strong critical stance on his experience in psychiatric hospitals. If we refer to his series of articles titled "La psychiatrie Suisse" and the biography by Andrée Yanacopoulo, we cannot help but see in them the wish to settle accounts with the psychiatric hospital of Schaffhausen canton (Breitenau), where he was head doctor of the women's section between 1943 and 1953 and was subjected to snubs from management. At the initiative of Jörg Püschel, the historical association of the canton (Historischer Verein des Kantons Schaffhausen) is preparing a history of the asylum. (*Ed.*)

15 I would like to express my deep gratitude to Ms Martha Reime of Oslo, who, with great dedication, translated from the Danish several articles by Bertelsen dealing with the pression work. Author's note: Henri Ellenberger.

16 The Ainu are a people who settled in the Japanese archipelago even before the Japanese, largely on the northern island of Hokkaïdo. They are the last representatives of the Jomon culture, which preceded the Yayoi culture (which goes back to the third century BC) developed by migrants from Southeast Asia, and which led to modern Japan. The Ainu do not have the Japanese physical type (they are taller and have more hair), and their language is somewhat similar to some Siberian languages. A peaceful people, they were forced to assimilate with the Japanese as the latter gradually occupied their territory. The Japanese conquest destroyed or banned their culture, which is now preserved in museums and other institutions. (*Ed.*)

17 It was this establishment that Kraepelin visited in the late nineteenth century in order to verify the universality of his nosology of mental disorders. (*Ed.*)

18 Carl G. Jung's theory of archetypes. (*Ed.*)

19 See H. Murphy, "Méthodologie de recherche." (*Ed.*)

20 On the issue of the revision of schizophrenic illness, note that the problem of boundaries in this vague category has been the subject of numerous controversies and attacks in postwar psychiatry: in France, we may refer to the discussions of the Société de l'Évolution psychiatrique and the Société médico-psychologique of the 1950s and 1960s, which their journals respectively published and which continued unabated in the decades

that followed, to then focus on the official American (*DSM-III* and subsequent) and international (*CIM* of *WHO*) classifications. In the United States, transcultural psychiatry played a role in the revision of categories by introducing a list of culture-bound syndromes in the appendix of the *DSM*. But we should also note that schizophrenia and its treatment have been the target of anthropological observations and works in English, outside the medical field. (*Ed.*)

21 *Berdache*, or two-spirited. This word is not of indigenous origin, but is actually French (*bardash*), and designates among North American Native peoples men who dress as women, who make up a society of a third sex with determined social roles. See Désy, "L'homme-femme." (*Ed.*)

22 The institutionalization of transsexuality has greatly evolved in the West and worldwide over the past fifty years; I refer to a recent historical analysis to place this remark of the author in context: P.-H. Castel, *La métamorphose impensable. Essai sur le transsexualisme et l'identité personnelle* (Paris: Gallimard, 2003). (*Ed.*)

23 Judge Daniel Paul Schreber (1842–1911). (*Ed.*)

24 The role is an operative concept in the analyses of Devereux; it is likely that Henri Ellenberger took this into account in this passage, even though he does not quote it here. However, another explanation exists for the condemnation of the semantic confusion: historical reflections that inspire its success and the popularization of Moreno's works in the United States. The creator of methods of group therapy, the best-known of which is psychodrama, Jakob Moreno Levy (1889–1974), appears several times in *The Discovery of the Unconscious* (1970), in which Henri Ellenberger considers him to be the inventor of the term *group psychotherapy*. In a critical tone, Ellenberger indicates that he had numerous "imitators."(*Ed.*)

25 A mental disorder involving psychological dissociation described by the German doctor J.M. Ganser in 1897 and today still a part of international classifications. See Allen, Postel, and Berrios, "The Ganser syndrome." (*Ed.*)

26 There were seven international congresses; Brussels came after Rome (1885) and Paris (1889). The proceedings were published in French. See Garnier, "Les congrès d'anthropologie criminelle." (*Ed.*)

27 This selection of four great representatives of dynamic psychiatry is in accordance with the chapters of Henri Ellenberger's book *The Discovery of the Unconscious.* (*Ed.*)

28 Pierre Janet, "L'évolution des conduites morales et religieuses," Cours du Collège de France, 1921–22 (unpublished). Ellenberger put this reference in his bibliography about the collective psychosis in 1967. But Janet's

lecture has never been published. For this reason, the reference is now in an endnote and not included in the bibliography. (*Ed.*)

29 The analytical framework of this interpretation of collective psychoses is once again Jung's theory of archetypes, which is explained at the beginning of the presentation (chapter "The Problem of Cultural Relativism"), and used in the explanation of the way that poisons ("Poisons Deemed Magic") and certain neuroses ("Windigo") work. Henri Ellenberger nevertheless criticized it in the introduction ("Generalities") due to the misuse Carl G. Jung's disciples made of it (*Ed.*)

30 Max Stirner (1806–1856) was a German philosopher, the author of *The Ego and Its Own* (*Der Einzige und sein Eigentum*, 1845). (*Ed.*)

31 Henri Ellenberger wrote an article on animal psychology, published in several languages (English, French, and Japanese): "Zoological Garden and Mental Hospital" (1964). (*Ed.*)

32 This title calls to mind another addressed in the conclusion: "Psychoses collectives à forme prolongée." Henri Ellenberger deals partly with the topic in an earlier article, "Les mouvements de libération mythique." Furthermore, Brian Murphy and Michel Tousignant published an update in the EMC titled "Psychoses" in 1978. (Ed.)

33 Léon Marillier (1862–1901) was a pioneer in French clinical psychology. (*Ed.*)

Bibliography

JOURNALS

As far as is known, there is only one international journal specializing in ethnopsychiatry. *Transcultural Psychiatric Research Review and Newsletter* was published twice yearly by E.D. Wittkower and colleagues in the Transcultural Psychiatry Research Unit at McGill University. The first series included fifteen issues and ended in October 1963. The second series began in April 1964 with volume 1, issue 1.*

CITED WORKS BY HENRI ELLENBERGER

"Die Ahnen der dynamischen Psychotherapie." *Psyche* 10 (1956): 551–67.
"The Ancestry of Dynamic Psychotherapy." *Bulletin of the Menninger Clinic* 20 (1956): 288–99.
"Aspects culturels de la maladie mentale." *Canadian Psychiatric Association Journal* 4 (1959): 26–37; reprinted in *Revue de psychologie des peoples* 15 (1960): 273–87.
"Cultural Aspects of Mental Illness." *American Journal of Psychotherapy* 14 (1960): 158–73.

---

* The full bibliography of *Ethnopsychiatry* (1965) is reproduced here, with corrections and some additions. A number of titles were incomplete or translated into French by the first publisher, a practice that was once commonplace but is no longer widely accepted. Henri Ellenberger himself objected about this to the editor of the series "Encyclopédie Médico–Chirurgicale." The bibliography of works on collective psychoses appeared in a separate section in the French edition of this book; these works have been integrated into the bibliography for the English edition. As for the McGill journal, *Transcultural Psychiatry*, it still exists though other journals in this field have been started. New translations in English and references to works in the editor's endnotes have been added to the bibliography.

The Discovery of the Unconscious: The History and Evolution of Dynamic Psychiatry. New York: Basic Books, 1970; *À la découverte de l'inconscient: histoire de la psychiatrie dynamique*, translated by Joseph Feisthauer. Villeurbanne: SIMEP, 1974; new edition: *L'histoire de la découverte de l'inconscient*, translated by Joseph Feisthauer, edited by É. Roudinesco. Paris: Fayard, 1994.

"À propos du 'Malleus Maleficarum.'" *Schweizerische Zeitschrift für Psychologie* 10 (1951): 136–48.

"Aspectos culturales de las enfermedales mentales." *Archivos de criminologia, neuro-psiquiatria y disciplinas conexas* 7, no. 25 (1959): 47–63 ; reprinted in *Revista de psiquiatria y psicologia medical* 4 (1960): 695–05.

"Les mouvements de libération mythique." *Critique* 19, no. 190 (1963): 248–67.

"Le professeur De Martino et le 'tarantisme.'" *Critique* 19, no. 190 (1963): 1008–11.

"Psychologische *Geschlechtsunterschiede*." *Der Psychologe* 3 (1951): 262–71.

"Die Putzwut." *Der Psychologe* 2 (1950): 91–4, 138–47.

"Der Selbstmord im Licht der Ethno-Psychiatrie." *Monatsschrift für Psychiatrie und Neurologie* 125 (1953): 347–61.

"The Syndrome of Depression" [1959]. [unpublished].

"Der Tod aus psychischen Ursachen bei Naturvölkern (Voodoo Death)." *Psyche* 5 (1951): 333–44.

BOOKS, PAMPHLETS, AND ARTICLES

Aall, Louise. *Epilepsie beim Wapogoro–Stamm in Tanganyika*. Thesis in medicine, Zurich, 1962 (50 typewritten pages, with illustrations).

Ackerknecht, Erwin H. "Psychopathology, Primitive Medicine and Primitive Culture." *Bulletin of the History of Medicine* 14 (1943): 3067.

Adler, Alfred. "Zur Massenpsychologie." *Zeitschrift für Individualpsychologie* 12, no. 3 (1934): 133–41.

Agresti, Enzo. "Studio delle varianti cliniche dei temi a dei contenuti deliranti in epoche diverse. Confronto dei vari tipi di deliro a distanza di circa un secolo." *Rivista di patologia nervosa e mentale* 80 (1959): 845–65.

Aliaga-Lindo. P. "Aspectos culturales de una población andina." *Boletin del departamento de higiene mental* (Lima) nos. 2–3 (1959): 1–7.

Allen, D.F., J. Postel, and G.E. Berrios. "The Ganser Syndrome." In

Memory Disorders in Psychiatric Practice, edited by G.E. Berrios, 443–55. Cambridge: Cambridge University Press, 2000.

Andics, Margarethe (von). *Ueber Sinn und Sinnlosigkeit des Lebens.* Vienna: Gerold, 1940.

Aubin, Henri. "Esquisse d'une ethno-psycho-psychopathologie." *L'Algérie médicale* nos. 5–6 (1945): 174–9.

Bachet, Maurice. "Étude sur les états de nostalgie." *Annales medico-psychologiques* 108, nos. 1–2 (1950): 559–87, 11–34.

Bachofen, Johann Jakob. *Das Mutterrecht. Eine Untersuchung über die Gynaikokratie der alten Welt nach ihrer religiösen und rechtlichen Natur.* Stuttgart: Kraiz und Hoffmann, 1861.

Baderot, Albert. *De l'influence du milieu sur le développement du délire religieux en Bretagne.* Paris: Jouve, 1897.

Barkley, Henri C. *Between the Danube and the Black Sea, or Five Years in Bulgaria.* London: John Murray, 1876.

Baschwitz, K. *Du und die Masse.* Leyden: E.J. Brill, 1951.

Basedow, Herbert. *The Austalian Aboriginal.* Adelaide: F.W. Preece & Sons, 1925.

Bastian, Adolf. *Reisen in Siam in Jahre 1863.* Jena: H. Costenoble, 1867.

Bateson, Gregory, and Margaret Mead. "Balinese Character: A Photographic Analysis." New York: New York Academy of Sciences, 1942.

Baumann, Hermann. *Das dopplte Geschecht. Ethnologische Studien zur Bisexualität in Ritus und Mythos.* Berlin: Dietrich Reimer, 1955.

Beaglehole, E., and P. Beaglehole. *Some Modern Maoris.* Wellington and London: New Zealand Council for Educational Research / Whitcombe and Tombs / Oxford University Press, 1946.

Begbie, Harold. *On the Side of the Angels: The Story of the Angel at Mons: An Answer to "The Bowmen."* London: Hodder and Stoughton, 1915.

Béguin, Albert. "Qui est fou?" *Esprit* 20, no. 12 (1952): 777–88.

Behr-Sigel, Élisabeth. "Les "fous pour le Christ" et la "sainteté laïque" dans l'ancienne Russie." *Irenikon* 15 (1939): 554–65.

Benedict, Paul King, and I. Jacks. "Mental Illness in Primitive Societies." *Psychiatry* 17 (1954): 377–89.

Benedict, Ruth. *Patterns of Culture.* Boston: Houghton Mifflin, 1934.

Benz, Ernst. "Heilige Narrheit." *Kyrios* 3 (1938): 33–55.

Bérard, Victor. *Les navigations d'Ulysses*, 2: *Pénélope et les barons des îles.* Paris: A. Colin, 1928.

Bermann, Gregorio. "Necesidad de la psiquiatría comparada y su metodología." *Archivos venezolanos de psiquiatría y neurología* 4 (1958): 92–107.

Berndt, Ronald M.A. "Devastating Disease Syndrome: Kuru Sorcery in the Eastern Central Highlands of New Guinea." *Sociologus* 8, no. 1 (1958): 4–28.

Bertelsen, Alfred. "Grönlandak medicinsk statistik og nosografl." *Meddelelser om Grönland* 117, no. 3 (1940): 176–90.

– "Om Kajak-Svimmelhed." *Bibliothek for Laeger* 97, nos. 1–2 (1905): 109–35, 280–335.

Bertogg, Hercli. "Aus der Welt der Bündner Vaganten." *Schweizerisches Archiv für Volkskunde* 43 (1946): 21–48.

Best, Elsdon. "Maori eschatologie." *Transactions and Proceedings of the New Zealand Institutes* 38 (1905): 148–239.

Bhandari, L.C. "Some Aspects of Psychoanalysis Therapy in India." *Progress in Psychotherapy* 5 (1960): 218–20.

Binder, Hans. "Das Verlangen nach Geschlechtsumwandlung." *Zeitschrift für die gesamte Neurologie und Psychiatrie* 143 (1933): 84–174.

Boas, Franz. *The Kwakiutl of Vancouver Island*. Leiden: E.J. Brill, and New York: G.E. Stechert, 1909.

Bogoras, Waldemar. *The Chuckchee: Social Organization*. Publications of the Jessup North Pacific Expedition, Memoirs of the American Museum of Natural History. Leiden: E.J. Brill, and New York: G.E. Stechert, 1909.

Boissier de Sauvages, François. *Nosologie méthodique, dans la quelle les maladies sont rangées par classe suivant le système de Sydenham, et l'ordre des botannites*, 10 vols. Paris: Hérissant le fils, 1770–71.

Borgoltz. "La psychiatrie en pratique rurale." *Transcultural Research in Mental Health Problems* 8 (July 1960): 46–7.

Boudin, Jean Christian Marc. *Traité de géographie et de statistiques médicales et des maladies endémiques*, 2 vols. Paris: J.-B. Baillière et fils, 1857.

Bowman, Karl M., and Bernice Engle. "Medicolegal Aspects of Transvestism." *American Journal of Psychiatry* 113, no. 7 (1957): 583–8.

Brisset, Charles. "Anthropologie culturelle et psychiatrie," fasc. no 37715A10. *Traité de psychiatrie*, 1–9. Paris: Éditions techniques (Encyclopédie médico–chirurgicale), 1960.

Brosin, Henry W. "Panic States and Their Treatment." *American Journal of Psychiatry* 100 (July 1943): 54–61.

Brousseau, Albert. *Essai sur la peur aux armées, 1914–1918*. Paris: Alcan, 1920.

Buck, Pearl. *L'enfant qui ne devait jamais grandir*. Paris: Stock, 1960.

Buckingham, Benjamin H., George C. Foulk, and Walter McLean. *Observations upon the Korean Coast, Japanese-Korean Ports, and Siberia, Made During a Journey from the Asiatic Station to the United States, Through Siberia to Europe, June 3 to September 8, 1882*. Washington, DC: US Navy Department, 1884.

Bühler, Alfred. "Kritische Bemerkungen zur Verwendung ethnographischer Quellen in der Psychologie." *Schweizer Archiv für Neurologie und Psychiatrie* 68, no. 2 (1952): 415–21.

Bürger-Prinz, Hans, Hans Albrecht, and Hans Giese, *Zur Phänomenologie des Transvestitismus bei Männern*. Stuttgart: Enke, 1953.

Burton, Robert. *The Anatomy of Melancholy*. Oxford: Lichfield, 1621.

Bush, Richard J. *Reindeer, Dogs and Snow-Shoes, a Journal of Siberian Travel and Explorations made in the years 1865, 1866, and 1867*. New York: Harper, 1871.

Bychowski, Gustav. "Disorders in the Body-Image in the Clinical Picture of Psychoses." *Journal of Nervous and Mental Disease* 97 (1943): 310–35.

Calmeil, Louis F. *De la folie considérée sous le point de vue pathologique, philosophique, historique et judiciaire*. Paris: J.-B. Baillière, 1845.

Cannon, Walter B. "Voodoo Death." *American Anthropologist* 44, no. 2 (1942): 169–81.

Cantril, Hadley. *The Invasion from Mars: A Study in the Psychology of Panic*. Princeton: Princeton University Press, 1940.

Carothers, John Colin. *The African Mind in Health and Disease: A Study in Ethno-Psychiatry*. Geneva: OMS Monograph Series (no. 17), 1953.

– "Culture, Psychiatry, and the Written Word." *Psychiatry* 22, no. 4 (1959): 307–20.

– "A Study of Mental Derangement in Africans and an Attempt to Explain Its Peculiarities, More Especially in Relation to the African Attitude to Life." *Journal of Mental Science* 93, no. 392 (1947): 548–97.

Carstairs, George Morrison. "Daru and Bhang: Cultural Factors in the Choice of an Intoxicant." *Quarterly Journal of Studies on Alcohol* 15 (1954): 220–37.

Castro De La Mata, R., G. Gingras, and E.D. Wittkower. "Impact of Sudden, Severe Disablement of the Father upon the Family." *Canadian Medical Association Journal* 82, no. 20 (1960): 1015–20.

Catrou, Jacques. "*Étude sur la maladie des tics convulsifs*." Thesis in medicine, University of Paris, no. 129. Paris: Jouve, 1890.

Cerletti, Ugo. "Sulle recenti concezioni dell'isteria e della suggestione a proposito di una endemia di possessione demoniaca." *Annali dell'Instituto psichiatrico della universita di Roma* 3 (1904): 92.

Cheyne, George. *The English Malady: Or a Treatise of Nervous Diseases of all Kinds*. London: S. Powell, 1733.

Clifford, Hugh. *Studies in Brown Humanity*. London: Grant Richards, 1898.

Codrington, Robert Henry. *The Melanesians. Studies in their Anthropology and Folk-Lore*. Oxford: Clarendon Press, 1891.

Collet, Octave J.A. *Terres et peuples de Sumatra*. Amsterdam: Elsevier, 1925.

Coolidge, Dane, and Mary Roberts. *The Navajo Indians*. Boston and New York: Houghton Mifflin, 1930.

Cooper, John M. "The Cree Witiko Psychosis." *Primitive Man, Quarterly Bulletin of the Catholic Anthropological Conference* 6, no. 1 (1933): 20–4.

Courchet, Jean-Louis, C. Bontron, and R. Perraut. "Sur cinquante cas de 'mania transitoria' de Krafft-Ebing d'une population ouvrière rurale." *Annales medico-psychologiques* 121, no. 2 (June 1963): 31–56.

Crawley, Ernest. *Dress, Drinks and Drums: Further Studies of Savages and Sex*. London: Methuen and Co., 1931.

Cromwell Cox, Oliver. "Caste, class, and race" [1948]. *Monthly Review Press* (1959): 548–54.

Delcambre, Étienne. *Le concept de sorcellerie dans le duché de Lorraine au xvie et au xviie siècle*, vol. 1. Nancy: Société d'archéologie lorraine, 1948.

Delille, Emmanuel. "Teaching the History of Psychiatry in the 1950s: Henri Ellenberger's Lectures at the Menninger Foundation." *Zinbun* 47 (2016): 109–28.

Delille, Emmanuel, and Marc Kirsch. "Le cours de Ian Hacking au Collège de France: la psychiatrie comme lieu d'observation privilégié de l'histoire des concepts scientifiques" [2000–2006]. *Revue de synthèse* 137, nos. 1–2 (2016): 89–117.

De Martino, Ernesto. "Fureurs suédoises." *L'arc* 5 (1962): 89–96.

Denig, Edwin T. "The Assiniboine." *American Anthropologist*, new series, no. 1 (1932).

Désy, P. "L'homme-femme. (Les berdaches en Amérique du Nord)." *Libre – politique, anthropologie, philosophie* 78, no. 3 (1978): 57–102.

Devereux, George. "Institutionalized Homosexuality of the Mohave Indians." *Human Biology* 9 (1937): 498–527.

– *Mohave Ethnopsychiatry and Suicide: The Psychiatric Knowledge and the Psychic Disturbances of an Indian Tribe*. Washington, DC: Smithsonian Institution, Bureau of American Ethnology, Bulletin 175, 1961.

– *Reality and Dream: The Psychotherapy of a Plains Indian*. New York: International University Press, 1951.

– "A Sociological Theory of Schizophrenia." *Psychoanalytic Review* 26, no. 3 (1939): 315–42.

Dhunjibhoy, Jal Edulji. "A Brief Resume of the Types of Insanity Commonly Met in India, with a Full Description of "Indian Hemp Insanity" Peculiar to the Country." *Journal of Mental Science* 76 (1930): 254–64.

Doi, Takeo. "Amae: A Key Concept for Understanding Japanese Personality Structure." *Psychologia* 5, no. 1 (1962): 1–7.

– "Morita Therapy and Psychoanalysis." *Psychologia* 5, no. 1 (1962): 117–23.

– "Psychopathology of Jibun and Amae." *Psychiatria et Neurologia Japonica* 61 (1959): 149–62.

– "Psychopathology of 'Shinkeishitsu,' Especially Regarding the Psychodynamics of Its 'Toraware.'" *Psychiatria et Neurologia Japonica* 60 (1958): 733–44.

– "Some Thoughts on Helplessness and the Desire to Be Loved." *Psychiatry* 26 (1963): 266–72.

– "Sumanai and Ikenai: Psychodynamics of Guilt in the Light of Japanese Concepts." *Japanese Journal of Psychoanalysis* 8 (1961): 1–5.

Douyon, Emerson. "Les techniques psychologiques en pays sous-développés." *Cahiers de psychologie clinique* 1 (1964): 31–7.

Dudan, L. "Observaciones sobre la orgía en el carnaval del norte argentine." *Revista de antropología y ciencias afines* 1 (1952): 43–8.

Dumézil, Georges. *Mythes et dieux des Germains*. Paris: Leroux, 1939.

Dupréel, Eugène. "Y-a-t-il une foule diffuse? L'opinion publique." In *La Foule. Quatrième semaine internationale de synthèse*, edited by Georges Bohn, 109–30. Paris: Alcan, 1934.

Eaton, Joseph W., and Robert J. Weil. *Culture and Mental Disorders*. Glencoe: The Free Press, 1955.

Ellis, Gilmore W. "The Amok of the Malays." *Journal of Mental Science* 39 (1893): 325–38.

– "Latah: A Mental Malady of the Malays." *Journal of Mental Science* 43 (1897): 32–40.

Ernst, Fritz. *Vom Heimweh*. Zurich: Fretz & Wasmuth, 1949.

Esquirol, Étienne. *Des maladies mentales*, 2 vols. Paris: J.-B. Baillière, 1838.

– *Mental Maladies: A Treatise on Insanity.* Translated by E.K. Hunt. New York: Hafner, 1965.

Faladé, Solange A. "Le développement psycho-moteur de l'enfant africain au Sénégal." *Le concours medical* (20 February 1960): 1005–13.

Faris, Robert E.L., and H. Warren Dunham. *Mental Disorder in Urban Areas: An Ecological Study of Schizophrenia and Other Psychoses.* New York: Hafner, 1939.

Félice, Philippe de. *Foules en délire. Extases collectives.* Paris: Albin Michel, 1947.

– *Poisons sacrés, ivresses divines. Essais sur quelques formes inférieures de la mystique divine.* Paris: Albin Michel, 1936.

Flacourt, Étienne de. *Histoire de la grande isle de Madagascar.* Troyes and Paris: N. Oudot / G. Clouzier, 1642–60.

Fletcher, William. "Latah and Crime." *The Lancet* 2 (1908): 254–5.

Forbes, Henry O. *A Naturalist's Wanderings in the Eastern Archipelago.* London: Low, Marston, Searle, and Rivington, 1885.

Foucault, Michel, ed. *I, Pierre Rivière, Having Slaughtered My Mother, My Sister, and My Brother.* Lincoln: University of Nebraska Press, 1973.

Freud, Sigmund. *Group Psychology and the Analysis of the Ego.* Translated by James Strachey. London and Vienna: International Psychoanalytical Press, 1922.

– *Massenpsychologie und Ich-Analyse.* Vienna: Internationaler Psychoanalytischer Verlag, 1921.

– *Totem and Taboo.* Translated by James Strachey. Mineola: Dover, 2018.

– "Totem und Tabu." *Imago* 1 (1912): 17–33, 213–27, 301–33; 2 (1913): 357–408.

Frick, J. "Körpergeruch als Krankheit." *Anthropos* 58 (1963): 477–84.

Fried, Jacob. "Acculturation and Mental Health among Indian Immigrants in Peru." In *Culture and Mental Health*, edited by M.K. Opler, 119–37. New York: Macmillan, 1959.

Garbe, E. "La psychiatrie en clientèle rurale." *Le concours medical* (1960): 1489–98.

Garnier, L. "Les congrès d'anthropologie criminelle et la naissance d'un patrimoine penal." *Crimino-corpus*, 2010. www.criminocorpus.cnrs.fr/article435.html.

Gillin, John Lewis. *Taming the Criminal.* New York: Macmillan, 1931.

Gillon, J.J., Henri Duchêne, and Yves Champion. "Pathologie mentale de la mobilitée géographique," fasc. nos. 37730C10 and 37730C20, 1–7 and 1–10. *Traité de psychiatrie.* Paris: Éditions techniques (Encyclopédie medico-chirurgicale), 1958.

Goldie, William H. "Maori Medical Lore." *Transactions and Proceedings of the New Zealand Institute* 37 (1904): 1–120.

Gorer, Geoffrey, and John Rickman. *The People of Great Russia, a Psychological Study.* London and New York: Cressett Press, 1949.

Grébert, Fernand. *Au Gabon (Afrique équatoriale française).* Paris: Société des missions évangéliques, 1928.

Guinard, Joseph E. "Witiko among the Tête de Boule." *Primitive Man* 3 (1930): 69–71.

Güntert, Hermann. *Über altisländische Berserker–Geschichten.* Heidelberg: Universitäts-Buchdruckerei J. Hörning, 1912.

Hagemann. Walter. *Vom Mythos der Masse. Ein Beitrag zur Psychologie der Offentlichkeit.* Heidelberg: Vowinckel, 1951.

Halbwachs, Maurice. *Les causes du suicide.* Paris: Alcan, 1930.

Hammond, William A. "Miryachit: A Newly Described Disease of the Nervous System and Its Analogues." *The New York Medical Journal* 39 (1884): 191–2.

– *Sexual Impotence in the Male.* New York: Bermingham, 1883.

– *A Treatise on Insanity in Its Medical Relations.* New York: D. Appleton, 1883.

Hansen, Joseph. *Quellen und Untersuchungen zur Geschichte des Hexenwahns.* Bonn: Carl Georgi, 1901.

– *Zauberwahn, Inquisition und Hexenprozess im Mittelalter.* Munich and Leipzig: R. Oldenburg, 1900.

Hecker, Justus F.C. *Die grossen Volkskrankheiten des Mittelalters.* Berlin: Adolph Enslin, 1865.

Heiberg, Johan Ludvig. "Geisteskrankheiten im klassischen Altertum." *Allgemeine Zeitschrift für Psychiatrie* 86 (1927): 1–44.

Hellpach, Willy. *Die geistigen Epidemien.* Frankfurt: Rütten & Loening, 1904.

Herskovits, Melville J. *Dahomey: An Ancient West-African Kingdom,* 2 vols. New York: J.J. Augustin, 1938.

Heun, E. "Nahrungsenthaltung bei Naturvölkern." *Thorraduran-Therapie* 34 (February 1963).

Hill, Williams Willard. "The Status of the Hermaphrodite and Transvestite in Navajo Culture." *The American Anthropologist* 37 (1935): 273–9.

Hippocrates. *Ancient Medicine. Airs, Waters, Places. Epidemics 1 and 3. The Oath. Precepts. Nutriment.* Cambridge, MA: Harvard University Press, 1923.

Hives, Frank. "Meine persönliche Bekanntschaft mit den Mayalls." *Die Garbe* 25 (1942): 726–9, 753–8.

Hoch, Erna. "Comments on Schizophrenia." *Transcultural Psychiatric Review and Newsletter* 11 (October 1961): 65–71.

– "Indische Christen, vom Psychiater gesehen." *Evangelisches Missionsmagazin* 3–4 (1959): 110–20, 149–58.
– "A Pattern of Neurosis in India." *American Journal of Psychoanalysis* 20, no. 1 (1960): 8–25.
– "Psychiatrie in Indien." *Praxis* 46 (1957): 1145–50.
– "Psychitrische Beobartungen und Erfahrungrn an indischen Patienten." *Praxis* 48 (1959): 1051–7.
– "Wunderdoktor wider Willen im Himalaya." *Schweizerische Aerztezeitung* (1964): 120–7.
Holder A.B. "The Bote: Description of a Peculiar Sexual Perversion found among North-American Indians." *The New York Medical Journal* 50 (1889): 623–5.
Hollingshead, August, and Frederick Redlich. *Social Class and Mental Illness*. New York: Wiley, 1958.
Horton, Walter M. "The Origin and Psychological Function of Religion According to Pierre Janet." *American Journal of Psychology* 35, no. 1 (1924): 16–52.
Ideler, Karl Wilhelm. *Versuch einer Theorie des religiösen Wahnsinns*, vol. 1: *Die Erscheinungen des religiösen Wahnsinns*. Halle: Schwetschke, 1848.
Israël, Lucien, and E. North. "Incidence médico–légale d'un délire de sorcellerie: exorcisme ayant entraîné la mort d'un enfant." *Cahiers de psychiatrie*. Supplement to *Strasbourg médical* 15 (1961): 72–85.
Jaco, Gartly E. *The Social Epidemiology of Mental Disorders*. New York: Russell Sage Foundation, 1960.
Janet, Pierre. "Un cas de possession et l'exorcisme moderne." *Bulletin de l'Université de Lyon* 8 (1894): 41–57.
– *Contribution à l'étude des accidents mentaux chez les hystériques*. Paris: Rueff, 1894.
Jaspers, Karl. "Heimweh und Verbrechen." *Archiv für Kriminal-Anthropologie und Kriminalistik* 35 (1909): 1–116.
Jochelson, Waldemar. "The Koryak." In *The Jesup North Pacific Expedition: Memoir of the American Museum of Natural History*, vol. 6, edited by F. Boas. New York: G.E. Strechert, 1908.
– "The Yukaghir and the Yukaghirized Tungus." In *The Jesup North Pacific Expedition*, vol. 9, pt. I, edited by F. Boas, 30–8. Leiden and New York: E.J. Brill / G.E. Stechert and Co., 1910.
Jörger, Josf. *Psychiatrische Familiengeschichten*. Berlin: Julius Springer, 1919.

Jourdan, Edmond. "Psychologie des Sarimbavy, perversion sexuelle observée en Imerina." *Archives d'anthropologie criminelle* 18 (1903): 808–12.

Julien, Félix. *Harmonies de la mer, courants et revolutions*. Paris: Plon, 1861.

Jung, Carl G. *Ein moderner Mythus. Von Dingen, die am Himmel gesehen warden*. Zurich: Rascher, 1958.

– "Wotan." *Neue Schweizer Rundschau* 3 (1935–36): 657–69.

Kaplan, Bert, and Thomas Plaut. "Personality in a Communal Society." In *An Analysis of the Mental Health of the Hutterites*. Lawrence: University of Kansas Publications, 1956.

Karsch-Haack, Ferdinand. "*Uranismus oder Päderastie* und Tribadie bei den Narurvölkern." *Jahrbuch für sexuelle Zwischenstufen* 3 (1901): 72–201.

Kiev, Ari. "Beliefs and Delusions of West Indian Immigrants to London." *British Journal of Psychiatry* 109 (1963): 356–63.

– "Brief Note: Primitive Holistic Medicine." *International Journal of Social Psychiatry* 8 (1962): 58–61.

– "Folk Psychiatry in Haiti." *Journal of Nervous and Mental Diseases* 132, no. 3 (1961): 260–5.

– "Primitive Therapy." *Psychoanalytic Study of Society* 1 (1960): 185–217.

– "Psychiatric Illness among West Indians in London." *Race and Class* 5 (1964): 48–54.

– "The Psychotherapeutic Aspect of Primitive Medicine." *Human Organization* 21, no. 1 (1962): 25–9.

– "Ritual Goat Sacrifice in Haiti." *American Imago* 19 (1962): 349–59.

– Subud and Mental Illness." *American Journal of Psychotherapy* 18 (1964): 66–78.

Klineberg, Otto. *Social Psychology*. New York: Henry Holt, 1940.

Kluckhohn, Clyde. *Mirror of Man*. New York: Whittlesey House, 1949.

Koch-Grünberg, Theodor. *Vom Roroima zum Orinoco. Ergebinsse einer Reise in Nordbrasilien und Venezuela in den Jahren 1911–1913*. 3 vols. Stuttgart: Strecker und Schröder, 1923.

Koritschoner, Hans. "Ngoma ya Sheitani: An East African Native Treatment for Physical Disorders." *Journal of the Royal Anthropological Institute of Great Britain and Ireland* 66 (1936): 209–19.

Koty, John. *Die Behandlung der Alten und Kranken bei den Naturvölkern*. Stuttgart: Hirschfeld, 1934.

Kraepelin, Emil. "Vergleichende Psychiatrie." *Centralblatt für Nervenheilkunde und Psychiatrie* 15 (1904): 433–7.

Kroeber, Alfred Louis. *Anthropology*. New York: Harcourt Brace, 1948.

Landy, David. "Cultural Antecedents of Mental Illness in the United States." *Social Service Review* 32, no. 4 (December 1958): 350–61.

Lang, Andrew. *Myth, Ritual, and Religion*, 2 vols. London: Longmans, Green, 1887.

Lasnet, Antoine. "Notes d'ethnologie et de médecine sur les Sakalaves du nord-ouest." *Annales d'hygiène et de médecine colonials* 2 (1899): 471–97.

Laubscher, Barent J.F. *Sex, Custom, and Psychopathology: A Study of South African Pagan Natives*. London: George Routledge & Sons, 1937.

Laurent, Émile. "Les Sharimbavy de Madagascar." *Archives d'anthropologie criminelle* 26 (1911): 241–8.

Le Bon, Gustave. *La psychologie des foules*. Paris: Alcan, 1895.

Le Hérissé, Auguste. *L'ancien royaume du Dahomey. Moeurs, religion, histoire*. Paris: Émile Larose, 1911.

Leighton, Alexander. "Mental Illness and Acculturation." In *Medicine and Anthropology*, edited by I. Galdston, 108–28. New York: International Universities Press, 1959.

Leighton, Alexander H., and J.M. Hughes. "Cultures as Causative for Mental Disorders." In *Causes of Mental Disorders: A Review of Epidemiological Knowledge 1959*, 341–83. New York: Milbank Memorial Fund, 1961.

Leriche, René. "Règles générales de la chirurgie de la douleur." *Anesthésie et analgésie* 2 (1936): 218–40.

Le Savoureux, Henri. *Contribution à l'étude des perversions de l'instinct de conservation: le spleen*. Paris: Steinheil, 1913.

Lévi, Jules. "Une épidémie psychique parmi les indigènes du Fezzan (Tripolitaine)." In *Comptes rendus du XXIIe Congrès des médecins aliénistes et neurologistes de France et des pays de langue française. Tunis 1er–7 avril 1912, comptes rendus publiés par le Dr Antoine Porot*, 196–8. Paris: Masson & Cie, 1913.

Lévi-Strauss, Claude. "Introduction à l'oeuvre de Marcel Mauss." In *Sociologie et anthropologie*, by Marcel Mauss, ix–lii. Paris: Presses universitaires de France, 1968.

– *Introduction to the Work of Marcel Mauss*. Translated by Felicity Baker. London: Routledge and Kegan Paul, 1987.

– *La pensée sauvage*. Paris: Plon, 1962.

– "Sorciers et psychanalyse." *Courrier de l'*UNESCO 9 (July–August 1956): 8–10.

Lewin, Bruno. "Differentialdiagnostische Probleme bei Schizophrenien in Ægyten." *IIe Congrès international de psychiatrie, Zurich, 1957* 3 (1959): 23–30.

– "Die Komfliktneurose der Mohammedanerin in Ægyten." *Zeitschrift für Psychotherapie und medizinische Psychologie* 8, no. 3 (1958): 98–112.

Lewin, Louis. *Die Gifte in der Weltgeschichte.* Berlin: Springer, 1920.

– *Phantastica: A Classic Survey on the Use and Abuse of Mind-Altering Plants* [1924]. Rochester: Park Street Press, 1998.

Linton, Ralph. *Culture and Mental Disorders.* Springfield: Charles Thomas, 1956.

Lippert, E. "Über Heimweh." *Zeitschrift für Kinder Psychiatrie* 17, no. 3 (September 1950): 79–84.

Listwan, I.A. "Mental Disorders in Migrants: Further Study." *Medical Journal of Australia.* 1, no. 17 (April 1959): 566–8.

– "Paranoid States: Social and Cultural Aspects." *Medical Journal of Australia* 1, no. 19 (May 1956): 776–8.

Lockhart, Bruce R.H. *Return to Malaya.* New York: G.P. Putnam's Sons, 1936.

López Ibor, Juan José. *Neurosis de Guerra.* Madrid: Editorial científico médica, 1942.

Lorant, Stefan, ed. *The New World: The First Pictures of America.* New York: Duell, Sloane, and Pearce, 1946.

Loursin, Jean-Marie. *Tahiti.* Paris: Éditions du Seuil, 1960.

Lovén, Sven. *Origin of the Tainan Culture, West Indies.* Göteborg: Elanders Bokfryckeri Akefiebolog, 1935.

Lowie, Robert Harry. "The Assiniboine." *Anthropological Papers of the American Museum of Natural History* 4, pt. 1, 1909.

– "Notes on a Shoahonean Ethnography." *Anthropological Papers of the American Museum of Natural History* 20, pt. 3, 1924.

– *Primitive Religion.* New York: Liveright, 1948.

– "Social life of the Crow Indians." *Anthropological Papers of the American Museum of Natural History* 9, pt. 2, 1912.

– "The Sun Dance of the Crow Indians." *Anthropological Papers of the American Museum of Natural History* 16, pt. 1, 1915.

Machen, Arthur. *The Angels of Mons: The Bowman and other Legends of the War.* London: Simpkin, Marshall, Hamilton, Kent & Co., 1915.

Mackay, Charles. *Memoirs of Extraordinary Popular Delusions,* 2 vols. London: Office of the National Illustrated Library, 1852.

MacMunn, George Fletcher. *Moeurs et coutumes des basses classes de l'Inde.* Paris: Payot, 1934.

Majoska, A.V. "Sudden Death in Filipino Men: An Unexplained Syndrome." *Hawaii Medical Journal* 7 (1948): 469–73.

Mandelbaum, David G. "The Plains Cree." *Anthropological Papers of the American Museum of Natural History* 37, pt. 2, 1940.

Manning, F.N. "Statistics of Insanity in Australia." *Journal of Mental Science* 25 (1948): 165–77.

Mannoni, Octave. *Psychologie de la colonization*. Paris: Éditions du Seuil, 1950.

Margetts, Edward L. "The Psychiatric Examination of Native African Patients." *Medical Proceedings, Mediese Bydraes* 4 (October 1958): 679–83.

Marillier, Léon. "Apparitions of the Virgin in Dordogne." *Proceedings of the Society for Psychical Research* 7 (1891–92): 100–10.

Mars, Louis. *La lutte contre la folie*. Port-au-Prince: Imprimerie de l'État, 1947.

–. "Nouvelle contribution à l'étude de la crise de possession." *Psyché* 60 (October 1951): 640–69.

– "La schizophrénie en Haïti." *Bulletin du bureau d'ethnologie* 15 (1958): 39–57.

Martin, Alexander R. "Nostalgia." *American Journal of Psychoanalysis* 14 (1954): 93–104.

Martin, Gustave. "La mentalité primitive indigène devant nos méthodes de prophylaxie et de thérapeutique modernes." *Les grandes endémies tropicales*, vol. 6, 93–106. Paris: Vigot, 1934.

– "Sur les troubles psychiques de quelques infections tropicales. Aperçus de l'assistance psychiatrique aux colonies." *Les grandes endémies tropicales*, vol. 7, 117–34. Paris: Vigot, 1935.

Maruyama, Michiro. *Anatahan*. New York: Hermitage House, 1954.

Matthews, Washington. 1902. *The Night Chant, a Navaho Ceremony*. New York: The Knickerbocker Press, 1902.

Mauss, Marcel. "Effet physique chez l'individu de l'idée de mort suggéré par la collectivité (Australie, Nouvelle–Zélande) [1926]." In *Sociologie et anthropologie*, 313–30. Paris: Presses universitaires de France, 1968.

– "The Physical Effect on the Individual of the Idea of Death Suggested by the Collectivity (Australia, New Zealand)." In *Cultural Psychiatry and Medical Anthropology: An Introduction and Reader,* edited by Roland Littlewood and Simon Dein. London and New Brunswick: Athlone Press, 2000.

Mazellier, Philippe. *Tahiti*. Lausanne: Éditions Rencontre, 1964.

McDougall, William. *The Group Mind: A Sketch of the Principles of Collective Psychology with Some Attempts to Apply Them to the Interpretation of National Life and Character*. Cambridge: Cambridge University Press, 1920.

Meerloo, Joost Abraham Maurits. *Patterns of Panic*. New York: International Universities Press, 1950.

Menninger, Karl. *Man against himself*. New York: Harcourt, Brace & Co., 1938.

Metzger, Emil. "Einiges über Amok und Mataglap." *Globus* 52 (1887): 107–10.

– "Sakit Latah." *Globus* 42 (1882): 381–3.

Mira, Emilio. *Psychiatry in War*. New York: W.W. Norton, 1943.

Miroglio, Abel. *La psychologie des peoples*. Paris: Presses universitaires de France, 1958.

Mishler, Elliot G., and Norman A. Scotch. "Sociocultural Factors in the Epidemiology of Schizophrenia." *Psychiatry* 26 (1963): 315–51.

Mitscherlich, Alexander. "Buchbesprechungen. Berndt, R.M.: "A 'Devastating Disease Syndrome.' Kuru Sorcery in the Eastern Central Highlands of New Guinea." *Sociologus* 8, no. 1: 4–28. Berlin, Duncker & Humblot)." *Psyche* 12 (1958): 784–6.

Montagu, Ashley. "Culture and Mental Illness." *American Journal of Psychiatry* 118, no. 1 (1961): 15–23.

Morita, Shoma. *Shinkeishitsu no hontai to ryoho* [*The nature and treatment of Shinkeishitsu*]. Tokyo: 1928.

Morselli, Giovanni Enrico. "Expérience mescalinique et vécu schizo-phrénique." *L'évolution psychiatrique* 24, no. 2 (1959): 275–82.

– "Le problème d'une schizophrénie expérimentale." *Journal de psychopathologie normale et pathologique* 33, nos. 5 and 6 (1936): 368–92.

– "Recherches expérimentales et délires." *Congrès international de psychi-atrie*. Paris: Hermann & Cie 1 (1950): 89–121.

Mühlmann, Wilhelm E. *Die geheime Gesellschaft der Arioi. Eine Studie über polynesische Geheimbünde, mit besonderer Berücksichtigung der Siebungs- und Auslesevorgänge in Alt-Tahiti*. Leiden: E.J. Brill, 1932.

Murphy, H. Brian M. "Le cannibalisme. Revue de la littérature psychiatrique récente." *Bulletin des stupéfiants* 15 (1963): 15–24.

– "Culture, Society, and Mental Disorder in South East Asia." MD thesis, Edinburgh University, 1959.

– "Méthodologie de recherche en socio-psychiatrie et en ethno-psychi-atrie," fasc. no 37720A10. *Traité de psychiatrie*, 1–14. Paris: Éditions techniques (Encyclopédie médico–chirurgicale), 1965.

– "Social Change and Mental Disorder in Singapore." In *Culture and Mental Health*, edited by Marvin K. Opler, 291–316. New York: Macmillan, 1959.

Murphy, H. Brian M., Eric D. Wittkower, Jacob Fried, and Henri

Ellenberger. "A Cross-Cultural Survey of Schizophrenic Symptomatology." *Transcultural Psychiatry* 9, no. 4 (1963): 327–49.

Musgrave, William E., and A.G. Sison. "Mali–Mali, a Mimic Psychosis in the Philippine Islands: A preliminary report." *Philippine Journal of Sciences*, B: *Medical Sciences* 5 (1910): 335–9.

Niceforo, Alfredo. *Les Classes pauvres : Recherches anthropologiques et sociales.* Paris : Giard & Brière, 1905.

Ninck, Martin. *Wodan und germanischer Schicksalsglaube.* Jena: Eugen Diederichs, 1937.

Obersteiner, Heinrich. "Geisteskrankheiten." *Vom Fels zum Meer* 2 (1889): 1399–403.

O'Brien, H.A. "Latah." *Journal of the Straits Branch of the Royal Asiatic Society* 11 (1883): 143–53.

Oesterreich, Traugott Konstantin. *Die Besessenheit.* Langensalza: Wendt & Klauwell, 1921.

Opler, Marvin E. *An Apache Life-Way: The Economic, Social, and Religious Institutions of the Chriricahua Indians.* Chicago: University of Chicago Press, 1941.

Opler, Marvin E., ed. *Culture and Mental Health.* New York: Macmillan, 1959.

Orelli, Andreas (von). "Der wandel des Inhaltes der depressiven Ideen bei der reinen Melancholie." *Schweizer Archiv für Neurorologie und Psychiatrie* 73 (1954): 217–87.

Ortega y Gasset, José. *La rebelión de las Masas.* Madrid: Revista de Occidente, 1930.

Palem, R.M. *Henri Ey et les congrès mondiaux de psychiatrie.* Canet: Trabucaire, 2000.

Palgi, Phyllis. "The Traditional Attitude towards Physically Handicapped Persons in Certain Middle-Eastern Jewish groups." *Transcultural Research in Mental Health Problems* 8 (July 1960): 58–9.

Pascal, Pierre. *Avvakum et les débuts du raskol. La crise religieuse au xviie siècle en Russie.* Paris: Liguré, 1938.

Payne, Robert. *Forever China.* New York: Dodd, Mead, 1945.

Pelikan, Eugen. *Gerichtlich-medicinische Untersuchungen über das Skopzentrum in Russland nebst historischen Notizen.* Saint Petersburg: Carl Ricker, 1876.

Pfister, Oskar. "Die Wahnideen der Jennischen." *Praktische Psychiatrie* 6 (1951): 109–11.

Pflanz, M. "Soziokulturelle Faktoren und psychische Störungen."

Fortschritte der Neurologie, Psychiatrie und ihrer Grenzgebiete 28 (1960): 472–508.

Piaschewsky, Gisela. *Der Wechselbalg: ein Beitrag zum Aberglauben der neordeuropäischen Völker.* Breslau: Maruschke & Berendt, 1935.

Pillai, K. Subrahmania. *Principles of Criminology.* Madras: n.p., 1924.

Pineau, A. "Médecine et psychiatrie rurale en Guadeloupe." *Le concours medical* (1960): 413–16, 533–44.

Pittard, Eugène. *La castration chez l'homme. Recherche sur les adeptes d'une secte d'eunuques mystiques, les Skoptzy.* Paris: Masson, 1934.

Powers, Stephen. "Tribes of California." *Contributions to North American Ethnology,* vol. 3. Washington, DC: Government Printing Office, 1877.

Radin, Paul. *Indians of South America.* Garden City: Doubleday, 1946.

Raper, Arthur Franklin. *The Tragedy of Lynching.* Chapel Hill: University of North Carolina Press, 1933.

Rapoport, A.M. "Transkulturalnye Issledovaniliia Po. Probleman Psikhicheakogo Zdorovia." *Transcultural Research in Mental Health Problems* 8 (July 1960): 53–4.

Rasch, Christian. "Ueber Amok." *Neurologisches Centralblatt* 13, no. 15 (1894): 550–4.

– "Ueber die Amok–Krankheit der Malayen." *Neurologisches Centralblatt* 14, no. 19 (1895): 856–9.

Ratanakorn, Prasop. *Selected Papers Presented at International Conferences From 1957 to 1962.* Bangkok: Phakdi Pradit Press, 1962.

– *Studies of Mental Illness in Thailand.* Bangkok: Prasat Hospital for Neurological Disorders, 1957.

Reiwald, Paul. *Vom Geist der Massen.* Zurich: Pan, 1946.

Reko, Viktor. *Magische Gifte, Rausch- und Betäubungsmittel der neuen Welt.* Stuttgart: Enke, 1936.

Rencurel, M. "Les Sarimbavy. Perversion sexuelle observée en Emyrne." *Annales d'hygiène et de médecine tropicale et colonial* 3 (1900): 562–8.

Répond, André. "Le Lattah: une psycho-névrose exotique." *Annales médico–psychologiques* 1, no. 4 (1940): 311–24.

Révész, Béla. "Die rassenpsychiatrischen Erfahrungen und ihre Lehren." *Archiv für Schiffsund Tropenhygiene* 15, Supplement no. 5 (1911).

Rigler, Johannes. *Über die Folgen der Verletzungen auf Eisenbahnen, insbesonderes der Verletzungen des Rückenmarks.* Berlin: G. Reimer, 1879.

Rin, Hsien. "Koro: A Consideration on Chinese Concepts of Illness and Case Illustrations." *Transcultural Psychiatric Research Review and Newsletter* 15 (October 1963): 23–30.

Róheim, Géza. "Racial Differences in the Neuroses and Psychoses." *Psychiatry* 2–3 (1939): 375–90.

Roscoe, John. *Twenty-Five Years in East Africa*. Cambridge: Cambridge University Press, 1921.

Roskoff, Gustav. *Geschichte des Teufels*, 2 vols. Leipzig: Brockhaus, 1869.

Roth, Henry Ling. *The Natives of Sarawak and British North Borneo*, 2 vols. London: Truslove and Hanson, 1896.

Ruffin, H. "Melancholie." *Deutsche Medizinische Wochenschrift* 82 (1957): 1080–92.

Scarfone, Marianna. "La psychiatrie coloniale italienne. Théories, pratiques, protagonistes, institutions 1906-1952." PhD diss., Ca' Foscari University of Venice and Lumière University Lyon 2, 2014.

Saindon, R.J.E. "Mental Disorders among the James Bay Cree." *Primitive Man: Quarterly Bulletin of the Catholic Anthropological Conference* 6 (1933): 1–12.

Sal y Rosas, Federico. "Milieu géographique et terrain convulsif." *L'encéphale* 47 (1958): 167–210.

– "El mito del Jani o Susto de la medicina indigena del Perú." *Revista de la sanidad de policía* 18 (1958): 167–210.

Schjelderup, Harald. *Das Verborgene in Uns*. Berne and Stuttgart: Huber, 1964.

Schroeder, Clarence W. "Mental Disorders in Cities." *American Journal of Sociology* 48 (1942–43): 40–7.

Schuler, Edgar A., and Vernon J. Parenton. "A Recent Epidemic of Hysteria in a Louisiana Hight School." *Journal of Social Psychology* 17 (May 1943): 221–35.

Schulte, Walter. "Die gesunde Umwelt in ihrer Reaktion auf Psychoses und Psychopathien." In *Psychiatrie und Gesellschaft*, edited by H. Erhardt, D. Ploog, and H. Stutte, 60–69. Berne and Stuttgart: Hans Huber, 1958.

Scriptor, Jean D. *Sous l'oeil d'Odin*. Levallois-Perret: Société industrielle d'imprimerie, 1953.

Seguin, Carlos Alberto. "Migration and Psychosomatic Disadaptation," *Psychosomatic Medicine* 18 (1956): 404–9.

Seligman, Charles Gabriel. "Temperament, Conflict, and Psychosis in a Stone-Age Population." *British Journal of Medical Psychology* 9 (1929): 187–202.

Shand, Alexander. "The Moriori people of the Chatham Islands." *Journal of the Polynesian Society* 3 (1894): 76–92.

– "The Occupation of the Chatham Islands by the Maoris in 1835." *Journal of the Polynesian Society* 1 (1892): 83–94, 154–63.

Shirley, Ralph. *The Angel Warriors at Mons*. London: Newspaper Publicity Company, 1915.

Shirokogoroff, Sergej M. *Social Organization in the Northern Tungus*. Shanghai: The Commercial Press, 1929.

Sighele, Scipio. *The Criminal Crowd and Other Writings on Mass Society*. Edited by Nicoletta Pireddu. Translated by Nicoletta Pireddu and Andrew Robbins. Toronto: University of Toronto Press, 2018.

– *La foule criminelle. Essai de psychologie collective*. Paris: Alcan, 1892.

Skinner, Alanson. "Notes on the Eastern Cree and Northern Saulteaux." *Anthropological Papers of the American Museum of Natural History* 9, pt. I (1911–12).

Sleeman, James L. *Thug, or a Million Murders*. London: Sampson Low, Marston & Co., 1933.

Sleeman, William Henry. *Ramaseeana, or a Vocabulary of the Peculiar Language Used by the Thugs, with an Introduction and Appendix, Descriptive of the System Pursued by that Fraternity and of the Measures Which Have Been Adopted by the Supreme Government of India for Its Suppression*, 2 vols. Calcutta: G.H. Huttmann, 1836.

– *The Thugs or Phansigars of India, Compiled from the Original and Authentic Documents Published by Captain W.H. Sleeman, Superintendent of Thug Police*. Philadelphia: Carey & Hart, 1839.

Soldan, Wilhelm Gottlieb, Heinrich Heppe, and S. Ries. *Geschichte der Hexenprozesse*, 2 vols. Stuttgart: Cotta, 1880.

Spiro, Melford E. "Cultural Heritage, Personal Tensions, and Mental Illness in the South Culture." In *Culture and Mental Health*, edited by M.K. Opler, 141–71. New York: Macmillan, 1959.

Sprenger, Jakob, and Heinrich Institoris. *Der Hexenhammer. Zum ersten Male ins Deutsche übertragen und eingeleitet von J.W. Schmidt*, 3 vols. Berlin: Barsdorf, 1906.

Sreenivasan, U., and J. Hoening. "Caste and Mental Hospital Admissions in Mysore State, India." *American Journal of Psychiatry* 117, no. 1 (1960): 37–43.

Staehelin, John. "Ueber Depressionszüstände." *Schweizerische medizinische Wochenschrift* 85 (1955): 1205–9.

Stainbrook, Edward. "A Cross-Cultural Evaluation of Depressive Reactions." In *Depression*, edited by P. Hoch and J. Zubin, 39–50. New York: Grune and Stratton, 1954.

– "Some Characteristics of the Psychopathology Behavior in Bahian Society." *American Journal of Psychiatry* 109 (1952): 330–5.

Stalcruz, J.Z. "The Pathology of Bangungui." *Journal of the Philippine Medical Association* 27 (1951): 476–81.

Stephanopoli, M. "Contribution à l'étude du folklore de la Corse." *Nouvelle revue des traditions populaires* 2, no. 5 (1950): 467–78.

Stewart, Kilton. "A Cross-Cultural Study of Dreams." Reviewed in *Transcultural Psychiatric Research Review and Newsletter* 11 (October 1961): 12–17.

Stieler, Georg. *Person und Masse.* Leipzig: Meiner, 1929.

Stoll, Otto. *Suggestion und Hypnotismus in der Völkerpsychologie.* Leipzig: Von Veit, 1904.

Stoller, Alan. *Assignment Report on Mental Health Situation in Thailand.* Bangkok: OMS Regional Office for South East Asia, no. 7, 1959.

Swanton, John Reed. "Aboriginal Culture of the Southeast." *42nd Annual Report of the Bureau of American Ethnology.* Washington, DC: Smithsonian Institution, 1924–25.

Taine, Hippolyte. *Les origines de la France contemporaine.* I. *L'Ancien Régime.* Paris: Hachette, 1876.

– *Les origines de la France contemporaine.* II. *La Révolution,* 3 vols. Paris: Hachette, 1876, 1881, 1885.

Tanzi, Eugenio. "Il Folk-lore nella patologia mentale." *Rivista di filosofia scientifica* 9 (1890): 385–419.

Tarde, Gabriel (de). *Les crimes des foules. Actes du IIIe Congrès international d'anthropologie criminelle, Bruxelles, août 1892.* Brussels: Hayez, 1892.

– *The Laws of Imitation.* Translated by Elsie Clews Parsons. New York: H. Holt, 1903.

– *Les lois de l'imitation.* Paris: Alcan, 1890.

– *L'opinion et la foule,* Paris: Alcan, 1901.

Tavernier, Jean-Baptiste. *Les six voyages de J.-B. Tavernier en Turquie, en Perse et aux Indes,* vol. 4. Rouen: J.-B. Machuel le père, 1713.

Teicher, Morton I. "Windigo Psychosis: A Study of a Relationship between Belief and Behavior among the Indians of Northeastern Canada." *Proceedings of the 1960 Annual Spring Meeting of the American Ethnological Society.* Seattle: University of Washington Press, 1960.

Teit, James A. "The Salishan tribes of the Western Plateau." *45th Annual Report of the Bureau of American Ethnology.* Washington, DC: Smithsonian Institution, 1927–28.

Terrien, Maxime. "De l'hystérie en Vendée." *Archives de neurologie* 26 (1893): 447–75.

– *De l'hystérie en Vendée.* Thesis in medicine, Toulouse, 1897.

Thomae, Hans. "Männlicher Transvestitismus und das Verlangen nach Geschlechtsumwandlung." *Psyche* 11, no. 2 (1957): 81–124.

Thornton, Edward. *Illustrations of the History and Practices of the Thugs.* London: Allen, 1837.

Tokarski, Ardalion. "Merjatschenie" [1890], analyzed in *Allgemeine Zeitschrift für Psychiatrie*, 48 (1892): 309; and in *Neurologisches Centralblatt* 9 (1890): 662–3.

Tooth, Geoffrey. *Studies in Mental Illness in the Gold Coast*, vol. 4. London: HMSO, 1950.

Turnbull, John. *Voyage fait autour du monde en 1800, 1801, 1802, 1803 et 1804.* Paris: Xhrouet, 1807.

Uchimura, Yushi. "Imu, eine psychoreaktive Erscheinung bei Ainu–Frauen." *Nervenarzt* 27 (1956): 535–40.

Vaerting, Mathias, and Mathilde Vaerting. *Neubegründung der Psychologie von Mann und Weib*, 2 vols. Berlin: Karlsruhe im Braunschweig, 1921–23.

Vallon, Charles, and Georges Génil-Perrin. "La psychiatrie medico-légale dans l'oeuvre de Zacchias." *Revue de pychiatrie* 16 (1912): 46–84, 90–106.

Van Bergen, Gerhard. "Betrachtungen über Amok, unter Berücksichtigung der eigengesetzlichen, schwer verständlichen seelischen Aeusserungsformen der Bevölkerung im Raum seines Auftretens." *Zeitschrift für Psychotherapie* 3 (1953): 226–31.

– "Zur Deutung des Amok-Lattah-Geschehens unter der hypothetischen Betrachtungsweise vergleichender Affektiverwertungsmechanismen." *Zeitschrift für Psychotherapie* 5 (1955): 83–6.

Van Brero, Pieter Cornelis Johannes. "Einiges über die Geisteskrankheiten der Bevölkerung des malaiischen Archipels." *Allgemeine Zeitschrift für Psychiatrie* 53 (1897): 25–78.

– "Koro, eine eigenthümliche Zwangsvorstellung." *Allgemeine Zeitschrift für Psychiatrie* 53 (1897): 569–73.

– "Über das sogenannte Latah, eine in Niederländisch-Ostindien vorkommende Neurose." *Allgemeine Zeitschrift für Psychiatrie* 51 (1895): 939–48.

Van Loon, Feico G. Herman. "Amok and Lattah." *Journal of Abnormal and Social Psychology* 21 (1926–27): 434–44.

Van Wulfften Palthe, Pieter Mattheus. "Amok." *Nederlandsch Tijdschrift voor Geneeskunde* 77, no. 1 (1933): 983–91.

– "Koro. Eine merkwürdige Angsthysterie." *Internationale Zeitschrift für Psychoanalyse* 21 (1935): 249–57.

– *Neurologie en psychiatrie*. Amsterdam: Wetenschappelijke, Uitgeverij, 1948.

Varagnac, André, et al. *L'homme avant l'écriture*. Paris: A. Colin, 1959.

Wallace, Alfred Russel. *The Malay Archipelago* [1869]. London: Macmillan & Co., 1898.

Welter, Gustave. *Histoire des sectes chrétiennes des origines à nos jours*. Paris: Payot, 1950.

Williams, Francis Edgar. *Orokaiva Magic*. Oxford: Oxford University Press, 1928.

Winge, Paul. *Der menschliche Gonochorismus und die historische Wissenschaft. Abhandlungen aus dem Gebiete der Sexualforschung* vol. 1, no. 3. Bonn: Marcus & Weber, 1918–19.

Winthuis, Josef. *Das Zweigeschlechterwesen bei den Zentralaustraliern und anderen Völkern. Lösungsversuch der ethnologischen Hauptprobleme auf Grund primitiven Denkens*. Leipzig: Hirschfeld, 1928.

Winiarz, Wiktor, and J. Wielawski. "Imu: A Psychoneurosis Occurring among Ainus." *Psychoanalytic Review* 23 (1936): 181–6.

Wisse, Jacob. *Selbstmord und Todesfurcht bei den Naturvölkern*. Zutphen: Thieme, 1933.

Wissler, Clark, "Social Organization and Ritualistic Ceremonies of the Blackfoot Indians." *Anthropological Papers of the American Museum of Natural History*, no. 7. New York: American Museum of Natural History, 1912.

– "Societies and Ceremonial Associations in the Oglala Division of the Teton-Dakota." *Anthropological Papers of the American Museum of Natural History*, vol. 11, pt. 1, 1912.

Wittkower, Eric D. "Aspectos transculturales de la psiconeurosis." *Revista psiquiátrica peruana* 3 (1960); *Revue de médecine psychosomatique* 2 (1960): 39–46; *Revista archivos de neurología y psyquiatría* 10 (1960): 213–22.

– "A Cross-Cultural Approach to Mental Health Problems." In *Neuroses*. I. *Congressus Psychiatricus Bohemoslovenicus Cum Participatione Internationali (1959)*, 67–76. Prague: Státní zdravotnické nakladatelství, 1961.

– "Interplay of Cultural and Scientific Values in Higher Education Today." *International Universities Bureau* 5 (1960): 69–81.

– "Psiquiatría social cultural y transcultural." *La revista de psiquiatría y psicología médica de Europa y América Latina* 4 (1960): 705–14.

Wittkower, Eric D., and L. Bijou. "Perspectives of Transcultural

Psychiatry." *Israël Annals of Psychiatry and Related Disciplines* 2, no. 1 (1964): 19–26.

– "Psychiatry in Developing Countries." *American Journal of Psychiatry* 120 (1963): 218–21.

– "Spirit Possession in Haitian Vodun Ceremonies." *Acta Psychotherapeutica* 12 (1964): 70–80.

Wittkower, Eric D., and Jacob Fried. "Some Problems of Transcultural Psychiatry." *International Journal of Social Psychiatry* 3, no. 4 (1958): 245–52.

– "A Cross-Cultural Approach to Mental Health Problems." *American Journal of Psychiatry* 116 (1959): 423–8.

Wittkower, Eric D., Jacob Fried, and Henri Ellenberger. "A Cross-Cultural Survey of Schizophrenic Symptomatology." In *Proceedings of the 3rd World Congress of Psychiatry, Montreal, Canada, 4–10 June 1961*, 1309–15. Toronto: University of Toronto Press; and Montreal: McGill University Press, 1961.

– "A Cross-Cultural Survey of Schizophrenic Symptomatology." *International Journal of Social Psychiatry* 9, no. 4 (1963): 237–49.

Wittkower, Eric D., et al. "Crosscultural Inquiry into the Symptomatology of Schizophrenia." *Annals of the New York Academy of Sciences* 84 (1960): 854–63.

Wrangell, Ferdinand (de), Fedor F. Matiouchkine, and Kozmine. *Le Nord de la Sibérie. Voyage parmi les peuplades de la Russie asiatique et dans la mer glaciale*, 2 vols. Paris: Amyot, 1843.

Yap, Pow-Meng. "A Diagnostic and Pronostic Study of the Schizophrenia in Chinese." In *Congrès international de psychiatrie, Zurich, 1957*, vol. 1, 354–64. Zurich: Orell Füssli Arts Graphiques S.A., 1959.

– "Koro or Suk-Yeong: An Atypical Culture-Bound Psychogenic Disorder Found in Southern Chinese." *Transcultural Psychiatric Research* 1, (April 1964): 36–8.

– "The Latah Reaction: Its Pathodynamics and Nosological Position." *Journal of Mental Science* 98, no. 413 (1952): 515–64.

– "Mental Diseases Peculiar to Certain Cultures: A Survey of Comparative Psychiatry." *Journal of Mental Sciences* 97 (1951): 313–27.

– *Suicide in Hong Kong*. Hong Kong: Hong Kong University Press, 1958.

Zigas, Vincent, and Daniel Gajdusek Carleton. "Kuru: Clinical Study of a New Syndrome Resembling Paralysis Agitans in Natives of the Eastern Highlands of Australian New Guinea." *Medical Journal of Australia* 2, no. 21 (November 1957): 745–54.

PART THREE
APPENDICES

Outline of Updated Booklets Published in 1978 in the *Traité de psychiatrie* of the *Encyclopédie médico-chirurgicale* (EMC) by Henri Ellenberger, Raymond Prince, Brian Murphy, and Michel Tousignant

ANTHROPOLOGICAL FOUNDATIONS OF ETHNOPSYCHIATRY

Personality and culture; influence of techniques of socialization: example of diachronic analysis; Oedipus and culture: example of synchronic analysis; the ego and defence mechanisms; the patient and his culture; stable environment and society in transition; anthropology and psychiatry: a necessary collaboration

PSYCHOSES

Schizophrenia (incidence, type and evolution, symptomatology); acute psychotic reactions; affective psychoses; other psychoses

NEUROSES AND MINOR CONDITIONS

States of anxiety; hysteria; *latah*-type conditions; obsessional states; phobias; sexual neuroses and escape roles

DRUG ADDICTIONS

The general problem; classification of drug addictions (alcoholism, stimulants of central nervous system activity, depressants of central nervous system activity, disruptors of central nervous system activity)

RESEARCH METHODOLOGY IN ETHNOPSYCHIATRY

The ethnographic approach in psychiatry; ethnopsychoanalysis; scales of measurement and standardized interviews

THERAPY AND CULTURE

Therapeutic variations and cultural characteristics; universal characteristics of therapy (endogenous factors, common exogenous factors, the use of dreams, mystical states and meditation, trances and dissociative states, shamanism and pharmacogenetic ecstasy); additional comments

Outline of an Unfinished Book by Henri Ellenberger, Excerpts of Which Have Been Published in Journals

ETHNOPSYCHIATRIC AND ETHNOCRIMINOLOGICAL STUDIES

Foreword

ETHNOPSYCHIATRY

1 Generalities
2 History
3 Mental diseases that have an organic cause
4 Intoxications: generalities
5 Drug addictions (published in *L'Union médicale du Canada*)
6 Alcoholism
7 Depressions (published in *L'Union médicale du Canada*)
8 Hysteria (published in *Confrontations psychiatriques*)
9 Phobia
10 Obsessions
11 Neuroses and imitation mania
12 Neuroses and delusions of metamorphosis
13 Non-aggressive reactions
14 Schizophrenia (chapter to be rewritten to incorporate recent data)

ETHNOCRIMINOLOGY

1 Aggressive reactions
2 Suicide
3 Self-sacrifice
4 Vendetta (published in the *Revue internationale de criminologie*)
5 Castration and eunuchs

6 Sexual mutilations inflicted upon women
7 Anthropophagy and cannibalism
8 Slaves and slavery
9 Headhunters
10 Crimes of witchcraft
11 Criminal sects and tribes
12 Ethnic types of criminals
13 Infanticides, senicide

"A Case of Peyote Drug Addiction": Unpublished Course Notes by Henri Ellenberger

Last week, our discussion focused on the transcultural aspects of alcoholism in perhaps a somewhat theoretical perspective. Now I would like to speak to you about another variety of drug addiction, taking a more directly clinical point of view.

Let me first sum up the clinical observation, which we will then be able to comment upon and discuss.

Let us take ourselves back to the year 1957 in the city of Topeka, Kansas, in the geographical centre of the United States. In those far-off days, I was interested in transcultural psychiatry, which led to my being given the honour to consult with Indian patients who entered the State Hospital. Most of these patients were Potawatomi,[1] and more rarely, a few Kickapoo[2] from the two Indian reserves located not far from Topeka. I was thus able to make very interesting observations, especially as I had visited these Indians several times on their reserves and had made friends among them. One of the facts that struck me the most was that these Indians basically had a split personality. Each of them had an American surname and first name and said they belonged to a Christian denomination: Baptist, Methodist, Catholic, and so on. But on the other hand, each had an Indian name and belonged to an Indian religion and these details never appeared in the medical observations. One day I noticed that this duality could even extend to the diagnosis: a thirty-three-year-old man who was born and had lived up to age twenty in the Potawatomi reservation had been diagnosed as suffering from a severe mental disability. His intelligence quotient had just been measured by the psychologist of the State Hospital at forty-three percent. This figure seemed implausible to me. Speaking with the Indian, I learned that he never attended school; he was born on the Mayetta Reservation[3] and never left until the age of twenty; he had only spoken Potawatomi. Afterwards he worked in road construction with a team of workers whose language was not in the least academic. So we understand why these verbal performances on tests were mediocre. A more in-depth investigation revealed that he was suffering from an organic cerebral syndrome, the cause of which could not be clearly determined.

In this case, the uncertainty of the diagnosis stemmed from the patient's difficulties in expressing himself verbally, but in other cases, I noticed that the Indians deliberately provided incomplete or unilateral anamneses, which leads us to our subject.

One day a Kickapoo Indian aged sixty-seven was admitted to the State Hospital. Sober until the previous year, he had suddenly begun drinking alcohol to excess following unclear circumstances in which disagreements with his wife appear to have played a role. The case was diagnosed as "alcoholic neurosis." The fact that an alcoholic neurosis could begin at age sixty-five may seem extraordinary. Fortunately, I knew one of his friends and neighbours whom I had visited on the reserve, and the patient, whose trust I had won, told me his whole story. He too had a kind of split personality, an American name and an Indian name, an "official" religion and an "Indian" religion. While nominally Protestant, he belonged to the peyote religion, to which he had converted at about the age of twenty-seven. He practised his Indian religion sincerely, but had ended up becoming addicted to peyote. His wife, who belonged to another Indian religion, that of the "Dream Drummers," was hostile to the peyote religion. One day there was no peyote to be found: the man suffered deeply, which led him to seek solace in alcohol. That was the real origin of this alcoholism late in life – but the man was loath to speak of peyote or of his religion, which he considered to be purely an Indian matter of no concern to doctors.

This observation is interesting on several levels. On one hand, it shows that, contrary to an opinion held by many authors, peyote is perfectly capable of leading to drug addictions, even if this is exceptional. Second, it illustrates the difficulties that arise when you practise transcultural psychiatry. The clinical image that we first have is a cover that masks the real clinical image. It is also very easy to miss very specific clinical characteristics that we do not notice if we are not aware of their possible existence. In other words, we don't notice things when we are unaware of their existence.

But, before going further in explaining the case in question, it is useful to digress to indicate some details related to the Indians in question here.

Potawatomi Indians are a branch of the large family of Algonquians, from whom they separated a long time ago. In the seventeenth century they, with the Chippewa and the Ottawa, still formed one same people, as reported by the Jesuit priests. Around 1800, under pressure from the invasions of the Whites, the dislocation of the Potawatomi people began. Today, it is estimated that approximately two thousand Potawatomi exist in Oklahoma and eleven hundred on the Mayetta Reservation, not far from Topeka, plus some isolated groups in Michigan, Wisconsin, and in several regions of Canada. As for the Kickapoo, they make up a branch that separated from the Potawatomi family. They are far less numerous than them and live on a small reservation located farther north than that of the Potawatomi. Their language may be considered a dialect stemming from the Potawatomi language, so much so that the two tribes can understand each other easily. One remarkable aspect of the Potawatomi is that even though their political and social organization was destroyed by white civilization, they maintain many traditions, the use of their language, and they are greatly attached to Indian religions.

From a religious point of view, the Potawatomi have maintained several of their ceremonial dances, even though these seem celebrated increasingly rarely. On the other hand, most of them have become followers of two relatively new forms of worship. On the Mayetta reservation, I have been told, about half the Indians belong to the religion of Dream Drummers, and the other half to the peyote religion.

The religion of the Drummers, according to ethnologists, arose in approximately 1870 among the Dakota (a Sioux tribe) and gradually extended to other tribes. The main ceremony consists of the "Dream Dance," celebrated regularly at the change of seasons, as well as in specific circumstances, such as to heal someone who is sick or at the funeral of a member of the group. This ceremony is long and complicated but also very colourful, as I was able to observe, having been invited to attend one of them by one of my Indian friends.

Completely different, the peyote religion seems to have been introduced among the Potawatomi shortly before 1900, most probably by the Indians of Oklahoma, who had received this religion following a chain of transmission starting in Mexico. The peyote religion consists of a more closed sect than that of the Drummers; here it is out of the question for an outsider to attend the ceremonies. We also note a more ardent religious zeal, coupled with proselytism, and can understand that the difference in religion between our patient and his wife could have played a role in their quarrels.

As for the Kickapoo, they had their own prophet, Kennekuk, who built a church and composed an alphabet. Nevertheless, many Kickapoo are part of the Drummers or belong to the peyote religion. Among them is our Indian, to whom I now return.

The patient agreed to explain to me in detail the way in which the ceremonies of his religion unfold. As among the Drummers, regular meetings are held on days of great celebration, but sometimes they take place at much closer intervals, and our Indian assured me that over twenty years, he had participated in ceremonies that took place one Saturday out of two. The meetings began at about eight o'clock in the evening and lasted the entire night till dawn. The average number of participants was approximately twenty, but on special occasions rose to thirty or forty. The meetings were extremely well structured, both from the point of view of the spatial arrangement of the participants and from the timing of the rites. On each side of the door of the room sat a "fire chief" in charge of lighting a fire on an altar. Opposite the door sat the "peyotl chief" (also called the leader) to whose left was the "cedar chief" and to whose right was the "drum chief." The other assistants sat in a circle around the altar. It was the peyotl chief who opened the ceremony by giving a brief speech followed by prayers. The cedar chief threw cedar branches into the fire and the drum chief was in charge of a small drum that circulated from time to time among those present. Songs, prayers, and various rites followed one another without interruptions during the entire night. Peyote, which had been brought from Oklahoma, was consumed – generally in the form of buttons – several times during the ceremony. In this way, none of the participants ever failed to have visions.

Questioned about his first experiences with peyote, our Indian told me about one of his very first visions, of which he retained a very vivid impression. He even agreed to illustrate it in a drawing.[4] The vision began with that of a mountain whose slopes were covered in rocks. It was an impressive sight; then clear, liquid water began to flow between the rocks and over top of them. In a third stage, it was no longer water that flowed but blood, which he experienced with deep horror. In a fourth stage, the rocks were transformed into the corpses of little children; the vision had become a horrible nightmare. He asked God through the intermediary of the peyotl chief why he had had this nightmare, and the divinity replied to him by the same means that it was because he had sinned, having had illicit sexual relations. Indeed, one of the most important conditions of the peyote religion consists in the obligation of purifying oneself beforehand, a purification which includes the confession of sins. Note that this involves a public confession, which naturally leads to embarrassing scenes when acts of adultery are involved.

The transcultural study of peyote would be incomplete without a comparison of the effects of the product among Indians and Whites. When the Spanish conquered Mexico, they were horrified to see that the native people of the country widely used drugs during their religious ceremonies. They also noticed that some of these drugs, including peyote, had been consumed according to rites that resembled those of Christian communion. That was all it took for the Spanish to declare that it was an act of the devil who gave himself as a sacrament to souls on the way to perdition. This was the point of departure for a ruthless persecution and apparently the use of peyote only persisted in the secret ceremonies of a few isolated tribes in virtually inaccessible regions, mainly the Tarahumara and the Huichol. It was only around the mid-nineteenth century that botanists began to become interested in peyote and identified it with a small, thornless cactus that grew in the most arid regions of northern Mexico, but for a long time botanists disagreed as to the exact identification of the plant, until Rouhier showed in 1927 that it was just one plant, despite its polymorphism.

The pharmacological effects of peyote had already been studied by several researchers. Pioneers of this research include Havelock Ellis[5] and Wier Mitchell.[6] More systematic experiments were conducted by Lewin[7] and by Beringer[8] in Germany, and by Rouhier[9] in France. Descriptions of a literary nature followed, among them those of Aldous Huxley[10] and Henri Michaux[11] are particularly well known.

We remind readers that Western experimenters noted, in the effects of peyote and mescaline, the following characteristics:

1   For the Western experimenter, it is above all an aesthetic spectacle, generally individual. It is a phantasmagoria of forms,

light, colour, and movement that fascinates by its incomparable beauty.

2 These are, strictly speaking, not hallucinations but "pseudo-hallucinations," that is, the subject remains perfectly aware that his hallucinations are unreal.

3 These hallucinations are very mobile; they are intermittent and unpredictable. Part of their charm stems from this element of constant surprise.

If we now look at the visions of the Indians, we note that they differ point by point from the preceding characteristics:

1 For them, it is basically a religious experience. The aesthetic element is not absent, but is subordinate to it. The experience begins with a deep sense of veneration and the believer comes out spiritually enriched. For the same reason, it has a communal character and reinforces ties among the individuals.

2 Unlike Europeans and North Americans, the Indian is persuaded that his visions are real; it is the divinity itself who appears through them.

3 The visions are not intermittent, but as they are mobile, they present a kind of temporal organization, in the way of a narrative or a drama.

PEYOTE ADDENDA[12]

– Sanford Unger, 1963;[13]

When mescaline is administered by Freudians; infantile experiences.

When mescaline is administered by Jungians; transcendent experiences.

When mescaline is administered Harvard students; philosophical problems (determinism, freedom, problem of evil).

The experience is *not*[14] an artificial psychosis.

– Henri Michaux; we are not unshackled from everything.

"these liberated people are prisoners."

"there exists a banality of the visionary world"

"the dizzying passage of images apparently unrelated among themselves or with the personality" – hence anxiety.

"banality within the extraordinary."

NOTES

1 Annotated by hand: "Cours et conférences inédits," Centre de documentation Henri Ellenberger. On the teaching of Henri Ellenberger in the United
   States, see Delille, "Teaching the History of Psychiatry." (*Ed.*)
2 This is a Plains Indians group (i.e, the Great Plains of North America) and
   is connected to the Algonquian group. The tribe is also connected to the
   Algonquian group. Their reserve is in northern Kansas. (*Ed.*)
3 Reservation located not far from Topeka (Kansas). (*Ed.*)
4 Drawing reproduced in E. Delille, "On the History of Cultural Psychiatry:
   Georges Devereux, Henri Ellenberger, and the Psychological Treatment of
   Native Americans in the 1950s," *Transcultural Psychiatry* 53, no. 3
   (2016): 402. (*Ed.*)
5 H. Ellis, "A Note on the Phenomenon of Mescal Intoxication," *The Lancet*
   75, no. 1 (1897): 1540–42. (*Ed.*)
6 Silas Weir Mitchell (1829–1914), an American neurologist and writer. See
   his "Remarks on the Effects of Anhelonium Lewinii (the Mescal Button),"
   British Medical Journal 2 (1896): 1625–29. (*Ed.*)
7 Louis Lewin (1850–1929), German scientist. See his *Phantastica: A Classic
   Survey on the Use and Abuse of Mind-Altering Plants* (Rochester: Park
   Street Press, 1998; originally published in German in 1924). (*Ed.*)
8 K. Beringer, "Experimentelle Psychosen durch Meskalin," *Zeitschrifte für
   die Gesamte Neurologie und Psychiatrie* 84 (1923): 426–33; Beringer, *Der
   Mezcalinrausch, seine Geschichte und Erscheinungsweise* (Berlin: Springer
   1927). (*Ed.*)
9 A. Rouhier, "Phénomènes de métagnomie expérimentale observés au cours
   d'une experience faite avec le peyotl," *Revue métapsychique* (1925): 144–45;
   Rouhier, *Monographie du peyotl*, PhD diss., Faculté de pharmacie de Paris,
   1926; Rouhier, *La plante qui fait les yeux émerveillés. Le peyotl (Echinocactus
   williamsii)* (Paris: Gaston Doin & Cie 1927; also published in Paris by G.
   Tredaniel, 1926); Rouhier, *Les plantes divinatoires* (Paris 1927). (*Ed.*)
10 Aldous L. Huxley (1894–1963), British writer. See his *The Doors of
   Perception*. (*Ed.*)
11 Henri Michaux (1899–1984), French poet of Belgian origin. See *Misérable
   miracle* (Monaco: Éditions du Rocher 1956). (*Ed.*)
12 This addendum was added on a manuscript page and written by Henri
   Ellenberger. (*Ed.*)
13 Unger, LSD, *Mescaline, Psilocybin, and Psychotherapy*; Unger, "Mescaline,
   LSD, Psilocybin and Personality Change." (*Ed.*)
14 Underlined word. (*Ed.*)

Correspondence between Henri Ellenberger
and Georges Devereux (1954–1974)

The professional correspondence of Henri Ellenberger is part of the archival material deposited at the Sainte-Anne Hospital in Paris following an agreement concluded between the Société internationale d'histoire de la psychiatrie et de la psychanalyse (International Society of History of Psychiatry and Psychoanalysis; SIHPP) and the Sainte-Anne Hospital shortly before the death of Henri Ellenberger. An agreement was signed to found a Centre de documentation Henri Ellenberger intended to hold this archival material, along with that of other psychiatrists and psychoanalysts, and all related documents. Address: 1, rue Cabanis, 75 674 cedex 14, Paris. In the transcription of the letters, the syntax and punctuation have been maintained; only minor spelling errors, and missing letters or accents (the correspondence was typewritten in the United States), have been corrected. The correspondence was compared to the identical one that is kept in the fonds Georges Devereux at IMEC.

Topeka, July 14, 1954

Dr George Devereux
Director of Research
Devereux Institute
Devon (Pennsylvania)

Dear Dr Devereux,
How are you doing? Several people here have asked me recently if I had news of you, and I had to reply no. Among these people, I must mention Dr Lythgoe, returned from a long trip to Europe, and Dr Ticho[1] who asked me to send his regards when I told him I would

be writing to you. Above all, I hope to have the pleasure of meeting you at a conference or at another occasion. Perhaps you will come by this way one of these days?

Allow me to send you an off-print of an article I wrote about three years ago that has been sound asleep in the drawers of the *Revue Int. De Criminologie*, which finally decided to publish it. Have you published something yourself during this time? Is your book on Ethno-Psychiatry progressing?

Cordially,
H. Ellenberger

19 July 1954

Dear friend,
Thank you so much for sending me your very interesting work on the relationships between the criminal and the victim, which has arrived at an opportune time, as I am writing a book in which I intend to address these types of questions in terms of primitive society. I am therefore most grateful to you.

I was sorry to not have seen you in St Louis, as I thought you would be there. Since I go to all the psychoanalytic conferences, we're bound to end up seeing one another.

Regarding stopping off in Topeka – it seems unlikely. What would I do there? I certainly have friends there, but I can see most of these friends at conferences – and I was not so happy in Topeka that I cannot wait to return there, even only briefly. I led a hard life there, truth be told!

Here, everything is going well. I am working – as always – like a maniac. I am writing two books – one book during office hours, and the book on ethnopsychiatry on evenings and weekends.

Otherwise, nothing new to report. I live very quietly, take care of my work, my dog, my house, and see friends that I have met in Philadelphia – and that's it. This evening I am going to a concert.

Please remember me to my friends.

Yours sincerely,
Georges Devereux

Director of Research
Devereux Foundation
Devon, Pennsylvania

Topeka, Sept. 12, 1954

Dr George Devereux
Devereux School
Devon, Pennsylvania

My dear friend,

Allow me to send you a copy of my work on Rorschach, which
you have perhaps already seen. It is, as you will be able to note, the
outline of a rather incomplete biography: for various reasons I was
able to use only part of my documentation; the rest may come out
in ten years or so!

Would you have, by any chance, an off-print of your article on
a sociological conception of schizophrenia that appeared in the
Psychanalytic Review in 1939 and which is of particular interest
to me?

Also, I wondered if you would be willing to write a review of my
book "La Psychiatrie Suisse," for an American journal other than the
American Journal of Psychiatry? This work of approximately two
hundred pages was an enormous undertaking for me, but I have not
been able to publish it in book form: Swiss publishers are asking a
hefty sum to bring it out in print; far from offering you fees, it is they
who ask for them to publish you! I could not do that and published
it in *L'évolution psychiatrique* as a series of seven articles. But the
printer neglected to give me the additional off-prints requested, so
I only received those provided by the journal. Which is to say that
the copies I do have are as rare as the Gutenberg Bible, although not
as well printed. This "Psychiatrie Suisse" contains: 1. A historical
presentation of the Swiss pioneers of this science. 2. A portrait of the
life in Swiss mental hospitals, in which I attempted a "sociology of
the psychiatric profession." 3. A presentation of eight adjacent territories: philosophy, biology, psychology, and so on, not to mention a
few forays into ethnology. – I can't really see who I could approach
for a review in an American journal: there are so few people here
who understand French. – My presentations of the systems of Jung,
Szondi, Binswanger, M. Bleuler, Binder, and so on have been read by

their protagonists and I have taken their observations into account; this is simply to say that they all guarantee objectivity and that it all constitutes a kind of textbook of psychopathology according to the main European theories. The "Psychoanalysis" chapter was read and approved by Pfister.

I hope to hear from you and see you at an upcoming event (perhaps in New York in early December).

Cordially,
H. Ellenberger

———

20 September 1954

My dear friend,
Thank you so much for your kind letter and for sending your study on Rorschach, which is wonderful.

Alas, I no longer have *even one* off-print left of my sociological study of schizophrenia!

Likewise, I am sorry not to be able to accept your very kind invitation to write a review of your study on Swiss psychiatry. I am working like a maniac, and am unable take on additional work. I am in the midst of writing TWO books. I am waiting at any moment for the proofs of another book that is soon to be released. I have agreed to prepare for the press (I mean, for the printer) the posthumous SALMON LECTURES of my late friend, Professor Ralph Linton of Yale. I have to prepare four lectures for various scholarly learned societies. To tell the truth, I am exhausted. I am so sorry, for the subject would have interested me, and I would have been delighted to have helped you out.

You too seem to be working hard and well. Good luck!

I look forward to seeing you in May in Atlantic City.

Yours sincerely,
George Devereux

———

Topeka, Dec. 28., 1954
Dr George Devereux
Devereux School, Devon, Pa.

Dear friend,

Mrs Morrison has decided to improve the journal she is preparing for the personnel of the Menninger Clinic; as proof, the Christmas issue, to which she asked several doctors and psychologists to contribute personally. She printed a hundred more copies than usual and generously gave me twenty, asking me to send them to people who could be interested in them. I thought that perhaps it would be interesting for you to glance at this issue, given the contributions on Christmas, Diwali, Chanukah, and so on, even if they are not scientific studies!

Just today I received a prospectus of the new journal *Archives of Criminal Psychodynamics*, and note that it will soon publish an article by you: "Cultural Anthropology and Criminal Psychodynamics." That is a most interesting subject, for which I myself gathered quite a bit of material at one time. Perhaps it would interest you to know that my article on the relationship between the criminal and the victim (which I sent you in the revised French translation) has finally been published, in its original text, in *Zeitschrift fuer Psychotherapie und medizinische Psychologie*,[2] by Kretschmer. The German text contains two examples of "reflexoid crime," one from Sarawak and the other from the Myall tribe in Australia; I am sorry I have no offprints, otherwise I would send you a copy.

I send you my best wishes for the New Year!

Sincerely,
H. Ellenberger

Devon, Pennsylvania
March 29, 1955

Dr H. Ellenberger
The Menninger Foundation
Topeka, Kansas

Dear Doctor Ellenberger:
My apologies for not having answered sooner your letter of December 28. I have been working seven days a week, 14 hours a day, trying to finish my book on therapeutic education, which is to come out this fall, and I didn't write any letters and hardly saw anyone.

Unfortunately, the ending of the book brought me little happiness. Almost within the minute when I put the final touch on the manuscript, Pupsie died through the stupidity of veterinarians who kept treating him for hepatitis while I kept telling them that he had a bone stuck in him. Yielding to my urging, they finally x-rayed his abdomen but did not think of x-raying his chest. The bone pierced his thoracic oesophagus and he died just a week ago today. I leave it to your imagination how I feel about it.

With kindest regards to you and your family

Cordially yours,
Georges Devereux, Ph.D.
Director of Research

---

18 October 1968
Mr Georges Devereux,
École des Hautes Études,
(Sorbonne) Paris 6e.

Dear colleague and friend,
Returning from a stay this summer in Europe, I found here your book *From Anxiety to Method in the Behavioral Sciences*. Thank you so much for sending me a copy.

The subject you deal with seems to me very original. You are looking at a subject that had been broached by Nietzsche. Perhaps you remember the passages where he speaks of the irrational and destructive nature of science, and how the scientist must, like Oedipus, be able to kill his father and possess his mother before managing to carry out his discoveries, how he also links the effort of the scientific researcher to the instinct for self-destruction. (I quote from memory.) But Nietzsche only touched upon this problem, whereas you tackle it directly and in various ways.

Your book is not a quick and easy read, and moreover we have serious concerns here: the students' strike, the occupation of the university buildings, and so on. But I would be happy to write an analysis of it as soon as I finish reading it.

I myself am very busy with finalizing the large *History and Evolution of Dynamic Psychiatry* which I have been working on for so many years, soon to be published by Basic Books in New York.

Your sincerely,

Henri F. Ellenberger, M.D.
Université de Montréal,
Département de Criminologie
Case Postale 6128, Montréal, Québec

Georges Devereux
Poste Restante
Bureau 115
Paris, France

7 November 1968

Dear Colleague and Friend:
Thank you for your kind letter. I am happy to know that my book interested you, and thank you in advance for the review you will write of it.

It is a difficult book and it is reassuring to know that a man *as scrupulous and as conscientious as yourself*[3] will review it. I understand so well the furious exclamation of the great Hellenist Willamowitz: *Kann man denn nicht lesen?* My experience would appear to indicate that the majority of people don't know how to read. I could give you examples of it! A doctoral thesis in French literature quotes some of my Mojave facts – *erroneously*. A recent article in the *American Anthropologist* discusses my theories – the author says he is in *partial* agreement. He indicates the points on which he "disagrees." Yet, had he taken the trouble to read, he would have quickly understood that he was *perfectly* in agreement regarding the details with which he *claims* he disagrees. A cursory reading? Negligence?

But there is worse! In 1940 I sent one of my off-prints to a famous professor at Harvard. The article began with the following sentence: "I am presenting *a* sociological theory of schizophrenia. I say clearly: *a* theory, and not "*the*" theory, for, according to Poincaré, if a fact is explainable in one way, it is explicable in other ways as well." That is clear, one would think! Well, sending me back my off-print, this illustrious (?) scholar criticized me for only having envisaged *just one* explanation, for having DENIED (!!!) the possibility of other explanations! In short, most people do not read what we write ... they read what they want to believe we have written.

I did not know that very interesting passage Nietzsche that you quote. Thank you for drawing my attention to it.

Congratulations on the upcoming publication of your book on the history of dynamic psychiatry!

Yours very sincerely,
Georges Devereux

Monsieur Georges Devereux
École des Hautes Études
(Sorbonne) Paris 6e.

Dear Colleague and Friend,
It has already been quite some time since we met, and, unsure of your home address, I am addressing this letter to you at the École des Hautes Études.

Excuse me for asking you about a detail that interests me. I remember that during a conference in Dakar you said that you were the one who introduced the term "transcultural psychiatry." Could you indicate to me what year that was, and in what publication, if you remember? I would really like to give credit to each author, even if it is a point of terminology.

As for the word "ethno-psychiatry," Dr Louis Mars says that he is the one who created it, but is he not mistaken? Do you know when the term was introduced and by whom?

I still read your publications with interest, even if I am not necessarily in agreement with you on all points. I hope that I will have the pleasure of seeing you again.

Yours sincerely,
Henri F. Ellenberger, M.D.
Faculty of Arts and Sciences
Université de Montréal
Case Postale 6128, Montréal
Canada

————————

19 Sept. 1974

Dear Dr Ellenberger:
Thank you for your kind letter. Please excuse the briefness of this note. I am in the middle of correcting proofs and preparing the indexes of my two books, and preparing the publicity for the two others, writing "commissioned" articles, etc. I am no longer saving minutes, but seconds.

ETHNOPSYCHIATRY: Louis Mars, "Introduction à l'Ethnopsychiatrie," *Bulletin de l'Association Médicale Haïtienne*, vol. 6, 2, 1953. I know no previous use of this word. It is I, actually, who insisted to Dr Mars that he claim priority of this term.[4]

TRANSCULTURAL PSYCHIATRY: G. Devereux, *Reality and Dream* (FIRST EDITION), 1951. It was somewhere in the first part of the book, but does not appear in the index. But "iatry" is used in the sense of healing, of therapy. Cross-cultural psychiatry: one that requires the therapist to know the culture of the patient. Transcultural psychiatry: the psychiatrist must be familiar with the notion of "Culture." Clark Wissler:[5] Universal Culture Pattern. Therefore I distinguish between two ways of healing, of caring for the patient. I never thought of making "transcultural" the name of a science – of a discipline – and I regret that this term was attributed to me (erroneously attributed and borrowed without naming the author), to designate the *science* of ethnopsychiatry in general.

Finally, in terms of the discipline, the priority of Mars is unquestionable: ethnopsychiatry. Transcultural: I invented it to designate a kind of treatment. It was "filched" from me (without naming me) to designate a science as a whole, which is actually contrary to the semantics of "trans": beyond. People thought of "transport" and not of "trans-Alpine." Beyond the culture of the patient's tribe, a treatment that uses the CONCEPT OF (anthropological) CULTURE in general, a concept applicable to all cultures.

As a last resort, I now call "transcultural" (therapy): metacultural (*Reality and Dream*, SECOND ED. 1969, new introduction).

To conclude, can I ask you if you have ever, as promised, completed the review of *From Anxiety to Method*?[6] Already published in Germany (where it will soon be printed in paperback), and to be released in France (Payot), the book deserves a review from a truly scientific mind such as yours.

In friendship and in haste,
G. Devereux

NOTES

1 Ernst Ticho. A correspondence exists between the two men. (*Ed.*)
2 German and Austrian journal (1951–1974), mouthpiece of both societies: Allgemeinen Ärztlichen Gesellschaft für Psychotherapie, and Österreichischen Ärztegesellschaft für Psychotherapie. (*Ed.*)
3 The elements in italics were underlined by hand in the original letter. Many corrections have been made in pen to the punctuation, spelling, and French accents. (*Ed.*)
4 In fact, Louis Mars had used the term previously in a French publication: Mars, "Nouvelle contribution." But today we can no longer attribute the origin of the word to him, as it has been established that it already existed in colonial medicine in the interwar period. See Scarfone, *La psychiatrie coloniale italienne*. (*Ed.*)
5 Clark David Wissler (1870–1947), American anthropologist. (*Ed.*)
6 This review has not been found. (*Ed.*)

Timeline: Reference Points for a Contextual History of Ethnopsychiatry (Emmanuel Delille)

1851 First International Sanitary Conference (Paris, 23 July) on health, generally considered to be the beginning of international cooperation in the struggle against epidemics.

1902 International Conference of American States founded in Washington, leading to the creation of the International Sanitary Bureau of the Pan American Health Organization.

1907–08 Creation of the International Office of Public Health in Paris.

1913 Freud publishes *Totem and Taboo*, an essay in which he compares primitive thought and neurosis, taking inspiration from evolutionary theory, naturalistic novels, anthropology, and the folklorists of his time.

1920 First meeting of the League of Nations in London on 10 January. First General Assembly in Geneva on 15 November, with the representatives of forty-one nations. US Congress refuses to join, though the project had been supported by American President Woodrow Wilson.

1922 The League of Nations Health Committee and Health Section takes action to control the spread of major epidemics of leprosy, malaria, yellow fever, and typhus, and to distribute health promotion information and foster education throughout the world.

1924 Creation of the Institut français de sociologie (French Institute of Sociology) at the École pratique des hautes études (Practical School for Higher Studies).

1925 Creation of the Centre international de synthèse by Henri Berr.

1933 Congress of Alienist Physicians and Neurologists of France and the French-Speaking countries in Rabat (Morocco).

1935 Project to create the *Encyclopédie française*, launched by France's Minister for National Education Anatole de Monzie (1932–34), directed by Lucien Febvre, which provided a panorama of the sciences on which psychologists, doctors, psychoanalysts, anthropologists, sociologists, and historians collaborated (six hundred collaborators, of whom approximately two hundred were academics).

1938 Congress of Alienist Physicians and Neurologists of France and the French-Speaking countries in Algiers.

1941 The Law of 11 February 1941 of the French Penal Code forbade false accusations, witchcraft, magic, and charlatanism.

1943 Creation of the Office de la recherche scientifique coloniale (ORSC, the future ORSTOM, then IRD).

1945 Fifth Pan-African Congress (Manchester, 15–21 October), which claimed Africa for Africans, adopted socialism as a policy direction, and proclaimed the right of Africans to win their freedom through force.

1946 Adoption at the UN (New York) of the World Health Organization (WHO), under the aegis of the UN.

1948 The WHO Constitution becomes effective on 7 April (a date that then became World Health Day). The sixth revision of the International Classification of Diseases is created under its aegis and for the first time includes a chapter devoted to mental disorders (Chapter 5).

1950 Roger Bastide publishes *Sociologie et psychanalyse*.

1952 Publication of *Peaux noirs, masques blancs*, by the French psychiatrist from Martinique, Frantz Fanon.

1955 Bandung Conference, condemning colonialism and imperialism and promoting the "Third World;" documentary film *Les maîtres fous* (The Mad Masters) by ethnologist Jean Rouch.

1956 Frantz Fanon participates in the First International Congress of Black Writers and Artists, organized by the journal *Présence africaine* (Paris, 19–21 September), bringing together sixty-three delegates from eighty-four countries, predominantly from the Caribbean and Africa, with an audience of more than six hundred people at the Sorbonne. Eric Wittkower organizes a panel devoted to transcultural psychiatry at the Second World Congress of Psychiatry (Zurich, Switzerland), which brings together representatives from about twenty countries.

1958 First All African Peoples' Conference (Accra, 8–12 December), in which, notably, psychiatrist Frantz Fanon (with a Tunisian passport, in the name of Omar Ibrahim Fanon) participates, representing the provisional government of Algeria (GPRA). Creation of the Communauté française d'Afrique. Bukavu Conference, under the aegis of WHO and the Scientific Council for Africa South of the Sahara / Commission for Technical Cooperation in Africa South of the Sahara, reports on traditional therapies and general recommendations on the inclusion of beliefs and traditional systems of care.

1959 Second congress of the journal *Présence africaine* (International Congress of Negro Writers and Artists, Rome, 26 March–1 April); delegates are granted an audience with Pope John XXIII. Frantz Fanon takes part in the Congress and at the end of the year publishes *L'an V de la révolution algérienne*. Roger Bastide founds with psychiatrist Henri Baruk and historian Charles Morazé the Centre de psychiatrie sociale (Centre for social psychiatry) in Paris, after obtaining a chair in social and religious ethnology at the Sorbonne; Bastide gives seminars there until 1968.

1960 Departure of the French Community from Africa. *Manifesto of the 121*, which declared the right to insubordination and called for the respect of the Algerian people. The journals *Tiers-Monde* and *Cahiers d'études africaines* are founded.

1961 Referendum on the independence of Algeria on 8 January. From 22 to 25 April, an attempted military coup in Algeria against de Gaulle by Generals Salan, Zeller, Jouhaud, and Challe; after it fails, soldiers and civilians led by Salan go underground and continue the struggle in the OAS (Secret Army Organization, created in February). Maurice Merleau-Ponty dies in May; in June, Jean-Paul Sartre, Simone de Beauvoir, and Claude Lanzmann, threatened by the OAS, leave for Rome in temporary exile; Frantz Fanon joins them. Fanon dies on 6 December in New York from acute leukemia; publication of *Damnés de la terre* (*The Wretched of the Earth*), preface by Jean-Paul Sartre, seized by police in Paris on the day of Fanon's death. First Pan-African Psychiatric Conference, Abeokuta, Nigeria, 12–18 November), organized by Thomas Lambo. Alexander Leighton organizes a panel on transcultural psychiatry at the Third World Congress of Psychiatry, organized in Montreal, connected to the section led by Eric Wittkower and Jacob Fried at McGill University.

1962 On 8 February, the Charonne Metro Station Massacre, when police suppress a demonstration against the OAS, at the call of the PCF (French Communist Party) and unions. In March, a ceasefire decreed by de Gaulle and the Evian Accords. In May, the departure of close to 100,000 *pieds-noirs* for France. Declaration of the Independence of Algeria on 3 July. On 17 October, bloody suppression by police of a peaceful demonstration in Paris protesting the curfew imposed upon Algerians in the city.

1963 US President John F. Kennedy signs into law the Community Mental Health Centers Act, whose goal is to avoid hospitalizations for chronic mental disorders.

1964 Posthumous publication of a collection of political articles by Frantz Fanon, *Pour la révolution africaine* (François Maspero), translated as *Toward the African Revolution*. The American Psychiatric Association establishes a Committee on Transcultural Psychiatry.

1965 Roger Bastide publishes *Sociologie des maladies mentales* (*The Sociology of Mental Disorder*). Moussa Diop and Henri Collomb found the journal *Psychopathologie africaine* in Dakar (Senegal). Publication of booklets by Henri Ellenberger on ethnopsychiatry in the *Encyclopédie médico-chirurgicale* (EMC), the first French-language synthesis in this field of knowledge.

1966 The Évolution psychiatrique group organizes a study devoted to psychiatric epidemiology (4 December). The Fourth World Congress of Psychiatry is held in Madrid on 5–11 September), where Henri Ellenberger presents a report titled "Intérêt et domaines d'application de l'ethnopsychiatrie" (Interest and areas of application of ethnopsychiatry).

1967 The Six-Day War is fought. Fanon's widow asks François Maspero to remove Sartre's preface to *Les Damnés de la terre* because in it Sartre defended the State of Israel; plans are launched for a posthumous paperback edition ("Petite collection Maspero"; Sartre's preface would be reinserted in 1985). The Canadian Psychiatric Association establishes a Committee on Transcultural Psychiatry.

1970 Georges Devereux publishes his *Essais d'ethnopsychiatrie générale* (translated as *Basic Problems of Ethnopsychiatry*). Brian Murphy creates the Transcultural Psychiatry section of the World Psychiatric Association (in charge of world congresses).

1972 Roger Bastide publishes *Le rêve, la transe et la folie*, a collection of articles that extends from the 1920s to the 1970s and supports a program of transcultural research.

1976 WHO's eighth revision of the International Classification of Diseases includes for the first time a glossary of mental disorders. The Ford Foundation launches the Prometra Project (Association of the Promotion of Traditional Medicine), an international association that promotes traditional medicine and the use of medicinal herbs in approximately twenty African countries.

1977 The Sixth World Congress of Psychiatry in Honolulu recommends that member countries make their classification of mental disorders compatible with WHO's international classification (ICD-9); the use of psychiatry as a tool for coercing political dissidents in the Soviet Union is condemned. American anthropologist Arthur Kleinman (Harvard University) founds the journal *Culture, Medicine, and Psychiatry.*

1978 Publication of *Orientalism* by Edward Said, widely viewed as the book that launched postcolonial studies.

1993 The tenth revision of the WHO's international classification of mental and behavioural disorders (ICD-10) designates in its category F48.8 ("other specified nonpsychotic mental disorders") "mixed disorders of behaviour, beliefs, and emotions which are of uncertain etiology and nosological status and which occur with particular frequency in certain cultures." Seven syndromes are listed: *koro*, *latah*, Dhat syndrome, occupational neurosis, psychasthenia, psychogenic syncope, and Briquet's disorder.

1996 The American Manual of Psychiatry establishes for the first time a glossary of "culture-bound syndromes" in the appendix of its fourth revision (DSM-IV). It lists twenty-seven syndromes, the terminology of which has roots in Spanish, English, French, and various Asian languages.

1999 International symposium: Culture and Diagnosis Across the World (Izmir, Turkey) under the aegis of WHO.

2009 Exposition at the Musée des Arts premiers du quai Branly (Paris) devoted to the journal *Présence africaine.*

Index